400 Anatomy SBAs for Medical Finals

This dynamic tool, designed to transform the way medical students and professionals approach anatomy, blends foundational concepts with real-world clinical relevance. This book bridges the gap between preclinical learning and practical application. The MCQs challenge critical thinking, and the inclusion of clinical cases and progressive difficulty levels ensures that readers master human anatomy and appreciate its indispensable role in diagnosis and patient management. Perfect for students, residents, and practicing physicians to build confident and informed medical practice globally.

Key Features

- Highlights the relationship between anatomical basics, function, and their application in emergency and operating room scenarios, bridging the gap between theory and practice
- Structured MCQs from basic to advanced levels, aligning with Bloom's taxonomy, to cater to medical students, residents, and practicing physicians, ensuring both foundational knowledge and advanced application
- Features MCQs that commence with basic human anatomy and progress to clinical scenarios and real-life simulated cases, challenging readers to apply anatomical knowledge effectively in practical and clinical contexts

MasterPass Series

Clinical Cases for the FRCA: Key Topics Mapped to the RCoA Curriculum
Alisha Allana

Spine Surgery Vivas for the FRCS (Tr & Orth)
Kelechi Eseonu, Nicolas Beresford-Cleary

MCQs, MEQs and OSPEs in Occupational Medicine: A Revision Aid
Ken Addley

ENT Vivas: A Guide to Passing the Intercollegiate FRCS (ORL-HNS) Viva Examination
Adnan Darr, Karan Jolly, Jameel Muzaffar

ENT OSCEs: A guide to your first ENT job and passing the MRCS (ENT) OSCE, 3E
Peter Kullar, Joseph Manjaly, Livy Kenyon

Plastic Surgery Vivas for the FRCS (Plast): An Essential Guide
Monica Fawzy

The Final FFICM Structured Oral Examination Study Guide
Eryl Davies

Neurosurgery: The Essential Guide to the Oral and Clinical Neurosurgical Exam, 2E
Vivian Elwell, Ramez Kirollos, Syed Al-Haddad, Peter Bodkin

Sport and Exercise Medicine: An Essential Guide
David Eastwood, Dane Vishnubala

Clinical Consultation Skills in Medicine: A Primer for MRCP PACES
Ernest Suresh

Refraction and Retinoscopy: How to Pass the Refraction Certificate, 2E
Jonathan Park, Leo Feinberg, David Jones

The Final FRCA Constructed Response Questions: A Practical Study Guide, 2E
Elizabeth Combeer, Mitul Patel

Diagnostic EMQs: A Comprehensive Collection for Medical Examinations
Syed Hussain, Umber Rind, Jawed Noori, Yasmean Kalam, Haseeb Ata, Emanuel Papageorgiou

Passing the Final FFICM: High-Yield Facts for the MCQ & OSCE Exams
Muzzammil Ali

Cases in Haematology: For the MLA and PLAB
Aaron Niblock

Postgraduate Ophthalmology Exam Success
Maneck Nicholson, Anjali Nicholson, Syed Faraaz Hussain

Pass the MRCP (SCE) Neurology Revision Guide
Dhananjay Gupta

100 Imaging Cases for the MRCP(UK) Neurology SCE
Osama Shukir Muhammed Amin

400 Anatomy SBAs for Medical Finals
Inyang Ukot

For more information about this series please visit: https://www.routledge.com/MasterPass/book-series/CRCMASPASS

400 Anatomy SBAs for Medical Finals

Inyang Ukot

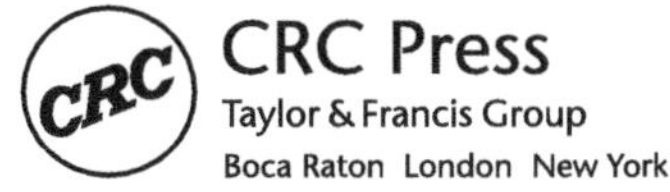

CRC Press is an imprint of the
Taylor & Francis Group, an **informa** business

Designed cover image: Shutterstock

First edition published 2027
by CRC Press
2385 NW Executive Center Drive, Suite 320, Boca Raton, FL 33431

and by CRC Press
4 Park Square, Milton Park, Abingdon, Oxon, OX14 4RN

CRC Press is an imprint of Taylor & Francis Group, LLC

Library of Congress Control Number: 2026937903

ISBN: 978-1-041-32684-7 (hbk)
ISBN: 978-1-041-30845-4 (pbk)
ISBN: 978-1-003-78396-1 (ebk)

DOI: 10.1201/9781003783961

Typeset in Minion
by KnowledgeWorks Global Ltd.

This book is dedicated to

My wife (Mrs. Sarah Inyang Ukot)

and to

My four adult daughters:

Grace Alegeh

Elor Ukot

Sarah Ukot

Joy Ukot

CONTENTS

FOREWORD

400 Anatomy SBAs for Medical Finals contains material that reasonably covers human anatomy in theory and clinical practice. In terms of size, it is unique, at least for the fact that it is a shift from the paradigm for most textbooks in human anatomy.

The book covers 400 multiple choice questions (MCQs) of the single best answer format. Each MCQ has an unambiguous stem that is further enhanced by making the font bold. The book makes a reasonable attempt to apply Bloom's taxonomy in the distribution of MCQs between the lower and upper segments of the ladder. This feature makes this MCQ book suitable for medical students and clinicians. Every MCQ in this book provides the reader with four options, of which only one is the best—making it the Answer. No matter how close any of the other options is, just one is the Answer and the reader should choose that one.

This book has answers that are backed with robust Notes; 75% of the Notes are between 300 and 350 words long; the remainder are either longer or slightly shorter. Many of the Notes are satisfactorily referenced using the Vancouver style; this book, therefore, has over 500 references; the references are chapter-based and so are numbered within the chapters, which contain Answers and Notes. This book goes further to include a comprehensive Index; these resources provide the reader with material for quick reference in the book and for further/deeper study.

Chapters 1 and 9 are on the abdomen. Chapters 2 and 10 cover the thorax. Chapters 3 and 11 are devoted to the back. Chapters 4 and 12 dwell entirely on the pelvis and perineum. Chapters 5 and 13 treat essential topics on the upper limb. Chapters 6 and 14 focus on the lower limb. Chapters 7 and 15 emphasize the head and neck. Chapters 8 and 16 are limited to topics on neuroanatomy. Each pair of chapters is crafted to be of benefit to medical students and practicing clinicians. The main foci are simplification, clarity, and applicability of the subject, contrary to the belief of many medical students that the only way to pass examinations is to memorize the facts.

I commend the author of this MCQ book for his painstaking production of a user-friendly text with essential theory and clinical relevance for the benefit of readers regardless of the number of years since they left medical school or wherever they are in studying medicine. This book will surely serve its target audience with good purpose. The book should be invaluable to medical students, general medical practitioners, residents in family medicine, general surgery, pathology, radiology, medicine, pediatrics, obstetrics and gynecology, and surgery.

Dr. Emmanuel Kunle Abudu
Professor of Pathology & Consultant Pathologist
University of Uyo & Teaching Hospital, Uyo

PREFACE

The need for **400 Anatomy SBAs for Medical Finals,** despite an abundance of standard textbooks in anatomy, is because there are still fewer books with multiple choice questions (MCQs) than textbooks on the entire subject or parts of it; there are even fewer books that concentrate on MCQs than journal articles that provide great details on various topics on human anatomy. Contending with this subject is the experience of many medical students. Human anatomy is so broad and deep that, in the early years in medical school, many students resort to memorization of facts, perhaps because they are unable to appreciate how fundamental human anatomy is to success in their medical school final examinations and eventual clinical practice.

The author was a medical student during the period when actual human cadavers were readily available in the anatomy laboratory for use for two years. Within the clinical years, he was fortunate to be engaged by the department as a practical demonstrator of the subject in the Human Anatomy Laboratory on a part-time basis; he was a guide to fellow medical students in their first two years during his last two years. He had the opportunity because he had shown consistent interest in the subject. He has maintained that consistency until today; that is why, forty-nine years after his first exposure to human anatomy, he has penned the contents of this book as one of his last books in medicine. Any author of a book on any aspect of the medical sciences would convincingly testify that it is easier for specialists to work as a team and produce a voluminous textbook in any area of medicine than to single-handedly craft an MCQ book with a global flair.

This book is written by a specialist in family medicine and not a professor in human anatomy. The book, in its entirety, is crafted to meet the needs of medical students in the clinical years, but for best benefits, it should be used from the early years. The book contains enough material to convince medical students in the first and second years of medical school that human anatomy is both a theoretical and very practical subject that transcends those initial years, which determine whether they will go through medical school or not. Prior to professional examinations in medical school, a student should have and use a variety of good sources of MCQs to test the level of their understanding of lectures and the contents of textbooks on human anatomy.

This book is also designed to fill an indispensable yet unbridged, or inadequately bridged, gap in clinical practice for many medical practitioners and other professionals who render care to patients whereby they need a proper transfer of knowledge to practice on their patients. This is because they had "burnt the bridge" of human anatomy, but the "ashes" of the subject still follow them; unfortunately, such practitioners hardly have time to read a standard textbook on human anatomy, although no professional examination awaits them.

Finally, this book is designed to allow the reader to self-test on the principles and practical applications of human anatomy. The contents of this book are well selected not only on the basis of its being representative of regional anatomy but also based on global relevance. The Notes are designed to help candidates fully cover the subject at least once before their medical finals.

ACKNOWLEDGMENTS

I hereby express appreciation to members of my immediate family who have joined me in enduring most of the stress involved in authoring this book—like for other books (previous and forthcoming). With their understanding and prayers in times of health, illness, and discouragement, they have formed impressive and reliable support that has led to the actualization of this dream project.

AUTHOR

Dr. Inyang Ukot is a 1981 graduate of the College of Medicine of the University of Lagos. He holds a diploma in Occupational Medicine from the Royal College of Physicians of London (2005). He is a family physician and holds two fellowships in the specialty from the West African College of Physicians (1995) and the National Postgraduate Medical College of Nigeria (1991). He is the author of multiple books in medicine, the most recent ones being *Understanding Diseases in Skin of Color* (2025) and *Ukot's Back to Basics MCQs – Volumes 1, 2, and 3* (2025).

INTRODUCTION

400 Anatomy SBAs for Medical Finals was conceived to have a relatively small size. This physically portable size makes it convenient for the user in the preclinical and clinical years in medical school to use. Any student or practitioner in the medical field and other healthcare professionals who render clinical services requiring a sound knowledge of the basics of this subject will enjoy using this book. Every reader has "in their hands" an invaluable resource with a well-thought-out mix of theory and practice in an orderly presentation. The book contains 400 multiple choice questions (MCQs) that have answers and robust notes that accompany them in the matching chapters.

The MCQs in this book are in the single-best answer (SBA) format. Specifically, every MCQ in this book comes as a unit; each unit consists of a number and a stem, both of which are in bold font. Every stem starts and ends as a standard question or starts as a statement (usually with a clinical bent) but ends as a question. The stem is followed by four options (A, B, C, D), of which only one is the best option and the Answer that the reader should choose.

The book contains 16 chapters crafted to meet the expectations of regional anatomy. The chapters are paired to create two sections: one section, Chapters 1 to 8, covers the MCQs, and a second section, Chapters 9 to 16, covers Answers and reasonably detailed Notes. The organization of the book is as follows:

- Chapters 1 and 9: Abdomen
- Chapters 2 and 10: Thorax
- Chapters 3 and 11: Back
- Chapters 4 and 12: Pelvis and Perineum
- Chapters 5 and 13: Upper Limb
- Chapters 6 and 14: Lower Limb
- Chapters 7 and 15: Head and Neck
- Chapters 8 and 16: Neuroanatomy

Everything about this book is deliberate, well thought out, and logically presented. For example, the choice of the abdomen as the first chapter is because it is the area that general practitioners must attend to; it is because of this that the chapter is assigned the highest number of MCQs—60.

There are over 500 essential chapter-based references (using the Vancouver style). The book also contains a representative index. The MCQs, Answers, Notes, References, and Index ensure that every reader (not just the "distinction student") has a sound understanding of the topics to pass medical finals or revisit anatomy during residency without grappling with the entire contents of a standard voluminous textbook on anatomy.

Part I
MCQs

CHAPTER 1

MCQs ON ABDOMEN

1. Which of the following statements about the skin is correct?

A. It has the epidermis and dermis as the inner and outer layers of tissue, respectively.
B. The epidermis consists of stratified squamous epithelium and elastic fibers.
C. Nervous tissue is absent in the dermis.
D. The hypodermis is synonymous with the subcutaneous layer of skin.

2. Regarding the surface anatomy of the abdomen, which of the following statements is correct?

A. The costal margins are formed by the costal cartilages of the 9th to the 12th ribs.
B. The linea semilunaris is a guide to the tip of the tenth costal cartilage.
C. The mid-inguinal point is a reference point for identifying the femoral pulse.
D. The inguinal ligament is attached to the anterior superior iliac spine and the symphysis pubis.

3. Which of the following statements is incorrect?

A. A midline incision below the umbilicus passes through the linea alba.
B. The position of the umbilicus is constant in all adults.
C. The subcostal plane passes through the inferior borders of the tenth costal cartilages.
D. Contraction of the rectus abdominis helps in identifying the linea semilunaris.

4. Which of the following relationships is correct?

A. The tip of the right tenth costal cartilage and gallbladder disease.
B. The transpyloric plane and the superior poles of the kidneys.
C. The origin of the common iliac arteries and the fourth lumbar vertebra.
D. The left 8th rib and the long axis of the spleen.

5. Which of the following statements about the abdomen is correct?

A. It is not involved in pleuritic pain.
B. Developmentally, the urachus links the bladder with the umbilicus.
C. The superficial inguinal ring is below and lateral to the pubic tubercle.
D. The broad ligament of the uterus passes through the superficial inguinal ring.

6. Regarding the abdomen, which of the following statements is correct?

A. Paramedian incisions should be made through the rectus abdominis.
B. Weakness of the abdominal muscles may lead to divarication recti.
C. Pararectal incision is preferred to a paramedian incision.
D. The rectus sheath receives no contribution from the transversus abdominis aponeurosis.

DOI: 10.1201/9781003783961-2

7. Which of the following statements about the inguinal canal is correct?

A. It lies between the deep and superficial inguinal rings.
B. It extends from the anterior superior iliac spine to the ipsilateral pubic tubercle.
C. It links a direct inguinal hernia with the scrotum.
D. An indirect inguinal hernia does not pass through the canal.

8. With respect to the inguinal canal, which of the following statements is correct?

A. The lateral end is the superficial inguinal ring.
B. The anterior wall is formed by the fascia transversalis.
C. The floor is formed by Poupart's ligament.
D. The roof is formed by the arching fibers of the transversus abdominis and external oblique.

9. Which of the following statements is incorrect?

A. The anterior wall of the inguinal canal is formed by the external oblique aponeurosis.
B. The concavity of the floor of the inguinal canal is downward.
C. The sharp edge of the lacunar ligament forms the medial relation of a femoral hernia.
D. The pubic tubercle is above and medial to the neck of a femoral hernial sac.

10. Which of the following relations is correct?

A. The conjoint tendon strengthens the medial part of Hesselbach's triangle.
B. The inferior epigastric artery is medial to a direct inguinal hernia.
C. Hesselbach's triangle is bounded laterally by the lateral border of the rectus sheath.
D. The deep inguinal ring is medial to the inferior epigastric artery.

11. Which of the following statements about the femoral ring is incorrect?

A. It is a part of the femoral canal.
B. Normally it contains fat and is a site for femoral hernia.
C. It is bounded laterally by the lacunar ligament.
D. It is bounded inferiorly by the pectineal ligament.

12. Which of the following is *not* expected on entering the abdominal cavity in a laparotomy?

A. Omentum covering intestine
B. Liver in the right hypochondrium and the epigastrium
C. Transverse colon at about the level of the umbilicus
D. Good view of the kidneys

13. Regarding contents of the abdominal cavity, which of the following statements is correct?

A. The duodenum has a mesentery.
B. The jejunum and ileum are immobile.
C. The ascending and the descending colon are not fixed.
D. The inferior vena cava provides significant physical support to the liver.

14. During surgery, which of the following is a reference for identification of the intestines?

A. The large intestine is always wider than the small intestine.
B. The longitudinal muscle layer forms a continuous layer a round the jejunum and ileum.
C. Appendices epiploicae are attached to the appendix.
D. The longitudinal muscle layer of the colon is arranged in three continuous bands.

15. Which of the following statements is not descriptive of pain arising from the abdomen?

A. Pain arising from the stomach is referred to the left iliac fossa.
B. Pain arising from parietal peritoneum is subserved by the anterior rami of the last six thoracic and first lumbar nerves.
C. Pain due to cholecystitis may be referred to the right shoulder.
D. Pain due to acute appendicitis may involve the whole abdomen.

16. Which of the following structures is *not* enclosed by the mesentery of the small intestines?

A. Adipose tissue
B. Inferior mesenteric vein
C. Lymph nodes
D. Nerve fibers

17. Which of the following statements is *not* characteristic of the alimentary canal?

A. The wall consists of three layers.
B. Of its layers, the innermost has lamina propria and a little smooth muscle.
C. The muscular layer is responsible for its movements.
D. Two coats of smooth muscle tissue comprise the muscular layer.

18. Which of the following is *not* a feature of the esophagus?

A. It transports food from the pharynx to the stomach.
B. It runs posterior to the trachea in the thorax.
C. It exits the thorax at the esophageal hiatus.
D. It has a pyloric sphincter that prevents regurgitation of stomach contents.

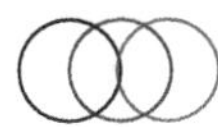

19. With respect to the stomach, which of the following is a correct statement?

A. It may be divided into three parts.
B. It has three valves.
C. The valve between it and the small intestine is the lower esophageal sphincter.
D. Inhibition of gastric secretions by the presence of food in the small intestine is a reflex activity.

20. Regarding the stomach, which of the following statements is incorrect?

A. It is C-shaped when empty and viewed in a vertical position.
B. It has rugae of mucosa and submucosa.
C. It is involved in the initial act of digesting proteins.
D. It has a third smooth muscle layer that is prominent close to the esophageal opening.

21. With respect to the stomach, which of the following statements is correct?

A. The fundus is sometimes filled with air, which is shown in radiographs of the abdomen.
B. The main part of the stomach is the cardia.
C. The pyloric canal becomes the pyloric antrum prior to the small intestine.
D. Mucous (goblet) cells are located at the deep portion of the gastric gland.

22. Pertaining to the pancreas, which of the following statements is correct?

A. It is located anterior to the parietal peritoneum.
B. It lies obliquely between the duodenum and the spleen.
C. The head lies on the spleen.
D. Its duct and the gallbladder's duct join at the ampulla of Vater.

23. Which of the following statements about the liver is correct?

A. It is the second largest internal organ.
B. It normally extends from the level of the second intercostal space to the subcostal margin.
C. Its lobes, right and left, are approximately equal in size.
D. It is divided into its major lobes by the falciform ligament.

24. Which of the following is a correct statement about the liver?

A. It is linked with the diaphragm by the falciform ligament.
B. The coronary ligaments are a fold of parietal peritoneum.
C. The functional units are the hepatic lobules.
D. A hepatic lobule of cells is arranged circumferentially around a central vein.

25. Regarding the liver, which of the following statements is incorrect?

A. It has sinusoids that separate plates of cells of functional liver units from one another.
B. It is completely surrounded by the lower ribs.
C. It has Kupffer cells in the endothelium of its sinusoids.
D. Hepatic ducts are a coalition of bile canaliculi.

26. Which of the following statements about the gallbladder is correct?

A. It is located on the anterior surface of the liver.
B. It is crescent-shaped.
C. Its duct and the liver duct join to form the common bile duct.
D. It is lined with cuboidal epithelial cells.

27. Regarding the gallbladder, which of the following statements is incorrect?

A. A capacity of 50 milliliters is abnormal.
B. Its strong muscular wall contracts in response to stimulus by cholecystokinin.
C. The hepatopancreatic sphincter is normally closed.
D. Gallstones in the bile duct may block bile flow, causing obstructive jaundice.

28. Which of the following statements about the small intestine is correct?

A. It may be up to 6 meters (20 feet) long in an adult cadaver.
B. It is the same length in a living or dead adult.
C. It is inverted U-shaped at the level of the duodenum.
D. It is about 25 cm in its first part.

29. With regard to the small intestine, which of the following statements is correct?

A. The ileum contains Brunner's glands.
B. The duodenum is anterior to the first three lumbar vertebrae and the right kidney.
C. Compared with the jejunum, the ileum is shorter.
D. The jejunum is retroperitoneal.

30. Which of the following relationships is incorrect?

A. Mesentery—double-layered peritoneal fold
B. Duodenum—mesenteric attachment
C. Omentum—stomach
D. Intestinal villi—increased mucosal surface area and absorption

31. With respect to the small intestine, which of the following statements is correct?

A. Segmentation is the movement that propels chyme through the small intestine.
B. Sympathetic impulses improve both mixing and propulsive movements.
C. Diarrhea is a result of a strong peristaltic rush.
D. The ileocecal valve is a sphincter muscle that normally stays open.

32. With respect to the large intestine, which of the following statements is correct?

A. It is about 3 meters in length.
B. It commences at the left side of the abdominal cavity.
C. It has the same diameter as the duodenum, although it is referred to as "large."
D. It lacks villi.

33. With respect to the large intestine, which of the following statements is incorrect?

A. The rectum is rigidly attached to the anterior part of the sacrum by peritoneum.
B. The colon has three parts.
C. The transverse colon is the longest and most mobile part of the large intestine.
D. There are six to ten longitudinal columns of mucosa in the anal canal.

34. Regarding the large intestine, which of the following statements is correct?

A. The transverse colon runs transversely from right to left.
B. The sigmoid colon is the C-shaped continuation of the descending colon at the brim of the pelvis.
C. The rectum continues below the tip of the coccyx.
D. The internal and external anal sphincter muscles are composed of skeletal muscles.

35. With regard to the stomach, which of the following statements is correct?

A. The greater curvature forms the superior aspect.
B. The orientation in tall and short persons is similar.
C. The mucosa is lined with simple columnar glandular epithelium.
D. Rugae are prominent in the full stomach.

36. Which of the following statements about gastric glands is correct?

A. Chief cells produce gastric lipase from infancy to adulthood.
B. Enteroendocrine cells stimulate gastric motility by producing histamine.
C. Neck cells produce mucus that protects mucosa from HCl.
D. Parietal cell intrinsic factor enhances vitamin B_{12} absorption by the colon.

37. A general surgeon makes an opening into the upper abdomen. Which of the following structures would the surgeon see when taking an anterior view of the liver?

A. Left lobe and falciform ligament
B. Quadrate lobe and ligamentum teres
C. Caudate lobe and gallbladder
D. Bare area

38. With respect to the liver, which of the following statements is correct?

A. The left lobe occupies most of the right hypochondrium.
B. Each hepatic lobule has a central vein surrounded by columnar cells—hepatocytes.
C. The hepatic triad consists of a bile ductule and two blood vessels.
D. It secretes bile directly into the right and left hepatic ducts.

39. With respect to the biliary tree, which of the following statements is correct?

A. The right and left hepatic ducts form the common hepatic duct on the superior surface of the liver.
B. The cystic duct arises from the head of the gallbladder.
C. As the bile duct enters the pancreas, it is joined by the pancreatic duct to form the hepatopancreatic ampulla.
D. The sphincter of Oddi lies within the major duodenal papilla.

40. Which of the following statements about the gallbladder and biliary tree is correct?

A. It is a continuation of the gallbladder fundus.
B. The interior of the gallbladder is lined with simple columnar epithelium.
C. It is abnormal to find the gallbladder fundus projecting below the liver margin.
D. The length of a normal gallbladder is about 15 cm.

41. Which of the following statements about the pancreas is correct?

A. Its body is encircled by the duodenum.
B. Ducts of secretory acini ultimately enter the pancreatic duct.
C. The accessory pancreatic duct opens into the minor duodenal papilla.
D. The pancreas is an intraperitoneal organ.

42. With respect to the small intestine, which of the following statements is correct?

A. The first part is approximately 15 cm long.
B. In a cadaver, the ileum is shorter than the jejunum.
C. During surgery, the ileum is identified among intestinal loops in the right lower abdominal cavity.
D. During surgery, the jejunum is identifiable just inferior to the liver.

43. With respect to the superior mesenteric artery, which of the following is *not* its usual direct branch?

A. Dorsal pancreatic artery
B. Ileocolic artery
C. Jejunal artery
D. Ileal artery

44. Which of the following statements about the appendix is correct?

A. Its blood supply is from an artery that runs in the greater omentum.
B. It is a structure with little significance to immunity.
C. A point 1/3 the distance along the spino-umbilical line marks the appendix.
D. During an appendectomy, the surgeon's instruments go through the rectus abdominis.

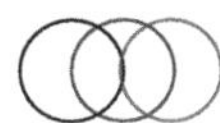

45. Which of the following structures in the abdominal cavity provides the origin of the greater omentum?

A. Transverse colon
B. Stomach
C. Jejunum
D. Ileum

46. With respect to the ascending colon, which of the following statements is correct?

A. It commences at the base of the appendix.
B. Its blood supply arises from the superior mesenteric artery.
C. It is intraperitoneal.
D. It terminates just inferior to the left lobe of the liver.

47. Which of the following statements about the appendix is correct?

A. Sympathetic afferent supply is via T12.
B. The appendicular artery is a branch of the ileocolic artery.
C. It is derived from embryologic hindgut.
D. Lymphatic drainage is into the right colic lymph nodes.

48. Which of the following statements about the descending colon is correct?

A. It terminates at the beginning of the rectum.
B. It is relatively mobile, being attached to the mesentery.
C. In its length, it is related to the groin.
D. Its blood supply is related to the inferior mesenteric artery.

49. Which of the following statements about the colon is correct?

A. Tenia coli are not found in the sigmoid colon.
B. The descending colon makes an inferomedial turn to form the sigmoid colon.
C. The arteries to the sigmoid colon run in the sigmoid mesocolon.
D. Venous drainage of the sigmoid colon is into the left colic veins.

50. Which of the following statements about the rectum is correct?

A. The longitudinal layer of the muscularis externa forms two bands.
B. Projections of the circular layer of muscles form two transverse folds.
C. The rectum is one of the sites of porta-caval anastomoses.
D. There is an absence of epiploic appendages.

51. With respect to the anal canal, which of the following statements is correct?

A. Its approximately 3–4 cm are divided into two halves by the pectinate line.
B. Internal and external anal sphincters consist of skeletal muscle.
C. Histologically, the anoderm part is made of stratified squamous keratinized epithelium.
D. The superior rectal vein provides venous drainage above the dentate line.

52. A 40-year-old para 6 woman with her last confinement 8 weeks previously develops features of weakness of the pelvic floor. Which of the following muscles is *not* expected to be primarily involved in exercises to strengthen the levator ani?

A. Puborectalis
B. Piriformis
C. Iliococcygeus
D. Pubococcygeus

53. Which of the following statements about the spleen is correct?

A. The splenic artery arises from the superior mesenteric artery.
B. Injury to the spleen is expected from a bullet entry wound at the left 9th rib.
C. It lies anterolateral to the stomach.
D. The white pulp contains lymphocytes, macrophages, and erythrocytes.

54. Regarding the kidney, which of the following statements is correct?

A. It is bean-shaped and has a rough surface.
B. Measuring about 20 × 10 × 5 cm in length, width, and thickness, respectively, is normal.
C. It is retroperitoneal and lies anterior to the vertebral column.
D. It changes position slightly with respiratory movement.

55. Which of the following statements about the kidney is correct?

A. When lying between the transverse processes of T12 and L3, it is within the normal size range.
B. The right kidney is higher than the left.
C. The medial surface is convex.
D. The calyx is the funnel-shaped part of the upper ureter.

56. With respect to the urinary system, which of the following relationships is correct?

A. Renal arteries—10% of cardiac output
B. Urinary bladder—posterior to the parietal peritoneum
C. Trigone—ureteric and urethral openings
D. Detrusor muscle—second layer (submucous coat) of the bladder wall

57. With respect to the kidneys, which of the following statements is correct?

A. The right kidney is at a slightly higher level than the left kidney.
B. A kidney measuring 15 cm in length is normal in size.
C. The lateral surface of the kidney is concave.
D. The two kidneys are retroperitoneal.

58. Which of the following structures is *not* in the hilum of the kidney?

A. Renal artery
B. Adrenal
C. Ureter
D. Lymphatics

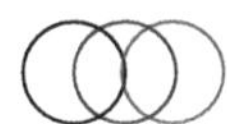

59. Macroscopically, which of the following structures is *not* identifiable in a cut frontal section of a kidney?

A. The cortex
B. The medulla
C. The nephron
D. The pelvis

60. Which of the following statements about the kidneys is correct?

A. The right adrenal rests on the superior pole of the kidney.
B. A normal kidney lies between T11 and L5.
C. From the outside in, the renal capsule is the first of the protective connective tissues.
D. Presence of fat in the renal sinus is abnormal.

Chapter 2

MCQs ON THORAX

1. Which of the following statements about membranes is correct?

A. Cutaneous, mucous, and serous membranes consist of epithelial tissues only.
B. At synovial joints, the covering membranes secrete very thin, colorless lubricating fluid.
C. Serous membranes provide lining for body cavities that do not communicate with the exterior.
D. Mucous membranes cover the outer surface of the heart.

2. Which of the following statements about the surface anatomy of the thorax is correct?

A. The angle of Louis lies at a level opposite the intervertebral disk between the second and third thoracic vertebrae.
B. The male nipple lies in the seventh intercostal space.
C. The clavicle is palpable throughout its length.
D. The 12th rib forms the lowest part of the costal margin.

3. With respect to the thorax, which of the following statements is correct?

A. The first two ribs are protected from fractures by the clavicle.
B. The seventh thoracic vertebral spine is at the same level as the superior angle of the scapula.
C. The root of the scapular spine is at the level of the fifth thoracic vertebral spine.
D. The position of the apex beat is normal when palpated at the anterior axillary line.

4. Regarding blood vessels of the thorax, which of the following statements is correct?

A. The axillary artery is susceptible to compression by a cervical rib.
B. The internal thoracic vessels are usually about 10 cm from the sternum.
C. There is no danger to the intercostal vessels when inserting a needle into the pleural cavity through the lower border of a rib.
D. Fractures of ribs rarely endanger the intercostal vessels.

5. With respect to the thorax, which of the following statements is correct?

A. Intercostal nerves do not supply parietal pleura.
B. The left intercostobrachial nerve is associated with referred pain of myocardial ischemia.
C. Lower rib fractures do not endanger the liver and spleen.
D. Inflammation of the central part of the diaphragmatic parietal pleura may cause referred pain to the umbilicus.

DOI: 10.1201/9781003783961-3

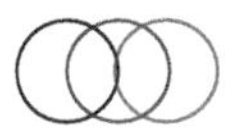

6. With respect to the thorax and its contents, which of the following statements is incorrect?

A. Mediastinal shift is demonstrable clinically by lateral deviation of the trachea in the suprasternal notch.
B. An infero-lateral displacement of the apex beat indicates enlargement of the heart.
C. A pulsatile swelling at the suprasternal notch may indicate aortic aneurysm.
D. Intercostal nerve block is done by infiltrating the local anesthetic agent just above the rib.

7. Which of the following relationships concerning ribs is incorrect?

A. Vertebrosternal ribs—true ribs
B. False ribs—the last 5 pairs of ribs
C. Floating ribs—11th and 12th pairs of ribs
D. Vertebrochondral ribs—9th and 10th pairs of ribs

8. With respect to the sternum, which of the following statements is correct?

A. It consists mainly of compact bone.
B. It consists of two parts.
C. It has a lower end that, in children, is actually cartilage.
D. The angle of Louis is at the level of the 4th ribs.

9. Regarding the bronchial tree, which of the following statements is correct?

A. It commences at the beginning of the trachea.
B. The left and right primary bronchi are its first branches.
C. The origin of the primary bronchi corresponds to the level of the sixth thoracic vertebra.
D. There are three left and two right secondary (lobar) bronchi.

10. Which of the following statements about the lungs is incorrect?

A. They are spongy, cone-shaped, and soft.
B. The visceral pleural lining of the lungs reflects at the diaphragm to become parietal pleura.
C. Large blood vessels and the bronchus suspend each lung in the thorax.
D. The right lung is larger than the left lung.

11. Which of the following statements about mature female breasts is incorrect?

A. They have mammary glands.
B. The nipple of a firm breast is at about the level of the sixth intercostal space.
C. They lie between the 2nd and 6th ribs.
D. Medio-laterally, they are between the sternum and axillae.

12. With regard to mammary glands, which of the following statements is correct?

A. In males and females, they are dissimilar up to puberty.
B. They are in the dermis.
C. Each consists of about fifty irregularly shaped lobes.
D. They are attached to the fascia of the pectoralis major.

13. Which of the following statements about bronchi is correct?

A. The main bronchi are of the same size.
B. The right main bronchus is more horizontal than the left.
C. The bronchial tree terminates at the alveoli.
D. Constriction of the bronchi plays a significant role in emphysema.

14. Which of the following statements about bronchi is correct?

A. An unconscious patient is more prone to aspiration via the right than the left primary bronchus.
B. The left main bronchus further divides into three bronchi.
C. The right main bronchus branches into two bronchi.
D. The left main bronchus is shorter than the right.

15. Which of the following statements pertaining to the lungs is correct?

A. The apices of the lungs are inferior to the level of the clavicles.
B. The mediastinal surfaces receive just bronchi and blood vessels.
C. The mediastinal and costal surfaces are of approximately the same size.
D. The cardiac impression diminishes the size of the left lung.

16. Which of the following statements about the bronchial tree within the lungs is correct?

A. Like the trachea and lobar bronchi, bronchioles have cartilage.
B. A bronchopulmonary segment is supplied by a secondary bronchus.
C. A pulmonary lobule is supplied by one bronchiole.
D. A terminal bronchiole is one of the 20–25 units formed by a bronchiole's branching.

17. Which of the following statements about terminal bronchioles is correct?

A. Terminal bronchioles have goblet cells.
B. Terminal bronchioles have mucous glands.
C. Terminal bronchioles have ciliated cells.
D. Terminal bronchioles are the commencement of the respiratory division.

18. A 32-year-old patient who within the past 10 days had fever, cough, and malaise with leukocytosis and marked neutrophilia develops sharp (pleuritic) right-sided chest pain and shortness of breath for 2 days. Which of the following parts is the most likely site of pathology?

A. The right main bronchus
B. The right costo-phrenic angle
C. The right ventricle
D. The right upper lobe of the lung

19. A medical student in the middle of the professional examination in the final year develops a runny nose, dry cough, and breathlessness that have become worse in the past 8 hours, preventing her from forming complete sentences without a break. She had a similar but significantly milder episode 2 years earlier. Where is the site of this pathology?

A. The bronchi
B. The trachea
C. The alveoli
D. Lung parenchyma

20. Which of the following muscles will a boxer use to give an opponent a knockout punch?

A. Rhomboideus (rhomboid) major
B. Serratus anterior
C. Trapezius
D. Rhomboideus (rhomboid) minor

21. With respect to the ribs, which of the following statements is correct?

A. Floating ribs are ribs 10–12.
B. False ribs are ribs 9–12.
C. The 1st rib is flat and vertically disposed.
D. True ribs are the first seven ribs.

22. Which of the following structures does *not* pass through the openings in the diaphragm?

A. Inferior vena cava
B. Esophagus
C. Central tendon of the diaphragm
D. Aorta

23. With respect to muscles of respiration, which of the following statements is correct?

A. Paralysis of the intercostal nerves affects the internal intercostals but not the external intercostals.
B. The diaphragm is innervated by the first intercostal nerves.
C. The internal intercostals are required to achieve forced expiration.
D. The external intercostal muscle fibers are parallel to those of the internal intercostals.

24. Which of the following statements about the esophagus is correct?

A. The length of the esophagus between the hiatus and cardia in an adult is 10 cm.
B. The lower esophageal sphincter is physiological rather than anatomical.
C. The muscularis externa consists of skeletal muscle in the proximal 2/3.
D. The submucosa consists of keratinized stratified squamous epithelium.

25. Which of the following blood vessels does *not* arise from the axillary artery?

A. Superior thoracic artery
B. Ulnar artery
C. Subscapular artery
D. Thoracoacromial artery

26. Which of the following statements about the heart is incorrect?

A. The heart is cone-shaped and a muscular pump.
B. The pericardium covers the heart and the proximal portion of its associated great vessels.
C. The pericardial cavity lies between the visceral and parietal layers of the pericardium.
D. The fibrous pericardium has no attachment to the sternum.

27. Which of the following relationships to the heart is incorrect?

A. Diaphragm—inferior
B. Spinal column—posterior
C. Lungs—medial
D. Second rib—base

28. With respect to the wall of the heart, which of the following statements is correct?

A. Purkinje fibers are specialized cells located in the myocardium.
B. The endocardium is continuous with the endothelium of the great vessels, which arise from the heart.
C. The endocardium is avascular.
D. The epicardium is devoid of nerve fibers and lymph capillaries.

29. Which of the following statements about the heart is incorrect?

A. The two heart chambers that receive blood to the heart are the auricles.
B. The ventricles lie beneath the atria.
C. The ventricles eject blood from the heart into the arteries.
D. Papillary muscles project from the walls of the ventricles.

30. With respect to cardiac valves, which of the following statements is incorrect?

A. Contraction of the right ventricle leads to tricuspid valve closure.
B. The pulmonary valve is semilunar and has three cusps.
C. Relaxation of the right ventricle leads to closure of the pulmonary valve.
D. The mitral valve prevents blood flow from the left atrium to the left ventricle.

31. Which of the following relationships pertaining to the heart is incorrect?

A. Aortic valve—three cusps; base of ascending aorta
B. Left ventricular contraction—closure of mitral valve
C. Left ventricular relaxation—closure of aortic valve
D. Right atrium—oxygenated blood

32. With respect to the heart, which of the following statements is correct?

A. The skeleton of the heart consists of rings of dense fibrous connective tissue.
B. The interventricular septum is not a part of the skeleton of the heart.
C. Blood from the coronary sinus into the right atrium is rich in oxygen.
D. The pulmonary trunk has three branches.

33. Which of the following statements pertaining to the heart is correct?

A. The atria and ventricles contract simultaneously.
B. Pressure within the ventricles remains constant.
C. Vibrations from valve movements are responsible for heart sounds.
D. Closure of the aortic and pulmonary valves is responsible for the first heart sound.

34. With respect to electrical activity of the heart, which of the following statements is correct?

A. An ECG/EKG records the electrical changes in the endocardium during a cardiac cycle.
B. The QRS complex in an ECG/EKG is a representation of ventricular repolarization.
C. The T wave of an ECG/EKG is an abnormal wave.
D. Ventricular repolarization occurs after ventricular depolarization.

35. Which of the following statements about capillaries is correct?

A. They link arterioles with venules.
B. The wall is a double layer of cells.
C. There is a loose arrangement of endothelial cells in brain capillaries.
D. The metabolic rate of a tissue has an inverse relationship with the density of its capillaries.

36. Which of the following statements about veins and arteries is incorrect?

A. Walls of veins contain less muscle and elastic tissue than arterial walls do.
B. The wall of a vein is thinner than the wall of a corresponding artery.
C. Veins are a merger of venules.
D. Arterial walls consist of endothelium, connective tissue, and skeletal muscle layers.

37. Which of the following artery-and-aorta relationships is incorrect?

A. Right coronary artery—ascending aorta
B. Left coronary artery—aortic arch
C. Left common carotid artery—aortic arch
D. Left and right common iliac arteries—abdominal aorta

38. Which of the following statements about the heart is correct?

A. Relaxation of the ventricle corresponds with diastolic blood pressure.
B. An increase in blood volume to the heart leads to a decrease in ventricular contraction.
C. The cardiac center is in the pons.
D. Central venous pressure is the pressure in the left atrium.

39. Which of the following blood vessels is *not* one of the great vessels?

A. Inferior vena cava
B. Jugular vein
C. Aorta
D. Pulmonary trunk

40. Which of the following is *not* considered a part of the circulatory system?

A. Heart
B. Arteries
C. Lymphatic vessels
D. Capillaries

41. With regard to the heart, which of the following relationships is incorrect?

A. Superior part—base
B. Anteroposterior diameter—shortest dimension
C. Inferior part—apex
D. Anterior surface—origin of the great vessels

42. With respect to blood vessels, which of the following is a correct relationship?

A. Pulmonary trunk—origin of right and left pulmonary arteries
B. Pulmonary arteries—oxygen-rich blood
C. Inferior vena cava—blood arising from the mediastinum
D. Pulmonary veins—oxygen-poor blood

43. With respect to the aortic arch, which of the following parts of the body does it *not* supply?

A. Head
B. Neck
C. Diaphragm
D. Both upper limbs

44. Which of the following statements pertaining to the wall of the heart is correct?

A. The myocardium is the thinnest layer.
B. The epicardium is synonymous with visceral pericardium.
C. The endocardium does not line the heart valves.
D. The fibrous skeleton site spares the origin of the great vessels.

45. Which of the following statements about heart valves is incorrect?

A. The mitral valve is synonymous with the tricuspid valve.
B. The right atrioventricular valve has three cusps.
C. The aortic valve is a semilunar valve.
D. Control of blood flow to the pulmonary trunk is effected by the pulmonary valve.

46. Regarding the pericardium, which of the following statements is incorrect?

A. Its various attachments maintain the position of the heart in the thorax.
B. Relative to the fibrous pericardium, the serous pericardium is thick.
C. The fibrous pericardium helps define middle mediastinal relationships.
D. The epicardium is the visceral pericardium.

 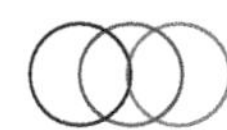

47. Which of the following statements about the pericardium is correct?

A. The serous pericardium has two layers.
B. The epicardium lines the inner surface of the fibrous pericardium.
C. The covering of the surface of the heart is the parietal pericardium.
D. Fluid accumulation in the pericardial cavity is between the serous and fibrous pericardium.

48. Pertaining to the distribution of fat tissue in the heart, which of the following statements is correct?

A. The pericardial cavity does not contain fat.
B. There is fat collection between the myocardium and epicardium.
C. The interventricular groove contains the least amount of fatty tissue.
D. It is uncommon in the acute angle of the right ventricle.

49. Which of the following statements about heart sinuses and recesses is incorrect?

A. On the right side, the transverse pericardial sinus forms the superior aortic recess.
B. The envelope of serous pericardial reflection has an inverted U-shape at the pulmonary veins.
C. The transverse pericardial sinus is anterior to the ascending aorta.
D. Pericardial reflections make the anterior and lateral surfaces of the ventricles accessible.

50. Pertaining to the heart, which of the following statements is correct?

A. The parietal pericardium comprises an outermost serosal layer with mesothelial cells.
B. The innermost layer of cells is the most distensible.
C. Pericardiocentesis is required whenever there is pericardial fluid in a patient.
D. Hemodynamic and clinical instability define cardiac tamponade.

CHAPTER 3

MCQs ON BACK

1. With regard to the epidermis, which of the following statements is incorrect?

A. The stratum basale receives nourishment from dermal blood vessels.
B. It does not have blood vessels.
C. The cells of the outermost layer are dead.
D. Keratinocytes are the main features of the deeper layer of cells.

2. Regarding the stratum granulosum of the epidermis, which of the following statements is correct?

A. The layer consists of at least ten layers of cuboidal cells.
B. The cells in this layer synthesize and store melanin.
C. Aggregation and cross-linkage are features of precursors in these cells.
D. Keratohyalin granules also synthesize bonding material for its keratin bundles.

3. With regard to the epithelium of the skin, which of the following statements is correct?

A. Defensins are products of lamellar bodies.
B. Keratohyalin produces keratinocytes.
C. Stratum lucidum is a feature of skin on the face in females.
D. The stratum corneum is made up of cuboidal cells.

4. Pertaining to heat loss from the body, which of the following statements is correct?

A. Sweat is a means of heat loss by evaporation.
B. Convection and radiation are responsible for approximately equal amounts of heat loss.
C. A person who lies on a cool floor loses heat to the floor by convection.
D. In conduction, cool air replaces warm air that has moved away from the surface of the skin.

5. Which of the following statements about the subcutaneous layer is incorrect?

A. It contains loose connective tissue fibers.
B. It has adipose tissue and skin blood vessels.
C. It contains the rete cutaneum.
D. It assists in conserving body heat.

6. Which of the following statements about somatic senses is incorrect?

A. They include the visceroception sense.
B. Meissner's corpuscles are receptors for the sensation of heavy pressure.
C. Pacinian corpuscles are receptors for the sensation of vibration.
D. Contraction of muscles stimulates muscle spindles.

DOI: 10.1201/9781003783961-4

7. Which of the following relationships is correct?

A. Thermoreceptors—free nerve endings
B. Muscle spindle—changes in muscle tension
C. Pacinian corpuscles—light touch
D. Meissner's corpuscles—heat and cold detection

8. Regarding cartilaginous joints, which of the following statements is incorrect?

A. The symphysis pubis is an example.
B. The intervertebral disk is in a symphysis.
C. A symphysis is an amphiarthrosis (amphiarthrotic joint).
D. Each of the seven costo-sternal joints is a synchondrosis.

9. Which of the following statements correctly describes a feature of a typical vertebra?

A. Intervertebral disks attached to smooth-surfaced vertebral bodies.
B. A drum-shaped posterior portion called the body.
C. Intervertebral foramina formed by the space between pedicles.
D. Weight-bearing action and cushioning effects by the vertebral bodies and intervertebral disks, respectively.

10. Regarding the vertebrae, which of the following statements is correct?

A. Vertebrae articulate with one another via the intervertebral foramina.
B. The number of intervertebral disks corresponds with the number of vertebrae.
C. Intervertebral disks compromise strength for the strength of the spinal column.
D. Articulation between an upper vertebra and a lower one involves the vertebral body indirectly.

11. Which of the following statements about vertebrae is incorrect?

A. Not all thoracic vertebrae articulate with ribs.
B. The spinal cord passes through the vertebral foramen of a vertebra.
C. The openings in a vertebra through which a spinal nerve pair passes are intervertebral foramina.
D. The bony tissue in a cervical vertebra is denser than in a lumbar vertebra.

12. Which of the following statements about the atlas is correct?

A. It has transverse foramina for the passage of nerves.
B. It is the first cervical vertebra.
C. It has a large body and two transverse processes bearing transverse foramina.
D. It is synonymous with vertebra prominens.

13. Regarding the axis, which of the following statements is correct?

A. It has an ovoid spinous process.
B. It is the third cervical vertebra.
C. It has the dens, a projection from the spinous process.
D. It enables turning of the head from side to side.

14. Which of the following bones does *not* belong to the axial skeleton?

A. The ribs
B. The clavicle
C. The sternum
D. The seventh cervical vertebra

15. Regarding the spine, which of the following statements is correct?

A. The spinal canal allows spinal nerves to exit.
B. The spinal canal is narrow in the cervical and lumbar regions.
C. The characteristic articulations allow rotation and bending movements.
D. Weight bearing is not a significant function of the spinal column.

16. Regarding blood supply to the spine, which of the following statements is correct?

A. Vertebral arteries are branches of the axillary artery.
B. Posterior intercostal arteries supply the spine.
C. Lumbar arteries arise from the lower part of the thoracic aorta.
D. The lateral sacral arteries branch from the external iliac arteries.

17. With respect to the venous drainage of the spine, which of the following statements is correct?

A. Blood from the internal and external vertebral veins enters the radicular veins.
B. Internal vertebral veins obtain their blood from intervertebral veins.
C. The venous system of the spine is a network of veins with valves.
D. The inferior vena cava primarily drains the cervical spine.

18. Which of the following statements about nerves pertaining to the spine is correct?

A. Cranial nerves are a part of the central nervous system.
B. Spinal nerves belong to the peripheral nervous system.
C. The spinal cord and spinal column are synonymous.
D. Meningeal nerves are direct branches from the spinal cord.

19. Which of the following statements pertaining to innervation of the spine is correct?

A. The spinal cord spans the distance between C1 and the tip of the coccyx.
B. The usual lower limit of the conus medullaris is L5.
C. Thirty-three pairs of spinal nerves pass through intervertebral foramina.
D. The filum terminale attaches to the dorsal surface of the coccyx.

20. Regarding the extrinsic muscles of the back, which of the following is *not* a superficial muscle?

A. Serratus posterior inferior
B. Trapezius
C. Latissimus dorsi
D. Levator scapulae

21. Regarding the intermediate muscles in the extrinsic group of muscles of the back, which of the following muscles is a member?

A. Serratus posterior superior
B. Serratus anterior
C. Deltoids
D. Subscapularis

22. Which of the following statements about the intrinsic muscles of the back is correct?

A. They are divided into two layers, referred to as superficial and deep.
B. The superficial group consists of one muscle, the splenius cervicis.
C. The splenius cervicis primarily serves in rotation movements of the spine.
D. The erector spinae are principal actors that enable extension movements of the spine.

23. Regarding the deep layer of intrinsic muscles of the back, which of the following statements is correct?

A. The muscles lie between the transverse processes and sides of the bodies of vertebrae.
B. The muscles are in two groups.
C. They are the paravertebral muscles.
D. The most superficial of the muscles is the semispinalis.

24. Which of the following muscles is *not* among the muscles that form the suboccipital triangle?

A. Rectus capitis posterior major
B. Obliquus capitis superior
C. Occipitalis
D. Obliquus capitis inferior

25. Regarding the suboccipital muscles, which of the following statements is correct?

A. Their location is the superficial part of the neck.
B. They form an important anatomical landmark, the suboccipital triangle.
C. Within a triangle that they create, the vertebral artery makes a turn to supply the cerebrum.
D. They primarily cause flexion of the head onto the upper chest.

26. Regarding the embryology of the vertebral column, which of the following statements is correct?

A. Formation of the notochordal process commences at about 12 weeks.
B. Notochordal plate arises from the floor of the notochordal processes.
C. The notochord plays little role in the formation of the vertebrae.
D. The rostral and caudal parts of the neural tube become, respectively, adult brain and spinal cord.

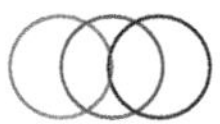

27. With regard to the development of vertebrae, which of the following statements is correct?

A. Gastrulation of the embryo commences at about 14 days.
B. Sclerotome in the mesodermal portion grows around the notochord and neural tube.
C. Formation of a vertebral body is by the process of aggregation.
D. Week 9 of embryogenesis is when cartilage formation first occurs.

28. Which of the following is *not* a vertebral defect that is associated with congenital defects of the spine?

A. Misshapen vertebrae
B. Fused vertebrae
C. Gibbus
D. Extra vertebrae

29. Regarding spina bifida, which of the following statements is correct?

A. Four types are recognized.
B. It is the result of incomplete closure of just the vertebral column.
C. The most severe form is spina bifida occulta.
D. Arnold–Chiari malformation is usually associated with myelomeningocele.

30. Regarding kyphosis, which of the following statements is correct?

A. It commonly affects the cervical spine.
B. There is exaggeration of the anterior concavity of the thoracic spinal level.
C. Obesity is the most significant risk factor.
D. It may result from osteosclerosis.

31. Which of the following statements about a patient with abnormal lordosis is correct?

A. The lumbar spine is an unusual site for this condition.
B. There is straightening of the normal curvature at the affected portion of the spine.
C. There is an increase in the anterior convexity of the affected vertebral bodies.
D. First-trimester pregnancy is a common cause.

32. Which of the following statements about scoliosis is correct?

A. There is abnormal lateral deviation and curvature of the spine.
B. It is hardly due to a genetic predisposition.
C. Disk herniation is a conspicuous cause.
D. It is common among elderly males

33. Regarding conditions that are associated with pathology in the vertebral column, which of the following statements is correct?

A. Spinal cord injury at the level of the C3 spine may result in paraplegia.
B. Exaggerated reflexes suggest a tear of the annulus fibrosus.
C. Pott's disease is from osteomyelitis of vertebral bodies and intervertebral diskitis.
D. Spondylolisthesis with posterior displacement of an upper vertebra over the lower one.

34. In a patient who suffers from back pain that is relieved by bending forward, which of the following is the most likely pathology?

A. Spinal canal stenosis
B. Osteoarthritis
C. Osteomalacia
D. Osteomyelitis

35. Which of the following conditions is *not* associated with the seronegative spondyloarthropathies?

A. Psoriatic arthritis
B. Reactive arthritis
C. Staphylococcal osteomyelitis
D. Ankylosing spondylitis

36. With respect to the sacrum, which of the following statements is correct?

A. It is part of the pelvis posteriorly.
B. It is a triangular bone made of seven fused vertebrae.
C. Its components normally fuse by age 12 years.
D. It has a promontory that indicates likely easy vaginal delivery if readily palpated on vaginal examination in an adult female.

37. With regard to lumbar vertebrae, which of the following statements is incorrect?

A. They have obliquely disposed spinous processes.
B. They have bodies that are stronger and larger than the lower thoracic vertebrae.
C. They are important in bearing weight.
D. They have transverse processes that project backward at sharp angles.

38. Which of the following statements about muscles that move the vertebral column is incorrect?

A. The iliocostalis lumborum extends the lumbar part of the vertebral column.
B. The iliocostalis cervicis extends the cervical region of the vertebral column.
C. The iliocostalis thoracis helps keep the spine erect.
D. The longissimus cervicis flexes the cervical vertebral column.

39. With respect to the vertebral column, which of the following statements is correct?

A. Kyphosis is exaggerated cervical curvature.
B. Scoliosis is exaggerated spinal curvature.
C. Gibbus is excessive thoracic angulation from wedge collapse.
D. Lordosis is a feature in newborns and not in adults.

40. Regarding the relationship between spinal nerve roots and vertebrae, which of the following statements is correct?

A. The first spinal nerve exits below the C1 vertebra.
B. The cervical enlargement serves the C4 and C5 spinal nerves.
C. There are eight cervical spinal nerves.
D. Cauda equina arises from lumbar enlargement.

41. Regarding the posterior triangle of the neck, which of the following statements is correct?

A. The semispinalis capitis and splenius capitis constitute its floor.
B. The trapezius is lateral to the sternocleidomastoid.
C. The great auricular nerve lies superior to the lesser occipital nerve.
D. The lesser occipital nerve and the great auricular nerve arise from the cervical plexus at C2 and C3.

42. Which of the following statements about vertebral ligaments in the lumbosacral region is incorrect?

A. The anterior longitudinal ligament attaches to the dorsal surface of the sacrum.
B. The posterior and lateral sacrococcygeal ligaments attach to the sacrum and the coccyx.
C. The posterior longitudinal ligament runs along the concave surface of vertebral bodies.
D. Supraspinous and interspinous ligaments extend to the coccygeal cornu.

43. Regarding the sacrum and the coccyx, which of the following statements is incorrect?

A. The apex of the sacrum is its proximal part.
B. The anterior sacral foramina are synonymous with pelvic sacral foramina.
C. The median sacral crest is the equivalent of a spinous process in other vertebrae.
D. The sacral hiatus is the inferior limit of the sacral canal.

44. Which of the following statements about the multifidus is incorrect?

A. Its proximal attachment includes the ilium.
B. Its principal action is rotation of the spine.
C. Blood supply of its cervical portion is by deep cervical arteries.
D. The dorsal rami of each region provide innervation to the multifidus.

45. A 61-year-old man developed severe left lower back pain after sitting on the edge of a bed for about 3 hours working on a laptop. The pain got worse on trying to roll out of bed on waking up the next morning. Which muscle must have gotten strained?

A. Serratus posterior
B. Quadratus lumborum
C. Multifidus lumborum
D. Semispinalis thoracis

CHAPTER 4

MCQs ON PELVIS AND PERINEUM

1. Which of the following relationships is correct?

A. Oral cavity—pseudostratified columnar epithelium
B. Small intestine—stratified squamous epithelium
C. Nasal cavity—stratified squamous epithelium
D. Reproductive tract—mucus secretion

2. Which of the following is *not* a feature of synovial joints?

A. The synovial membrane is avascular.
B. The inner layer of the joint capsule consists of loose connective tissue.
C. The synovial membrane encloses the synovial cavity.
D. Synovial fluid is clear and viscous.

3. Which of the following statements about the human pelvis is correct?

A. The postero-lateral and antero-medial surfaces of the ilium are smooth.
B. The ilium is the second largest of the pelvic bones.
C. Posterior superior iliac spines correspond to two skin dimples in some individuals.
D. The true pelvis and false pelvis are separated by the pelvic outlet.

4. Which of the following describes the pelvis in an adult female?

A. The false pelvis is deeper.
B. The pubic arch has an angle that is >90°.
C. The coccyx is less moveable.
D. The pelvic inlet has the shape of the heart.

5. Which of the following statements about the pelvis is incorrect?

A. The sacral promontory, ileo-pectineal lines, and symphysis pubis are boundaries of the true pelvis.
B. The widest diameter of the female pelvic inlet is antero-posterior.
C. The upper limit of the rectum is at the third piece of the sacrum.
D. The right ureter is expected anterior to the bifurcation of the right common iliac artery.

6. Regarding the bony framework of the pelvis, which of the following is *not* a part of the iliac crest?

A. Intermediate zone
B. Tubercle
C. Outer lip
D. Inner lip

DOI: 10.1201/9781003783961-5

7. With regard to measurements of the pelvis, which of the following is an incorrect description?

A. The plane of the pelvic outlet joins the inferior margin of the pubic symphysis and the tip of the coccyx.
B. The diagonal conjugate is the distance between the inferior margin of the pubic symphysis and the sacral promontory.
C. The plane of the pelvic inlet is the true conjugate diameter of the pelvic inlet.
D. The transverse diameter of the pelvic outlet is the narrowest distance of the pelvic outlet.

8. Which of the following parts of the bony framework of the pelvis does *not* contribute to the outline of the pelvic inlet?

A. Ischial spine
B. Pecten pubis
C. Arcuate line
D. Sacral promontory

9. Regarding the pelvic bones, which of the following statements is incorrect?

A. The sacrum has five segments and four foramina.
B. The ilium and pubis contribute to the anatomy and surgery of inguinal hernias.
C. The ilium makes the major contribution to the obturator foramen.
D. The lesser sciatic notch is closely related to the ischial spine.

10. Which of the following statements about the bony structure of the pelvis is incorrect?

A. The ischial spine separates the greater sciatic notch from the lesser sciatic notch.
B. The pubic arch is formed by the inferior pubic rami linked by the inferior pubic ligament.
C. The subpubic angle helps in forensic identification of the sex of a deceased person using the pelvis.
D. The transverse process of the third lumbar vertebra articulates with the iliac tuberosity.

11. Regarding the false pelvis, which of the following statements is incorrect?

A. The arcuate line forms its upper limit.
B. The greater sciatic notch is between the posterior inferior iliac spine and the ischial spine.
C. The anterior gluteal line is on the posterior equivalent of the iliac fossa.
D. The iliopubic eminence is a part of the boundary between the false and true pelves.

12. Which of the following statements about the true pelvis is inaccurate?

A. The greater sciatic foramen is posterosuperior to the obturator canal.
B. The greater and lesser sciatic foramina are separated by the sacrospinous ligament.
C. The obturator canal pierces the obturator membrane.
D. The sacrotuberous ligament attaches to the ischial tuberosity inferiorly.

13. Which of the following statements about the structure of the bony pelvis is correct?

A. During pregnancy, there is strengthening of the ligaments and cartilages, especially in the pubic bone.
B. The ischiopubic ramus is superior to the superior pubic ramus.
C. The posterior sacral foramina are lateral to the supraspinous ligament.
D. The anterior longitudinal ligament extends to the convex surface of the sacral bones.

14. Which of the following statements about the pelvic bones is correct?

A. The obturator membrane is attached to the symphyseal surface of the pubic bone.
B. The acetabulum is notched at its anterolateral margin.
C. The transverse acetabular ligament is inferior to the acetabular notch.
D. There is no articulation at the lunate surface of the acetabulum.

15. With regard to the ligaments of the pelvis, which of the following is *not* located on the posterior aspect of the pelvic bones?

A. The two ligaments on the concavity of the sacrum
B. The supraspinous ligament
C. The posterior sacroiliac ligament
D. The sacrotuberous ligament

16. Regarding the pelvic diaphragm in females, which of the following statements is correct?

A. The deep dorsal vein of the clitoris lies between the pubic bone and the urethra.
B. From the posterior to anterior, the correct order of structures is the vagina, rectum, and urethra.
C. The tendinous arch of the levator ani muscle links the pubic bone with the sacral promontory.
D. The iliococcygeus muscle is posterior to the ischiococcygeus muscle.

17. Which of the following statements about the pelvic floor in males is correct?

A. The deep dorsal veins of the penis lie lateral to the urethra.
B. The coccygeus lies inferior to the sacrospinous ligament and sacrotuberous ligament.
C. The levator ani muscle consists of the puborectalis muscle and iliococcygeus muscle.
D. The puborectalis is the most anteriorly positioned component of the levator ani muscles.

18. With regard to the levator ani muscle in males, which of the following statements is correct?

A. The body of the pubic bone constitutes the proximal attachment.
B. The distal attachment is at three sites.
C. The arterial blood supply is via the inferior gluteal artery and internal pudendal artery.
D. Innervation is by the dorsal rami of the lower sacral nerves and the perineal nerve.

19. Regarding the pelvic diaphragm in females, which of the following is not a midline structure?

A. Levator plate of levator ani muscle
B. Tendinous arch of levator ani muscle
C. Interdigitating fibers of the perineum
D. Transverse perineal ligament

20. Which of the following statements about pelvic viscera in females is correct?

A. The pouch of Douglas is a peritoneal reflection over the uterus.
B. An ovary lies anterior to the external iliac artery and external iliac vein.
C. The vesicouterine pouch is at a higher level than the rectouterine pouch.
D. The ureter is an intraperitoneal structure.

21. When viewing the pelvis from the abdominal cavity, which of the following statements is correct?

A. The fundus of the non-pregnant uterus is in the abdominal cavity.
B. The round ligament of the uterus takes a course posterior to the fallopian tube.
C. The ovary is on the anterior wall of the broad ligament.
D. The rectouterine folds are at a higher level than the rectouterine pouch.

22. Which of the following statements regarding the female reproductive organs is correct?

A. The uterine cervix is not enveloped but lined anteriorly by the uterovaginal fascia.
B. The cardinal ligament is synonymous with Mackenrodt's ligament.
C. The transverse ligaments run transversely from the fundus and body of the uterus.
D. The sacrouterine ligament is a single ligament that links the uterus to the sacrum.

23. With respect to the uterus, which of the following statements is correct?

A. Like the bladder in a child, it is an abdominopelvic organ.
B. When retroverted, it may present as painful coitus.
C. It is anteverted and anteflexed in the minority of women.
D. It is linked to the labia by the ligament of Trietz.

24. Which of the following statements about female genital organs is correct?

A. An acutely inflamed fallopian tube becomes gangrenous without early intervention.
B. Ovarian vessels are structures normally found in the suspensory ligament of the ovary.
C. The fimbriae are at the mid-portion of the fallopian tubes.
D. The level of the pouch of Douglas is higher than that of the utero-vesical peritoneal reflection in the erect position.

25. Which of the following statements about the female reproductive system is incorrect?

A. Each ovary is ovoid and lies in an ovarian fossa.
B. An ovary is considered normal in size if it is about $3.5 \times 2.0 \times 1.0$ cm in length, width, and thickness, respectively.
C. The suspensory ligament contains ovarian blood vessels and nerves.
D. The ovarian ligament is a part of the suspensory ligament.

26. Which of the following is a female internal accessory organ?

A. Oviducts
B. Vestibule
C. Labium majus
D. Vagina

27. Regarding the testes, which of the following statements is incorrect?

A. They are the primary sex organs in males.
B. They are spherical structures.
C. They are enclosed in tunica albuginea.
D. They have at least 250 lobules each.

28. Which of the following statements about the male reproductive organ is incorrect?

A. A testicular lobule may have up to four seminiferous tubules.
B. A seminiferous tubule is about 25 cm long.
C. The epididymis is made up of ducts of the rete testis.
D. The rete testis is in the mediastinum testis.

29. Which of the following is *not* an internal accessory organ of the male reproductive system?

A. The seminal vesicle
B. The prostate gland
C. The scrotum
D. The bulbourethral glands

30. Which of the following statements about the male reproductive organs is correct?

A. Seminal vesicles are in close relationship with the anterior surface of the urinary bladder.
B. Seminal vesicles are within the rectovesical space.
C. A seminal vesicle lies superior to the ipsilateral ureter.
D. The ductus deferens courses around the inferior surface of the bladder toward the ipsilateral seminal vesicle.

31. Regarding the parts of the urinary bladder, which of the following is incorrect?

A. Fascia lines its external surface
B. The fundus is the posterior part
C. The neck is just superior to the prostate
D. The apex points upward

32. Which of the following statements about the urinary bladder is correct?

A. The trigone is bounded by ureteric and urethral openings.
B. A full normal bladder accommodates up to 1.2 liters of urine.
C. It fills up by expanding postero-inferiorly.
D. The mucosa has epithelial characteristics of the ureters.

33. With respect to the prostate, which of the following statements is correct?

A. Penetrating injury above the symphysis pubis by a narrow and sharp-pointed object would involve it significantly.
B. The prostatic venous plexus is located posterior to the prostate.
C. The prostatic venous plexus is superior to the transverse perineal ligament.
D. The lateral lobes of the prostate are most commonly implicated in bladder outlet obstruction.

34. A 65-year-old man complains of gradual onset of urinary frequency, urgency, terminal dribbling, and spending a longer time than usual to urinate. There is no dysuria, hematuria, or weight loss, and the volume of urine that he passes has not increased. To which of the following does the symptomatology primarily point?

A. The pancreas
B. The urethra
C. The prostate
D. The urinary bladder

35. Regarding the rectum, which of the following statements is correct?

A. Supero-inferiorly, the structures anterior to it are the rectovesical pouch, seminal vesicle, prostate, and Denonvilliers' fascia.
B. The ampulla of the rectum is the proximal portion.
C. It has two characteristic folds: the superior rectal valve and inferior rectal valve.
D. It is the site of absorption of vitamin B_{12}.

36. Which of the following is *not* a function of the rectum?

A. Storage of contents of the gut delivered by the sigmoid colon
B. Secretion of digestive enzymes
C. Delivery of fecal material to the anal canal
D. Secretion of mucus to lubricate feces

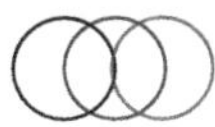

37. Which of the following statements about digital rectal examination is correct?

A. It is relevant in making clinical diagnosis of benign prostatic enlargement.
B. It is painless in patients with anal fissure.
C. It helps in diagnosing carcinoma of the colon.
D. It should not be carried out on a patient suspected of having a rectal neoplasm.

38. Which of the following veins is *not* a tributary of the inferior vena cava?

A. Common iliac veins
B. Right suprarenal vein
C. Hepatic veins
D. Left gonadal vein

39. Which of the following veins does *not* drain into the great saphenous vein?

A. Deep external iliac vein
B. Deep circumflex iliac vein
C. Superficial epigastric vein
D. Lateral accessory vein

40. Which of the following statements about the urethra in the adult female is correct?

A. It is about 10 cm in length.
B. For catheterization, it is identified between the vaginal orifice and the clitoris.
C. It extends from the internal urethral sphincter to the external urethral sphincter.
D. Its length naturally protects it from involvement in infections.

41. Regarding fasciae and ligaments in the female perineum, which of the following statements is correct?

A. The levator ani lies between the superior and inferior fasciae of the pelvic diaphragm.
B. The anococcygeal body lies anterior to the external anal sphincter body.
C. The location of the perineal body is between the bladder and vagina.
D. Colles' fascia forms the superior border of the superficial perineal space.

42. Which of the following statements about the female perineum and external genitalia is correct?

A. In the space formed by the ischiocavernosus, superficial transverse perineal, and bulbospongiosus muscles, the bulbospongiosus muscle makes the lateral wall.
B. Gallaudet's fascia is the deep perineal fascia.
C. The suspensory ligament of the clitoris and round ligament of the uterus are midline structures.
D. From the anterior to posterior, the structures are the perineal raphe, posterior commissure of labia majora, and hymenal caruncle.

43. Which of the following statements regarding the male urethra is correct?

A. The male's control of urine involves the internal and external urethral sphincters.
B. The prostatic urethra is the shortest of the three regions.
C. When doing instrumentation of the urethra, the C-shape should be considered.
D. The terminal part of the urethra is lined by stratified squamous epithelium.

44. With regard to the male perineal spaces, which of the following statements is incorrect?

A. Covered by the perineal membrane, the dorsal nerve of the penis runs lateral to the internal pudendal artery.
B. The internal pudendal artery gives off the artery of the bulb of the penis and the dorsal artery of the penis.
C. The bulbospongiosus muscle is external to the corpus spongiosum.
D. The external urethral sphincter muscle is lateral to the bulbourethral glands.

45. Which of the following statements about the perineum in a male is incorrect?

A. The lateral superficial vein is lateral to the deep dorsal vein and the dorsal artery.
B. The dartos fascia of the penis lies between the penile skin and Buck's fascia of the penis.
C. The penile urethra traverses the corpus spongiosum and its tunica albuginea.
D. A cross-section of the penis shows the intercavernous septum of deep fascia ventral to the urethra.

CHAPTER 5

MCQs ON UPPER LIMB

1. **Which of the following statements about the epidermis is incorrect?**

   A. Melanocytes are found in the mid-portion of the epidermis.
   B. By the process of cytocrine secretion, melanin granules may be introduced into non-melanocyte epidermal cells.
   C. Melanocytes are the only cells that produce melanin.
   D. Melanocytes play a role in protecting the skin from the ill effects of sunlight.

2. **Which of the following is *not* a feature of the dermis?**

   A. It contains collagenous fibers.
   B. Both smooth and striated muscle fibers may be present, depending on the site.
   C. It contains Pacinian corpuscles and Meissner's corpuscles, which appreciate light touch and heavy pressure, respectively.
   D. Sebaceous glands and sweat glands are in the dermis.

3. **Which of the following statements about nails is incorrect?**

   A. They are produced by specialized epithelial cells.
   B. They have a whitish, half-moon-shaped portion called the nail plate.
   C. They grow most actively at the base of the nail plate.
   D. They have keratinized cells.

4. **Which of the following statements about hair follicles is incorrect?**

   A. They are not present on the nipples and portions of the external reproductive organs.
   B. They produce hairs that are replaced by new hairs with time.
   C. They have a bundle of skeletal muscle cells called arrector pili muscle attached to them.
   D. They have a hair root.

5. **With respect to sweat glands, which of the following statements is incorrect?**

   A. The external part found on the skin surface is called the pore.
   B. They are responsible for certain people's hands being moist.
   C. The type called apocrine glands produces secretions with a scent.
   D. Apocrine sweat glands are common on the back, neck, and forehead.

6. **Which of the following statements about long bones is incorrect?**

   A. The diaphysis is synonymous with the shaft.
   B. The periosteum is fibrous tissue with no blood supply.
   C. The epiphysis is at the ends of the bone.
   D. The part of the bone that participates in a joint is covered with hyaline cartilage.

DOI: 10.1201/9781003783961-6

7. Which of these statements about bones is incorrect?

A. Vitamin D deficiency leads to poor small intestinal absorption of calcium and osteomalacia in adults.
B. Vitamin C is required for collagen synthesis in bone.
C. Androgens and estrogens play no role in the growth of long bones during puberty.
D. Exercise tends to strengthen bones.

8. With respect to synovial joints, which of the following statements is correct?

A. They are a minority in the skeletal system.
B. They have a synovial membrane but lack articular cartilage.
C. They do not possess a joint capsule.
D. They are more complex than cartilaginous joints.

9. Which of the following statements about a synovial joint is correct?

A. A thin layer of hyaline cartilage on articular ends of bones limits friction during movement.
B. There is a subchondral plate of cortical bone.
C. Injury to the subchondral plate produces more elasticity on healing.
D. The inner layer of the joint capsule has dense connective tissue.

10. Which of the following relationships pertaining to joint movements is correct?

A. Pronation—turning the hand so that the palm faces upward
B. Inversion—turning the foot, making the sole face laterally
C. Adduction—lifting the upper limb to a horizontal position and making a 90° angle with the side of the body
D. Elevation—shrugging the shoulders

11. Which of the following statements about joints is incorrect?

A. The shoulder joint is a ball-and-socket joint, like the hip joint.
B. The fibro-cartilage, acetabular labrum, makes the acetabulum deeper.
C. The capsule of the elbow joint does not cover the radioulnar joint.
D. The knee joint is not only the largest but also the most complex synovial joint.

12. Which of the following statements about the shoulder joint is correct?

A. The glenoidal labrum is too thin to contribute to the depth of the glenoid cavity.
B. The rotator cuff consists of tendons of several muscles that blend with the capsule.
C. The rotator cuff is a poor support of the joint.
D. The only bursa associated with it is the subscapular bursa.

13. Which of the following statements about the shoulder joint is correct?

A. Muscles are not important in maintaining stability of the joint.
B. The capsule covers the joint incompletely.
C. Falling on an outstretched arm hardly overcomes the supporting structures of the joint.
D. Acromio-clavicular and coraco-clavicular articulations further enhance the range of shoulder movements.

14. Which of the following statements about the elbow joint is incorrect?

A. It is an articulation between the humerus and both the ulna and radius.
B. It is a hinge joint that allows flexion and extension movements.
C. It is a pivot joint that allows pronation and supination.
D. By the articulation between the humerus and ulna, it forms a gliding joint.

15. Which of the following anatomic structures is *not* a lymphatic organ?

A. Thymus
B. Skin
C. Spleen
D. Mucous membranes

16. Which of the following relationships for lymphatic vessels is correct?

A. Superficial lymph vessels—origin in the dermis
B. Deep lymph vessels—accompany deep veins
C. Lymph channels—origin of lymphatic vasculature
D. Collecting vessels—drainage into lymph nodes

17. Regarding the lymph nodes of the upper extremities, which of the following relationships is incorrect?

A. Posterior nodes—drainage of the posterior thoracic wall and the scapular area
B. Lateral nodes—primary lymphatic drainage of the upper limb
C. Anterior nodes—lymphatic drainage of the breast
D. Central nodes—identified in close relationship with the first part of the axillary artery

18. Regarding lymph nodes in the upper limbs, which of the following statements is incorrect?

A. The axillary lymph nodes are in the axillary pad of fat.
B. Pectoral lymph nodes are synonymous with anterior lymph nodes.
C. Lymph from the breast goes to the posterior lymph nodes.
D. Lymph from the arm drains into the lateral lymph nodes.

19. Regarding the axilla, which of the following relationships is correct?

A. Medial wall—the brachium
B. Anterior wall—serratus anterior muscle
C. Posterior wall—latissimus dorsi muscle
D. Lateral wall—anterior surface of the clavicle

20. Which of the following structures is *not* in the axilla?

A. Bifurcation of brachial artery
B. Axillary artery
C. Lymph nodes
D. Axillary vein

21. A flatmate rushes an extremely weak patient to the emergency room; he says he heard him shout, "My arm, my arm!" and met him drenched in sweat and holding his left arm. With no history of a fall, what investigation must you carry out to find the cause of this sudden illness?

A. Chest X-ray
B. Complete (Full) blood count
C. Electrocardiography
D. Liver function tests

22. Considering the nerve network in the brachial plexus, which of the following is *not* an applicable term?

A. Trunks
B. Roots
C. Branches
D. Chords

23. Which of the following correctly describes the order of the brachial plexus from its proximal part toward the distal part?

A. Rami, cords, divisions, trunks, terminal branches
B. Trunks, rami, cords, divisions, terminal branches
C. Roots, trunks, divisions, cords, terminal branches
D. Cords, rami, trunks, divisions, terminal branches

24. Which of the following statements about the brachial plexus is correct?

A. The ventral rami are from the C4 to T1 spinal nerves.
B. Continuation of the C6 root forms the middle trunk.
C. The trunks have anterior and posterior divisions that form three cords.
D. The posterior cord has fibers from C6 to T1.

25. Which of the following relationships about the nerve supply of the indicated muscles is correct?

A. The radial nerve—pronator teres
B. Ulnar nerve—supinator
C. Ulnar nerve—extensor carpi ulnaris
D. Radial nerve—triceps brachii

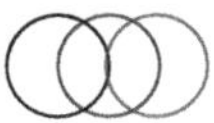

26. Which of the following associations between muscles and their nerve supply by the brachial plexus is correct?

A. Long thoracic nerve—serratus anterior
B. Dorsal scapular nerve—pectoralis major
C. Medial antebrachial cutaneous nerve—pectoralis minor
D. Middle subscapular nerve—teres major

27. Which of the following actions at the shoulder joint is the trapezius *not* involved in?

A. Medial rotation
B. Depression
C. Retraction
D. Elevation

28. Which of the following is *not* a part of the proximal portion of the humerus?

A. The surgical neck
B. The greater tubercle
C. The deltoid tuberosity
D. The intertubercular sulcus

29. With respect to the venous system, which of the statements below is correct?

A. Veins return only deoxygenated blood to the heart.
B. A brachiocephalic vein is formed by an axillary and a jugular vein uniting.
C. Major veins maintain a path different from the corresponding main arteries.
D. The median cubital vein is a usual site for venipuncture.

30. Which of the following is a superficial vein?

A. Subclavian vein
B. Basilic vein
C. Azygos vein
D. Superior mesenteric vein

31. In the upper limb, which of the following is correct?

A. The medial portion of a fractured clavicle is depressed by the sternocleidomastoid.
B. The deltoid convexity is reduced or obliterated in shoulder dislocation.
C. The first part of the axillary artery is palpable in the axilla.
D. The brachial artery is palpable on the lateral part of the arm.

32. Which of the following statements about the bones of the upper limb is correct?

A. The clavicle is one of the least commonly fractured bones.
B. The proximal part of the humerus is adducted when the humeral fracture line is below the insertion of the deltoid.
C. Involvement of the radial nerve in fracture of the humeral shaft results in wrist drop.
D. The posterior border of the ulna is palpable proximally only.

33. Regarding the nerves of the upper limb, which of these statements is correct?

A. Damage to the deep branch of the radial nerve causes wrist drop with flaccidity.
B. Injuries to the ulnar nerve are unlikely in fractures of the humeral medial epicondyle.
C. A stab wound causing injury to the ulnar nerve at the wrist results in paralysis of the muscles of the thenar eminence.
D. Injury to the median nerve proximal to the flexor retinaculum makes thumb opposition impossible.

34. By virtue of its relationship with the retinaculum, which of the following structures is *not* vulnerable to injury at the level of the flexor retinaculum?

A. Ulnar artery
B. Palmar cutaneous branch of the median nerve
C. Pronator teres tendon
D. Ulnar nerve

35. Which of the following statements is incorrect?

A. The radial artery is palpable in the "anatomical snuffbox."
B. The ulnar artery is palpable medial to the flexor carpi ulnaris tendon.
C. The median nerve innervates all the muscles of the thenar eminence.
D. The radial artery is palpable lateral to the flexor carpi radialis tendon.

36. With respect to the scapula, which of the following statements is correct?

A. It has a spine posteriorly that ends at the head, which bears two processes.
B. It bears the coracoid process, which meets the outer (lateral) end of the clavicle.
C. It has the coracoid process, which forms the tip of the shoulder.
D. It is a flat triangular bone with an anterior convexity.

37. Which of the following statements about clavicles is correct?

A. The lateral ends are attached to the manubrium.
B. The medial ends are the acromial ends.
C. Some muscles of the back and upper limbs are attached to the clavicles.
D. They are prone to fracture at the inner third.

38. Which of the following features applies to the humerus?

A. Muscles that move the upper limb at the shoulder are attached to the greater and lesser tubercles.
B. The greater tubercle is located on the anterior portion of the upper part of the humerus.
C. A nerve passes in the groove between the greater and lesser tubercles.
D. The surgical neck is the site where fractures least occur.

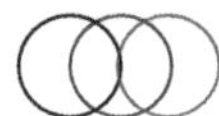

39. With respect to the humerus, which of the following statements is correct?

A. The coronoid fossa is at the posterior part of the lower end of the humerus.
B. The deltoid, which raises the arm horizontally, is attached to a medially located tuberosity.
C. The olecranon fossa receives a process of the radius.
D. The trochlea and capitulum are condyles and so help with movements at the elbows.

40. Which of the following statements about the radius and ulna is correct?

A. The radius is slightly shorter than the ulna.
B. The radial tuberosity is the proximal attachment of the biceps brachii tendon.
C. Supination of the hand results in the radius crossing over the ulna.
D. Both flexion and extension movements at the elbow involve the trochlea and capitulum.

41. Which of the following statements about the hands is incorrect?

A. The presence of fourteen phalanges in one hand is normal.
B. The wrist has two rows of four metacarpals, making eight bones.
C. The palm has bones that normally correspond to the number of fingers.
D. The first metacarpal is the most freely movable, allowing opposition movement.

42. Which of the following statements about muscles that move the arm is correct?

A. The deltoid is an adductor.
B. The coracobrachialis flexes the arm.
C. The pectoralis major and pectoralis minor are flexors.
D. The supraspinatus is an adductor.

43. With respect to muscles that move the arm, which of the following relationships is incorrect?

A. Coracobrachialis—median nerve
B. Teres major—extension and adduction
C. Latissimus dorsi—thoracodorsal nerve
D. Supraspinatus and infraspinatus—suprascapular nerve

44. Regarding the muscles that move the arm, which of the following statements is incorrect?

A. The deltoid and teres minor have the same nerve supply.
B. The pectoralis major and teres major rotate the arm laterally.
C. The latissimus dorsi and pectoralis major have the same insertion.
D. The coracobrachialis and pectoralis major cause flexion.

45. Which of the following relationships is incorrect?

A. Brachialis—strongest flexor of elbow
B. Brachioradialis—flexion
C. Biceps brachii—musculocutaneous nerve
D. Supinator—medial rotation of forearm

46. With respect to muscles that move the forearm, which of the following statements is correct?

A. The radial nerve supplies just the extensor muscles.
B. The pronator quadratus lies between the proximal ends of the radius and ulna.
C. The brachialis has more than one nerve supply.
D. The triceps brachii has the olecranon process of the ulna as its origin.

47. Which of the following is *not* a part of the proximal portion of the humerus?

A. The surgical neck
B. The greater tubercle
C. The deltoid tuberosity
D. The intertubercular sulcus

48. You direct a house officer (fresh medical graduate) posted to your department within the week to do a phlebotomy for laboratory investigations using blood from any of the patient's veins between the antecubital fossa and the wrist. Which of the following veins should *not* be used?

A. Median antebrachial vein
B. Median cubital vein
C. Accessory cephalic vein
D. Brachial vein

49. Which of the following arteries is useful for the measurement of pulse and blood pressure at the level of the arm of a patient?

A. Axillary artery
B. Brachiocephalic trunk
C. Brachial artery
D. Radial artery

50. Regarding having a good grip with the fingers, which of the following statements is incorrect?

A. The action of the wrist extensors is not required.
B. Thumb opposition is essential.
C. Both intrinsic and extrinsic hand muscles are in use.
D. The thumb provides a counterforce.

CHAPTER 6

MCQs ON LOWER LIMB

1. **Pertaining to the layers of the epidermis, which of the following statements is correct?**

   A. The stratum corneum consists of many layers of nucleated cells.
   B. The stratum granulosum is just beneath the stratum corneum in the soles of the feet.
   C. The stratum lucidum has cells that are clear.
   D. The stratum basale has five rows of cuboidal or columnar cells.

2. **With respect to temperature regulation, which of the following statements is incorrect?**

   A. The set point for body temperature is controlled by the hypothalamus.
   B. The liver and skeletal muscles produce insignificant amounts of heat.
   C. In a hot environment, the deeper blood vessels constrict to divert blood to the skin.
   D. Vasodilatation takes place in blood vessels of the skin to release heat from the body.

3. **Which of the following statements about sebaceous glands is incorrect?**

   A. They are present on the palms and soles.
   B. They are usually connected to hair follicles.
   C. They are holocrine glands.
   D. They produce fatty material.

4. **Which of the following is *not* a feature of sweat glands?**

   A. They arise from the superficial part of the dermis.
   B. They have both a tubular portion and a coiled, ball-shaped deeper end.
   C. They are synonymous with sudoriferous glands.
   D. The secretory portion consists of epithelial cells.

5. **Which of the following statements about the lymphatic system is incorrect?**

   A. The thoracic duct drains the mirror image of the body part drained by the right lymphatic duct.
   B. The right lymphatic duct and the thoracic duct empty into the subclavian veins.
   C. A typical lymph node consists of densely packed B and T cells.
   D. Lymph enters lymph nodes via vessels that are narrower than the ones by which they exit nodes.

6. **Regarding the blood supply and lymphatic drainage of the lower limb, which of the following statements is incorrect?**

   A. Genicular arteries are branches of the femoral artery.
   B. Venous cutdown for patients in shock can be done using the great saphenous vein.
   C. The position of the great saphenous vein is constant in front of the medial malleolus.
   D. The vertical superficial lymph nodes drain lymph from only part of the lower limb.

DOI: 10.1201/9781003783961-7

7. A patient in incipient shock from severe hemorrhage requires venous cutdown. Which of the following veins is suitable for the emergency procedure?

A. Great saphenous vein
B. Small saphenous vein
C. Popliteal vein
D. Femoral vein

8. Which of the following statements about the femoral artery is incorrect?

A. It plays an insignificant role in the etiology of intermittent claudication.
B. In the thigh, it passes through the femoral triangle.
C. It is a common site of cannulation for various procedures.
D. It is the main provider of arterial blood to the lower limb.

9. Which of the following arteries is a branch of the femoral artery?

A. Sural artery
B. Popliteal artery
C. Descending genicular artery
D. Anterior tibial artery

10. Which of the following blood supply relationships is incorrect?

A. Knee—femoral artery
B. Gastrocnemius—popliteal artery
C. Upper lateral thorax—axillary artery
D. Scalp—external carotid artery

11. Which of the following arteries does *not* supply the ankle joint?

A. Anterior tibial artery
B. Posterior tibial artery
C. Fibular artery
D. Genicular artery

12. Which of the following relationships correctly describes the bone?

A. Trapezoid—long bone
B. Cuneiform—flat bone
C. Frontal bone—short bone
D. Patella—sesamoid bone

13. Which of the following statements is representative of the anatomy of the lower extremities?

A. The greater trochanter of the femur is palpable on the medial surface of the thigh.
B. The landmark of the sciatic nerve is midway between the ischial tuberosity and the greater trochanter.
C. The femoral nerve lies medial to the pulsation of the femoral artery.
D. The rectus femoris does not insert into the patella.

14. Which of the following statements is correct?

A. Open fractures of the shaft of the tibia are unusual.
B. The distal part of the femur is pulled upward when there is a fracture of the neck of the femur.
C. The sciatic nerve is not at risk of injury in posterior dislocation of the hip.
D. The tibia is subcutaneous in its entire length laterally.

15. With respect to the lower limb, which of the following statements is correct?

A. The Achilles tendon lies lateral to the calcaneus.
B. The dorsalis pedis artery is palpable between the tendons of the extensor hallucis longus and extensor digitorum longus.
C. The medial malleolus is at the distal end of the fibula.
D. Midway between the medial malleolus and the Achilles tendon, the anterior tibial pulse is palpable.

16. Which of the following relationships of lower limb bones is incorrect?

A. Fibula—shinbone
B. Tibia—medial to the fibula
C. Patella—knee cap
D. Femur—longest bone in the body

17. Regarding the hip joint, which of the following statements is accurate?

A. The ligamentum capitis is essential to the union between the femoral head and the acetabulum.
B. The joint capsule is reinforced by other ligaments.
C. The capsule extends from the head of the femur to the acetabular rim.
D. The blood supply to the head of the femur is through the joint capsule.

18. When soldiers march during a parade, which of the following muscles plays an important role in flexing the femur at the hip joint?

A. Flexor digitorum superficialis
B. Iliopsoas
C. Soleus
D. Gastrocnemius

19. Regarding the glutei, which of the following statements is correct?

A. The gluteus medius originates from the inner aspect of the ilium.
B. The gluteus medius receives innervation from the superior gluteal nerve.
C. The gluteus medius inserts into the linea aspera.
D. The gluteus medius, acting alone, abducts the thigh at the hip joint.

20. With regard to the gluteus maximus, which of the following statements is correct?

A. Proximal attachment is the anterior surface of the ilium.
B. It has three points of insertion.
C. The sole arterial supply is by the superior gluteal artery.
D. Paralysis allows normal movement on a plane surface.

21. Which of the following is *not* a hip muscle?

A. Gemellus inferior
B. Piriformis
C. Adductor magnus
D. Gluteus minimus

22. With regard to the femur, which of the following statements is incorrect?

A. The greater trochanter is below the head of the femur.
B. Muscles are attached to the lesser trochanter.
C. A ligament is attached to the fovea capitis.
D. The patella does not articulate with the femur.

23. With regard to the muscles that move the thigh, which of the following statements is correct?

A. The psoas major and iliacus belong to the anterior group.
B. The tensor fasciae latae adducts.
C. The pectineus is one of the abductors.
D. The gracilis is a long, strap-like muscle of knee extension.

24. With respect to the muscles that move the leg, which of the following statements is correct?

A. The biceps femoris is at the front of the femur.
B. The semitendinosus flexes and rotates the leg laterally.
C. The semimembranosus is a part of the quadriceps femoris.
D. The sartorius flexes both the leg and thigh.

25. Which of the following is a part of the shaft of the femur?

A. Medial condyle
B. Lateral epicondyle
C. Greater trochanter
D. Linea aspera

26. A 40-year-old man complains of difficulty in flexing the left knee following vigorous exercise that led to a fall 2 days previously. Which of the following muscles is ruled out from involvement in the accident?

A. Sartorius
B. Semimembranosus
C. Vastus lateralis
D. Popliteus

27. A 53-year-old woman notices that she has *not* been able to cross her legs with ease following a trip and fall during which she hit her knee on the side of a heavy wooden stool. Which of the following muscles was most likely injured?

A. Semitendinosus
B. Biceps femoris
C. Vastus intermedius
D. Sartorius

28. Which of the following statements about the patella is incorrect?

A. It is a sesamoid bone.
B. It lies within a tendon that crosses over the knee anteriorly.
C. It may be dislocated from its position secondary to trauma.
D. It is a dispensable superficial bone.

29. Which of the following statements about the knee joint is incorrect?

A. It has two condyloid joints.
B. It has a gliding joint.
C. It has four menisci that separate the articulating surfaces of the tibia and femur.
D. It allows mainly flexion and extension.

30. Which of the following bursae associated with the knee joint is anatomically close to the largest sesamoid bone?

A. Suprapatellar bursa
B. Iliotibial bursa
C. Pes anserine bursa
D. Fibular collateral ligament bursa

31. Regarding bursae, which of the following are the most important weight-bearing locations?

A. Fingers
B. Shoulders
C. Knees
D. Toes

32. Which of the following statements is correct?

A. Rotation is possible at the fully extended knee.
B. The heavy joint capsule at the hip makes reinforcements by ligaments unnecessary.
C. The tibial collateral ligament is synonymous with the lateral collateral ligament.
D. Forceful twisting of the knee when the leg is flexed may lead to a tear of the meniscus.

33. Which of the following statements about the knee's synovial joints is incorrect?

A. Synovial fluid has the consistency of uncooked egg albumin.
B. The knee joint normally accommodates 5–10 mL of synovial fluid.
C. Menisci are within synovial joints.
D. Bursae are related structures.

34. With regard to the popliteal fossa, which of the following statements is correct?

A. The popliteal pulse is easily felt with the knee flexed.
B. The common peroneal nerve is not a content.
C. The popliteal artery is a superficial structure.
D. The gastrocnemius forms the upper boundaries.

35. Which of the following associations reflects the boundaries of the femoral triangle?

A. Floor—inguinal ligament
B. Superior—inguinal canal
C. Lateral—medial border of sartorius
D. Medial—medial border of adductor longus

36. Regarding the adductor canal, which of the following relationships is correct?

A. Medial border—vasto-adductor membrane
B. Anterolateral border—adductors (magnus and longus)
C. Proximal border—superior border of the femoral triangle
D. Posterolateral border—vastus medialis muscle

37. Which of the following relationships regarding the popliteal fossa is correct?

A. Deepest component of the roof—superficial fascia
B. Superolateral wall—semimembranosus and semitendinosus
C. Superomedial wall—biceps femoris (short and long heads)
D. Inferolateral wall—the plantaris muscle

38. Which of the following statements about the tibia and fibula is correct?

A. The distal and proximal ends of the fibula are, respectively, the head and lateral malleolus.
B. The articulation between the tibia and fibula proximally is just below the medial condyle.
C. The lateral malleolus is readily palpable through skin.
D. The medial and lateral condyles of the tibia have convex surfaces.

39. Regarding the tibia, which of the following statements is correct?

A. It has expanded proximal portions known as epicondyles.
B. It is not articulated with the medial condyle of the femur.
C. It has a tuberosity on its posterior surface.
D. It has a relationship with Osgood–Schlatter disease.

40. Which of the following statements about the tibia is incorrect?

A. It has convex upper surfaces.
B. It has an intercondylar eminence.
C. It provides an attachment anteriorly for the patellar ligament.
D. The talus has a direct articulation with the tibia.

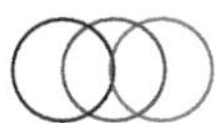

41. Which of the following statements about the fibula is correct?

A. It is at the medial side of the leg.
B. The upper part is called the condyle.
C. It does not partake in weight bearing.
D. The upper part articulates with the tibia at the condyle.

42. Regarding the fibula, which of the following statements is incorrect?

A. It articulates with the ankle at the medial malleolus.
B. It does not enter the knee joint.
C. It has the tibia medial to it.
D. It is the slenderer of the two leg bones.

43. With respect to foot phalanges, which of the following statements is correct?

A. Most of the toes have two phalanges.
B. They are shorter than finger phalanges.
C. The great toe has three phalanges.
D. They articulate with tarsals.

44. With respect to the foot, which of the following statements is correct?

A. The instep is the location of the phalanges.
B. The heads of the metatarsal bones are at the proximal ends.
C. The calcaneus is useful for body weight support.
D. The talus is fixed.

45. Which of the following statements about the foot is correct?

A. There are five tarsal bones.
B. The talus articulates with both the tibia and fibula.
C. The talus is not a tarsal bone.
D. The tarsus is the mid-portion of the foot.

46. With respect to the foot, which of these statements is incorrect?

A. The metatarsus lies between the ankle bones and toes.
B. The talus is at the same level as the other ankle bones.
C. The calcaneus is the largest of the tarsal bones.
D. The cuboid is on the lateral side of the foot.

47. Regarding the foot, which of the following statements is correct?

A. The metatarsus articulates distally with the tarsal bones.
B. The base of the heel is formed by the calcaneus.
C. The head of a metatarsal bone is the proximal part of the bone.
D. The navicular does not articulate with the talus.

48. With regard to the foot, which of the following statements is incorrect?

A. Movement of most of the tarsal bones is limited.
B. The talus is the only ankle bone that is freely movable.
C. Each metatarsal aligns with its corresponding phalanx.
D. The transverse arch does not extend across the foot.

49. Which of the following relationships with muscles that move the foot is incorrect?

A. Gastrocnemius—plantar flexion
B. Extensor digitorum longus—dorsal flexion
C. Peroneus longus—eversion
D. Soleus—inversion

50. A 42-year-old male warehouse worker with obesity complains that in the past 6 months he has experienced recurrent pain on stepping on the bare floor after waking up in the morning. The pain has become worse in the past 3 days, necessitating the consultation. Which of the following is the most likely affected part?

A. The calcaneus
B. The navicular
C. The fifth metatarsal
D. The fifth metacarpal

CHAPTER 7

MCQs ON HEAD AND NECK

1. Which of the following bones is *not* rich in red marrow?

A. Vertebrae
B. Ossicles
C. Ribs
D. Pelvis

2. Which of the following statements about joints is incorrect?

A. They are synonymous with articulations.
B. A synarthrosis is a freely movable joint.
C. They may be classified by the degree of movements possible.
D. They make bone growth possible.

3. Which of the following statements about fibrous joints is incorrect?

A. They typically lie between bones that do not make close contact.
B. Syndesmosis is the type with an interosseous ligament.
C. Suture is the type found only between flat bones of the skull.
D. Gomphosis is the type found between the root of a tooth and the jawbone.

4. Which of the following relationships is incorrect?

A. Ball-and-socket joint—spheroidal joint
B. Gliding joints—most wrist and ankle joints
C. Pivot joint—anterior arch of atlas and dens of axis
D. Condyloid joint—rotational movement

5. Which of the following statements pertaining to the neck is correct?

A. The sternocleidomastoid is not palpable in its whole length.
B. The cricoid cartilage is at the level of the fourth cervical vertebra.
C. The suprasternal notch is at the level of the first thoracic vertebral body.
D. The supraclavicular fossa is a part of the posterior triangle.

6. Which of the following statements about the cervical region is correct?

A. Skin incision should be transverse and lie along Langer's lines.
B. The trachea is palpable behind the lower part of the manubrium sterni.
C. The trapezius divides the neck into anterior and posterior triangles.
D. The axillary artery is palpable on the superior surface of the 1st rib.

DOI: 10.1201/9781003783961-8

7. Which of the following statements about the venous drainage and lymphatic drainage of the head and neck is correct?

A. The external jugular vein is in the anterior triangle of the neck.
B. The occipital lymph nodes are located in the base of the posterior triangle.
C. The superficial cervical nodes are found along the internal jugular vein.
D. A large boil located between the eye and the upper lip may cause cavernous sinus thrombosis.

8. Which of the following relationships is correct?

A. Inability to shrug the shoulders and paralysis of the eighth cranial nerve
B. The posterior cervical chain of lymph nodes and Winterbottom's sign
C. The facial artery pulse and the posterior border of the masseter
D. The thyroglossal duct and the posterior triangle of the neck

9. Regarding midline structures in the neck, which of the following is *not* included?

A. Isthmus of the thyroid gland
B. Internal jugular vein
C. Thyroid cartilage
D. Body of the hyoid bone

10. Which of the following is *not* a part of the structures in the anterior triangle of the neck?

A. Thyroid gland
B. Superior thyroid artery
C. Sternohyoid
D. Supraclavicular lymph nodes

11. Which of the following muscles does *not* play a part in facial expression?

A. Buccinator
B. Platysma
C. Mylohyoid
D. Levator labii superioris alaeque nasi

12. Which of the following relationships is correct?

A. Facial skin sensation and the facial nerve
B. The superficial temporal artery and pulse monitoring during anesthesia
C. The facial nerve branches and the submandibular gland
D. Sagging of the right angle of the mouth and left facial nerve palsy

13. Which of the following is *not* among the muscles of mastication?

A. Orbicularis oculi
B. Temporalis
C. Masseter
D. Lateral pterygoid

 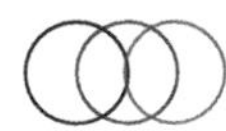

14. Which of the following statements about the muscles that move the pectoral girdle is incorrect?

A. The levator scapulae connects cervical vertebrae to the upper scapula and elevates the scapula.
B. The serratus anterior helps in making a thrusting motion.
C. The pectoralis minor helps make forceful inhalation by raising the upper ribs.
D. The trapezius, by its lower fibers, is important in making a shrugging movement.

15. Which of the following muscle versus nerve supply relationships is incorrect?

A. Trapezius—accessory nerve
B. Levator scapulae—dorsal scapular nerve
C. Serratus anterior—long thoracic nerve
D. Rhomboid major—eleventh cranial nerve

16. Which of the following statements about the sternocleidomastoid is correct?

A. It is found in the midline of the neck.
B. It has a dual origin, from the anterior and superior parts of the sternum and clavicle, respectively.
C. Its fibers run superoinferiorly, inserting at the base of the skull.
D. Contraction of the muscle turns the face to the ipsilateral side.

17. Which of the following statements about the trachea is correct?

A. It lies posterior to the esophagus.
B. It is cylindrical and rigid.
C. It is about 20 cm in an adult.
D. It has cartilaginous rings that protect it from collapsing.

18. Which of the following statements about the trachea is correct?

A. It extends between the end of the pharynx and the two primary bronchi.
B. It has eight tracheal rings, which are C-shaped.
C. Tracheostomy enables upper respiratory obstruction to be bypassed.
D. Full neck extension does not affect its length in an adult.

19. Which of the following statements about the trachea is correct?

A. The diameter of the trachea in an adult is at least 4 cm.
B. Trachealis allows modulation of airflow through the trachea.
C. The inner surface is lined with cuboidal epithelium.
D. Primary bronchi branch off the trachea at the same level.

20. Which of the following actions at the shoulder joint does *not* involve the trapezius?

A. Medial rotation
B. Depression
C. Retraction
D. Elevation

21. Regarding the air sinuses, which of the following is *not* included?

A. Frontal sinus
B. Cavernous sinus
C. Sphenoidal sinus
D. Maxillary antrum

22. Which of the following statements about muscles of mastication is incorrect?

A. The masseter inserts on the lateral surface of the mandible.
B. The masseter elevates the mandible.
C. The temporalis distal attachment is the temporal bone.
D. They include the medial pterygoid and lateral pterygoid.

23. Which of the following muscles is *not* involved in movements associated with facial expression?

A. Orbicularis oculi
B. Platysma
C. Epicranius
D. Occipitalis

24. Which of the following relationships is incorrect?

A. Orbicularis oris—blinking
B. Zygomaticus—smiling
C. Buccinator—facial nerve
D. Epicranius—surprise

25. Which of the following relationships is correct?

A. Frontalis and occipitalis—digastric
B. Platysma—elevation of the floor of the mouth
C. Levator palpebrae superioris alaeque nasi—constriction of the nostril
D. Lateral pterygoid—pulling jaw from side to side

26. Which of the following bones does *not* contain a paranasal sinus?

A. Frontal bone
B. Mastoid process
C. Ethmoid bone
D. Maxillary bone

27. Which of the following statements about paranasal sinuses is correct?

A. The sphenoid bone has a sinus that opens into the nasal cavity through the middle meatus.
B. Their mucous membranes have characteristics different from the nasal cavity mucous membrane.
C. Their structure helps increase the weight of the skull.
D. They have an effect on human voice quality.

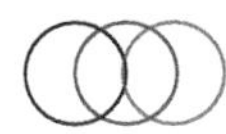

28. A newborn has anterior and posterior fontanels. Which of the following statements about the cranial bones that form the anterior fontanel is correct?

A. There is one temporal bone and one parietal bone.
B. There is one frontal bone and one parietal bone.
C. There is a frontal bone and the nasal bone.
D. There are two frontal bones and two parietal bones.

29. A vehicle is involved in a road traffic accident; there is impact with a stationary object. The front seat passenger's head hits the windscreen (windshield); the passenger did not wear a seat belt. Which of the following bones is likely to be fractured?

A. Parietal bone
B. Temporal bone
C. Frontal bone
D. Occipital bone

30. Which of the following statements about the cheeks and lips is correct?

A. The buccinator is in the lips.
B. The vermilion is located between the tongue and the hard palate.
C. The vestibule is the space between the lips and the teeth.
D. The superior labial frenulum is found in the upper and lower lips.

31. With regard to the tongue, which of the following statements is correct?

A. It is more of a fibrous than muscular structure.
B. The body forms 40% of its size.
C. Vallate (circumvallate) papillae are anterior to the fungiform papillae.
D. Lingual glands contribute both serous and mucous secretions to saliva.

32. Which of the following statements about human dentition is correct?

A. Canine teeth are for cutting food.
B. Incisors are best for puncturing food.
C. Molars crush food efficiently.
D. Premolars assist the action of the incisors.

33. Which of the following relationships is incorrect?

A. Medial squint and paralysis of the medial rectus
B. Lacrimal gland and the superolateral wall of the orbit
C. Fracture of the floor of the orbit and "dislocation" of the eyeball into the maxillary sinus
D. Ptosis and paralysis of the levator palpebrae superioris

34. Which of the following statements about the eye is correct?

A. Ciliary muscles are skeletal muscles.
B. The levator palpebrae superioris closes the eye.
C. The lateral rectus rotates the eye toward the midline.
D. The inferior oblique rotates the eye upward and away from the midline.

35. Which of the following relationships is incorrect?

A. Radial muscle fibers of the iris—sympathetic nerve fiber supply
B. Superior rectus—oculomotor nerve supply
C. Inferior and medial recti—similar nerve supply
D. Superior oblique—abducens nerve supply

36. Regarding muscles that are associated with the eyes and eyelids, which of the following statements is correct?

A. The levator palpebrae superioris has the same innervation as the inferior oblique.
B. The inferior rectus rotates the eye both downward and laterally.
C. The suspensory ligaments are put under tension by ciliary muscles.
D. The circular muscles of the iris dilate the pupil.

37. Which of the following statements about the eye is correct?

A. Aqueous and vitreous humors help maintain the shape of the eye.
B. The choroid is avascular and forms the middle layer of the wall of the eye.
C. The lens is normally translucent.
D. The cornea is not a part of the sclera.

38. Which of the following statements about visual pigments and visual receptors is correct?

A. There are four sets of cones.
B. Cones are responsible for color vision.
C. In dim light, colorless vision is provided by both rods and cones.
D. The retina contains fewer rods than cones.

39. Regarding the eyes and ears, which of the following statements is correct?

A. Tenderness when applying pressure to the tragus is an indicator of inflammation of the middle ear.
B. Superolateral movement of the right eye is caused by the ipsilateral superior oblique.
C. Horizontal movement of the two eyes to look at an object at the left involves the left lateral and the right medial recti.
D. The helix is the soft inferior end of the pinna.

40. Which of the following statements about the eyes, ears, and nose is correct?

A. Tears pass through the nasolacrimal duct into the nose via the middle meatus.
B. The central retinal artery and vein emerge from the optic disk.
C. In accommodation, the pupils of the convergent eyes are dilated.
D. Pulling the auricle upward and forward at auroscopy (otoscopy) straightens the external auditory meatus, thus facilitating examination of the tympanic membrane.

41. With respect to ear examination, which of the following statements is correct?

A. A hyperemic, bulging tympanic membrane indicates acute otitis externa.
B. The handle of the malleus normally runs an antero-inferior course.
C. The finding of a cone of light below the tip of the handle of the malleus is abnormal.
D. The mastoid bone should also be examined in cases of otitis media.

42. Which of the following statements about the nose and throat is correct?

A. Injury to the recurrent laryngeal nerve(s) during thyroidectomy affects phonation.
B. The middle ethmoidal sinus opens into the inferior meatus.
C. The superior turbinate is the largest turbinate.
D. The laryngeal orifice is posterior to the esophagus.

43. The parents of a pupil receive a telephone call that their 9-year-old son fell just after playing with classmates. They had held hands, creating a circle, and had run in a circular direction. The affected child was unwilling to join the group for this physical exercise. Where is the likely site of dysfunction?

A. Utricle
B. Saccule
C. Semicircular ducts
D. Medulla oblongata

44. A member of a church choir develops weakness, dry cough, and hoarseness of the voice, all in the past 3 days. Where is the most likely site of infection?

A. Nasopharynx
B. Trachea
C. Larynx
D. Bronchi

45. Which of the following statements about the palate is correct?

A. The soft palate is within the hard palate.
B. The palatine tonsils lie between the palatopharyngeal and palatoglossal arches.
C. The palatoglossal arch is posterior to the palatopharyngeal arch.
D. The uvula is the conical midline structure at the posterior end of the hard palate.

46. Which of the following statements about the pharyngeal muscles is correct?

A. The superficial layer consists of smooth muscle.
B. The deep layer has circularly disposed longitudinal muscle.
C. There are two pharyngeal constrictors, superior and inferior.
D. The pharyngeal constrictors force food downward during deglutition.

47. Which of the following correctly describes the actions of the superficial muscles in the anterior part of the neck?

A. Subclavius—elevation of the clavicle at the sternoclavicular joint
B. Platysma—relaxation of skin over the anterior neck
C. Sternocleidomastoid—elevation of the clavicle
D. Sternocleidomastoid—ipsilateral extension of the neck at the cervical spine

48. Regarding arterial blood supply to the head and neck, which of the following arteries is *not* derived from the common carotid artery?

A. Superior thyroid artery
B. Facial artery
C. Thyrocervical trunk
D. Superficial temporal artery

49. With respect to the grouping of muscles in the neck, which of the following is a correct relationship?

A. Strap muscles—muscles superior to the hyoid bone
B. Trapezius—innervation by the seventh cranial nerve
C. Prevertebral muscles—superficial muscles
D. Scalene muscles—deep to the sternocleidomastoid

50. Regarding the visceral compartment of the neck, which of the following structures is *not* a part?

A. Thyroid
B. Carotid artery
C. Esophagus
D. Larynx

CHAPTER 8

MCQs ON NEUROANATOMY

1. Which of the following relationships is incorrect?

A. Astrocytes—between neurons and blood vessels
B. Oligodendrocytes—phagocytosis
C. Ependyma—ventricles
D. Bipolar neurons—eyes, ears

2. With respect to the structure of a neuron, which of the following statements is correct?

A. A cell body is present in every neuron.
B. The nucleus is cylindrical.
C. The nucleolus is a conspicuous cytoplasmic (axoplasmic) structure.
D. There is one dendrite per axon.

3. Which of the following is *not* a part of a neuron cell body?

A. Mitochondria
B. Axon terminals
C. Microtubules
D. Golgi apparatus

4. Which of the following statements about the human nervous system is incorrect?

A. The two parts are the peripheral and sympathetic nervous systems.
B. There are blood vessels, neural tissue, and connective tissue.
C. Neurons are both structural and functional units.
D. The synapse is the interneuronal space essential in information exchange.

5. Which of the following is a correct relationship?

A. Pia mater—internal periosteum of skull bones
B. Falx cerebri—longitudinal fissure
C. Arachnoid mater—highly vascular membrane
D. Spinal cord—shallow anterior median fissure

6. With respect to the spinal cord, which of the following statements is correct?

A. It extends between the foramen magnum and the L3/L4 intervertebral disk levels.
B. It has two enlargements, the cervical and thoracic enlargements.
C. The filum terminale is of the same structure as spinal nerves arising from the conus medularis.
D. Nerve tracts run in the three funiculi of the spinal cord.

DOI: 10.1201/9781003783961-9

7. Which of the following relationships about the nerve tracts of the spinal cord is correct?

A. Fasciculus gracilis—anterior column
B. Spinocerebellar tracts—descending tracts
C. Corticospinal tracts—motor impulses
D. Reticulospinal tracts—pyramidal tracts

8. Which of the following relationships about the cerebral cortex is correct?

A. Primary motor areas—postcentral gyrus
B. Postcentral gyrus—touch, temperature, pain, and pressure
C. Visual area—temporal lobe
D. Association areas—two lobes of the brain

9. Which of the following relationships is correct?

A. Aqueduct of Sylvius—largest ventricle
B. Diencephalon—structures between the cerebral hemispheres and below the brainstem
C. Brainstem—midbrain, pons, and cerebellum
D. Hypothalamus—heart rate and arterial blood pressure regulation

10. With respect to the cranial fossae, which of the following statements is incorrect?

A. The frontal lobe occupies the anterior frontal fossa.
B. The cerebellum is found in the posterior cranial fossa.
C. The temporal lobe is in the middle cranial fossa.
D. The spinal cord occupies the middle cranial fossa.

11. Which of the following statements about the nervous system is incorrect?

A. Only the central nervous system performs sensory, integrative, and motor functions.
B. Effectors are non-nervous system structures, such as muscles and endocrine glands, which are stimulated by nerve impulses.
C. There are two types of neural tissue cells, e.g., neuroglia and neurons.
D. Schwann cells are peripheral nervous system neuroglia.

12. Which of the following statements about the sixth cranial nerve is incorrect?

A. It terminates in the medial rectus.
B. It passes through the superior orbital fissure.
C. Its paralysis causes medial rotation of the eye.
D. It arises from the inferior pons.

13. Which of the following cranial nerves is *not* directly related to the medulla oblongata?

A. Glossopharyngeal nerve
B. Accessory nerve
C. Facial nerve
D. Vagus nerve

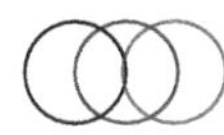

14. Which of the following cells is *not* a glial cell?

A. Oligodendrocyte
B. Schwann cell
C. Astrocyte
D. Neuron

15. Regarding the support cells in the central nervous system, which of the following statements is correct?

A. Microglia are derived from plasma cells.
B. Astrocytes take the shape of a star.
C. A Schwann cell myelinates at least five axons.
D. Ependymal cells are confined to the lateral ventricles.

16. Regarding the function of glial cells, which of the following relationships is correct?

A. Oligodendrocytes and Schwann cells—myelination of axons in the central nervous system
B. Astrocytes—provision of substrates for synthesis of ATP in neurons
C. Ependymal cells—resident macrophages in the central nervous system
D. Microglia—source of neural stem/progenitor cells

17. Which of the following statements about glial cells is correct?

A. Microglia are the most abundant cells in the central nervous system.
B. Ependymal cells and subependymal astrocytes form ependymal granulations.
C. Astrocytes provide the layer of cells that create a semi-permeable layer in the CNS.
D. Unlike oligodendrocytes, Schwann cells do not express myelin basic protein.

18. Regarding the structure of glial cells, which of the following relationships is incorrect?

A. Microglia—the smallest of the glial cells
B. Astrocytes—elongated nuclei with little cytoplasm
C. Ependymal cells—epithelial cells.
D. Schwann cells—equivalent of oligodendrocytes

19. Which of the following statements about the sympathetic nervous system is correct?

A. The preganglionic neurons arise from the T2 to L1 segments.
B. Cell bodies are distributed in two regions of the gray matter in the spinal cord.
C. Prior to synapsing, the first-order neurons are long.
D. The neurotransmitter at the preganglionic synaptic junction is acetylcholine.

20. Which of the following statements applies to the effector sites of postganglionic nerve fibers of the sympathetic autonomic nervous system?

A. In a few sites, they release epinephrine and norepinephrine.
B. Alpha-2 adrenergic receptors operate via the IP3/Ca^{2+} pathway.
C. Acetylcholine is the neurotransmitter released at sweat glands.
D. Beta-2 adrenergic receptors work by decreasing the cAMP pathway.

21. Regarding the actions of the sympathetic autonomic nervous system, which of the following is incorrect?

A. It inhibits glucose output induced by glucagon.
B. It increases renin secretion in the kidneys.
C. It reduces motility in the gastrointestinal tract.
D. It increases cardiac output.

22. Which of the following constitutes the sympathetic trunk?

A. Celiac ganglia
B. Superior mesenteric ganglia
C. Paravertebral ganglia
D. Inferior mesenteric ganglia

23. Which of the following is *not* a result of the actions of the sympathetic nervous system?

A. Immune system suppression
B. Ejaculation
C. Bronchodilation
D. Contraction of the detrusor muscle of the bladder

24. Which of the following statements about the parasympathetic division of the autonomic nervous system is correct?

A. The preganglionic neurons are in the brainstem and sacral portion of the spinal cord.
B. The ganglia of motor neurons are located distant from the structures they subserve.
C. The motor neurons respond to three neurotransmitters.
D. Regulation of the visceral motor system is by motor feedback.

25. Regarding impairment in or damage to the hypothalamus, which of the following is an incorrect relationship?

A. Paraventricular nucleus—decrease in the secretion of oxytocin
B. Posterior nucleus—excessive heat dissipation
C. Lateral nucleus—increase in appetite
D. Suprachiasmatic nucleus—circadian rhythm dysfunction

26. With respect to the craniosacral outflow of the parasympathetic autonomic nervous system, which of the following is *not* a component?

A. Seventh cranial nerve (CN VII)
B. Twelfth cranial nerve (CN XII)
C. Third cranial nerve (CN III)
D. Second sacral nerve (S 2)

27. Which of the following statements about the enteric nervous system is incorrect?

A. Multifunctional enteric neurons work alone.
B. Confocal microscopy is useful in visualizing enteric glial cells.
C. There is a relationship between the gut neurology and the brain.
D. Enteroendocrine cells modulate blood glucose levels and appetite.

28. Which of the following about examination of the cranial nerves is correct?

A. Identifying a familiar object by its mild smell with the eyes closed for cranial nerve 1 (CN I)
B. Vision screening by examining the eyes with just an ophthalmoscope for CN II
C. Assessing pupillary light reflex, eyelid and some extraocular muscle movements, and accommodation for CN III
D. Assessing eye movement downward and outward for CN IV

29. Which of the following statements about examining the integrity of the trigeminal nerve is correct?

A. It entails examination of motor functions of the V1.
B. Pinprick should be carried out before testing for light touch.
C. Jaw clenching tests the V3 division of the trigeminal nerve.
D. Eliciting sharp pain over the cheeks tests the largest of the divisions.

30. Which of the following statements about testing the facial nerve is incorrect?

A. It does not accurately test the umami taste.
B. The motor portion innervates all muscles of the face.
C. Testing the stapedius muscle is a part of testing CN VII.
D. Testing a person's ability to blow a balloon assesses CN VII integrity.

31. Regarding testing for CN VI, CN VIII, and CN IX in the consulting room, which of the following statements is incorrect?

A. CN VI evaluation must include movements by the lateral rectus muscle.
B. In the Rinne test, the mastoid process is tested after the external auditory meatus.
C. In normal hearing, the Weber test indicates equal hearing with both ears.
D. CN IX evaluation entails assessing the gag reflex, swallowing, and movement of the palate.

32. With respect to testing a patient for CN X, CN XI, and CN XII in the consulting room, which of the following statements is correct?

A. Assessing the trapezius suffices in evaluating CN XI function.
B. Percussion of the sternocleidomastoid and trapezius helps assess CN XI function.
C. Inspecting a protruded tongue provides the essential information about CN XII integrity.
D. In CN X paralysis, the uvula deviates to the unaffected side.

33. Which of the following statements about the sense of pain is incorrect?

A. Awareness of pain is at the level of the thalamus.
B. The cerebral cortex is able to judge the intensity of pain.
C. Appreciation of the exact source/location of pain is by the cerebellum.
D. Pain impulses ascend in the spinothalamic tract.

34. With respect to the sense of taste, which of the following statements is correct?

A. The gustatory cortex is in the frontal lobe.
B. There are three primary kinds of taste cells.
C. Impulses arising from taste receptors travel in facial nerve fibers.
D. Receptors for sweetness predominate at the back of the tongue.

35. With respect to the sense of smell, which of the following statements is incorrect?

A. Olfactory receptors are in the nasal cavity.
B. Olfactory receptors are chemoreceptors.
C. Olfactory receptors adapt gradually to smell.
D. Olfactory impulses are interpreted in the limbic system.

36. With respect to innervation of the alimentary canal, which of the following statements is correct?

A. The contribution by the sympathetic system is sparse.
B. The muscular layer is adequately supplied by fibers of sympathetic and parasympathetic nerves.
C. Impulses from the parasympathetic nerves reduce activities of the digestive system.
D. The lumbar region of the spinal cord contributes to the parasympathetic supply.

37. Which of the following statements about salivary glands is incorrect?

A. The major salivary glands are in pairs.
B. They produce saliva through serous cells and mucous cells.
C. Parasympathetic stimulation of the glands results in viscous saliva secretion.
D. The submandibular and sublingual glands are major salivary glands.

38. An adolescent with a history of brain damage displays poor social judgment and lack of motivation. Which part of the cerebrum must have been impacted adversely?

A. Parietal lobe
B. Frontal lobe
C. Occipital lobe
D. Temporal lobe

39. An individual has hearing loss and an inability to smell attributable to cerebral damage. Which part of the brain was affected?

A. Temporal lobe
B. Frontal lobe
C. Occipital lobe
D. Parietal lobe

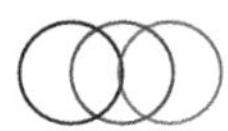

40. A 60-year-old man develops difficulty controlling motor activities. The physician determines that the pathology has to do with a part of the brain. Which part of the brain is most likely to have been involved?

A. Medulla oblongata
B. Insula
C. Basal nuclei
D. Occipital lobe

41. A patient has difficulty in appreciating heat, pressure, movement, and pain on the left side of the body. Which of the following parts of the brain is this somatosensory challenge test related to?

A. Precentral gyrus
B. Left temporal lobe
C. Right post-central gyrus
D. Left post-central gyrus

42. A patient desires to contract the elbow flexor muscles as part of the process of taking food from the plate to eat. Which part of the brain is utilized?

A. Premotor area
B. Angular gyrus
C. Broca's area
D. Post-central gyrus

43. A 65-year-old male develops tremors when he is at rest; getting up from a chair is slow and clumsy. The attending physician makes a tentative diagnosis pertaining to the affected part of the brain. Which part of the brain would the physician be considering as the site of the lesion?

A. Basal nuclei
B. Cerebellum
C. Primary motor cortex
D. Occipital lobe

44. A child develops hydrocephalus from bacterial meningitis. Which part of the brain is the pathology related to?

A. Putamen
B. Ventricular system
C. Dura mater
D. Gray matter

45. A recently well adult, but currently unconscious patient, is found to have pinpoint pupils bilaterally during physical examination by the attending physician in the emergency room. When considering the differential diagnoses, which part of the brain should be the focus?

A. Midbrain
B. Frontal cortex
C. Pons
D. Thalamus

46. A patient gradually develops a clumsy, awkward gait that makes it difficult to move the lower limbs when walking up uniform stairs; the patient also has difficulty playing the piano, quite unlike previously. In which part of the brain could the patient have a lesion?

A. Cerebellum
B. Temporal lobe
C. Occipital lobe
D. Frontal lobe

47. A patient develops gigantism. The endocrinologist determines that the organ that produces the affected hormone in excess is affected. Where is the location of this organ?

A. Posterior cranial fossa
B. Sphenoidal bone
C. Hypothalamus
D. Parietal lobe

48. A 22-year-old female wakes up and notices drooping of the right side of the face. She is alarmed and presents to the hospital, where she consults a young doctor in the general outpatient clinic later in the day. Where is the most likely site of the pathology responsible for this presentation?

A. Corticospinal tract
B. Mastoid bone
C. Stylomastoid foramen
D. Internal auditory meatus

49. A patient has difficulty in opening their mouth against resistance during examination in the outpatient clinic. Which of the following statements is correct?

A. The facial nerve is paralyzed.
B. Two of the branches of the seventh cranial nerve are paralyzed.
C. The mandibular division of the fifth cranial nerve is paralyzed.
D. The affected nerve is wholly composed of motor fibers.

50. A patient develops difficulty in shrugging the right shoulder. Which of the following is the result of injury to the eleventh cranial nerve?

A. The right serratus anterior is paralyzed.
B. The left trapezius is paralyzed.
C. The right trapezius is paralyzed.
D. Swallowing is impaired.

PART II
ANSWERS AND NOTES FOR MCQs

CHAPTER 9

ANSWERS AND NOTES FOR MCQs ON ABDOMEN

1. D The hypodermis is synonymous with the subcutaneous layer of skin. The location of the hypodermis is between the dermis and underlying organs. Apart from being a source of hormones and stem cells, the hypodermis serves the purposes of storage of energy in the form of fat, body insulation, and a link between the overlying skin and underlying bones, muscles, and other structures; it also functions as a "shock absorber" [1]. The epidermis is the outer layer, and the dermis, the inner layer. The elastic fibers are in the dermis. Nervous tissue is present in the dermis. The epidermis and dermis are separated by the basement membrane. The skin in its full thickness is the largest organ in the body; it covers the body in its entirety and forms the first protective barrier to the human body from ultraviolet radiation, chemicals, all types of pathogens, and mechanical injury. Although its skin lacks stratum lucidum, the human back is still a part of the parts of the body that have thin skin; however, it has the thickest skin of the thin-skinned parts because it has a thick epidermis [2]. The skin is essential in temperature regulation; it plays a major role in releasing water to the external environment via sweating (active perspiration) and insensible water loss (passive diffusion by evaporation) [3].

2. C The mid-inguinal point is a reference point for identifying the femoral pulse; the mid-inguinal point is the midpoint between an imaginary straight line that joins the anterior superior iliac spine and the pubic tubercle [4]. At this location, the femoral artery enters the pelvis from the abdominal cavity. The costal margin is formed by the costal cartilages of the 7th to 12th ribs. The inguinal ligament does not get to the symphysis pubis but to the pubic tubercle, where its fibers diverge to form two ligaments—the lacunar (Gimbernat's) ligament and the pectineal (Cooper's) ligament. A disruption of this important ligament results in the sportsman's groin [4]. Poupart ligament is an alternative name for inguinal ligament. The linea semilunaris (Spigelian line) is a fibrous line formed at the lateral borders of the rectus abdominis on the right and on the left sides; it presents as a longitudinal, slightly curved line (akin to a half-moon) [5]. With similar but transversely disposed fibrous connective tissue across the rectus abdominis muscles, some people show a demonstrable "six pack." The entire length of the iliac crest is palpable.

3. B The position of the umbilicus is inconstant in adults [6]. Factors that may make the position of the umbilicus deviate from the approximately L3/L4 intervertebral disk level are aging and body type [6]. Some medical conditions may also alter the position of the umbilicus; they may be congenital or acquired conditions. Such medical conditions include obesity, large hernias, ascites, abdominal tumors, and in women, pregnancy.

Congenital conditions that may change the position of the umbilicus are gastroschisis and omphalocele. Malrotation of the abdominal contents results in an omphalocele. In omphalocele, abdominal contents spill out of the abdominal wall; they are covered only by peritoneum. In patients with gastroschisis, the intestines are outside the abdominal wall; there is no membranous covering. Gastroschisis results from an embryonic failure of fusion of the lateral body wall folds.

DOI: 10.1201/9781003783961-11

 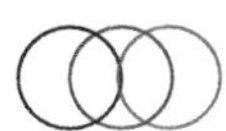

During abdominoplasty, the surgeon chooses and relocates the umbilicus to a most suitable and aesthetically appealing position following removal of excess fat in the patient undergoing plastic surgery [6].

A midline incision below the umbilicus passes through the linea alba. The subcostal plane passes through the inferior borders of the tenth costal cartilages. Contraction of the rectus abdominis muscles helps in identifying the linea semilunaris, particularly in non-obese individuals.

4. C With respect to surface anatomy relationships, the origin of the common iliac arteries and the fourth lumbar vertebra are related; the origin of these arteries is at the bifurcation of the abdominal aorta. The common iliac artery is a significant landmark for patients with peripheral artery disease who require endovascular stent placement or in patients for whom angiography is to be performed [7]. The tip of the ninth costal cartilage is related to gallbladder disease. The transpyloric plane relates to the hili of the kidneys. The left 10th rib and the long axis of the spleen are related.

5. B Developmentally, the urachus links the bladder with the umbilicus [8]. The abdomen is involved in pleuritic pain because of referred pain through the intercostal nerves. The superficial inguinal ring is superior and lateral to the pubic tubercle. It is not the broad ligament but the round ligament of the uterus that passes through the superficial inguinal ring. An incision through the linea alba causes minimal or no damage to muscles and nerves, as there are no muscles and nerves in the midline of the linea alba.

6. B Weakness of the abdominal muscles may lead to divarication recti. The linea alba is the tendinous band that represents the interweaving of collagen fibers of the aponeuroses of the anterior abdominal wall muscles at the midline. The linea alba runs from the lower border of the xyphoid process superiorly to the superior surface of the pubic symphysis inferiorly. The linea alba, by its structural peculiarity, provides an intrinsic stability to the abdominal wall even when there is a degree of chronic separation of the medial borders of the rectus muscles, like in obesity and during pregnancies. When there is abnormal separation of these muscles, diastasis recti abdominis (DRA) results, with consequent protrusion or bulging of the anterior abdominal wall. This occurs in the original anatomical position of the linea alba, which has succumbed to increased intraabdominal pressure and a volume increase [9]. Paramedian incisions are not made through the rectus abdominis, but the muscle is retracted laterally to get to the peritoneum. Pararectal incision is not preferred because of the smaller space—unless nerves and blood vessels are sacrificed to increase space. In the suprapubic region, the rectus sheath has no posterior wall, as the aponeuroses of all the muscles form the anterior layer of the rectus sheath at this level.

7. A The inguinal canal does not span between the anterior superior iliac spine and the pubic tubercle but from the deep to the superficial rings; what extends from the anterior superior iliac spine to the ipsilateral pubic tubercle is the inguinal ligament. A direct inguinal hernia does not pass through the inguinal canal. A direct inguinal hernia does not leave the abdomen at the deep inguinal ring. Although an indirect inguinal hernia passes through the inguinal canal, this does not always occur; when it does not occur, the indirect inguinal hernia does not exit the inguinal canal through the superficial inguinal ring. An inguinoscrotal hernia invariably passes through the two rings (deep, then superficial). Giant inguinoscrotal hernias frequently contain bowel, but having a part of, or the entire, stomach is a rarity. A case has been reported and it highlights, among other things, the danger of encountering an unusual organ or subjecting the patient to the risks of abdominal compartment syndrome, which may eventuate in multiorgan failure if decompressive laparotomy is not performed [10].

8. C The superficial inguinal ring is not the lateral but the medial end of the inguinal canal. The posterior wall is formed by the fascia transversalis. The roof is formed by the arching fibers of the transversus abdominis and the internal oblique muscles. The floor of the canal continues medially as the lacunar and pectineal ligaments.

9. B The anterior wall of the inguinal canal is formed by the external oblique aponeurosis. The sharp edge of the lacunar ligament forms the medial relation of a femoral hernia. The concavity of the floor of the inguinal canal is upward. The femoral vein is lateral to a femoral hernia. The pubic tubercle is above and medial to the neck of a femoral hernial sac.

10. A The conjoint tendon (Henle's ligament, inguinal aponeurotic falx) strengthens the medial part of Hesselbach's triangle. The conjoint tendon, also known as the inguinal aponeurotic falx or Henle's ligament, is derived from the common aponeurosis of the internal oblique muscle and transversus abdominis. The conjoint tendon constitutes a significant part of the medial portion of the posterior wall of the inguinal canal. When there is weakness in the conjoint tendon, a direct hernia may be the result [11]. A weakness in the conjoint tendon is anterior to intraperitoneal structures. The synonym of conjoint tendon is inguinal aponeurotic falx. This tendon (formed by the aponeuroses of the internal oblique and transversus abdominis muscles) lies medial to the inferior epigastric artery, making the weakness sited within Hesselbach's triangle. When the weakness in the tendon within Hesselbach's triangle is severe, an intraperitoneal structure may herniate (push into) the area of weakness and form a bulge medial to the inferior epigastric artery and vein; this differentiation to conclusively diagnose a direct inguinal hernia is best achieved during surgical intervention. Tentatively (during a clinical examination in the consulting room), a direct inguinal hernia still produces a bulge when the deep inguinal ring is occluded by using the examining hand to exert pressure over the midpoint of the inguinal ligament and the patient coughs as requested. This is unlike an indirect inguinal hernia that ceases to herniate in response to an increase in intraabdominal pressure created by the patient coughing after the indirect hernia was reduced prior to the test; this is because the hernia's point of entry from the posterior abdominal wall becomes occluded by this simple examination. The test is not conclusive in some patients. A direct hernia does not enter the inguinal canal but bulges directly through a weak area in the posterior wall of the inguinal canal; this occurs medial to the inferior epigastric artery and inferior epigastric vein. This is unlike an indirect hernia, which lies lateral to the inferior epigastric artery and can enter (and even pass through) the inguinal canal. An indirect inguinal hernia enters the canal from the deep inguinal ring, and if it exits the canal, it does so through the superficial inguinal ring. A large indirect inguinal hernia may extend into the scrotum and be called an inguinoscrotal hernia. A rare variant of direct inguinal hernias through a weakened conjoint tendon in otherwise athletic young individuals is referred to as Gill-Ogilvie hernia or Busoga herniation [11]. This type of direct inguinal hernia has a high potential to become strangulated. Hesselbach's triangle (the inguinal triangle) has the following borders: Superolateral—inferior epigastric vessels; inferior—inguinal ligament; medial—linea semilunaris [11].

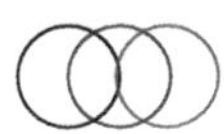

The inferior epigastric artery is lateral to a direct inguinal hernia. Hesselbach's triangle is bounded medially by the lateral border of the rectus sheath. The deep inguinal ring is lateral to the inferior epigastric artery. The inferior portion of the conjoint tendon is in Hesselbach's triangle.

The medical student or clinician should consider the fact that other conditions that may have features similar to the inguinal hernia are femoral hernia, lipoma, saphena varix, and inguinal lymphadenopathy; these could mimic a direct or indirect inguinal hernia. When a lump is in the scrotum, other conditions that should be considered are hydrocele, varicocele, torsion of the testis, orchitis, and testicular tumor. In females, it could be a cyst of the canal of Nuck.

11. C The femoral ring is a part of the femoral canal. It is a site for femoral hernia. Fat is a normal content of the femoral ring. The lateral boundary of the femoral ring is the fibrous septum on the medial aspect of the femoral vein. Medially, the boundary is the base of the lacunar ligament, which takes the shape of a crescent. Anteriorly, the boundary is the inguinal ligament, while posteriorly, the boundary is the pectineus muscle and its fascia. It is bounded inferiorly by the pectineal ligament.

12. D On entering the abdominal cavity, the omentum, liver and transverse colon are easily viewed, with the omentum covering the intestines. Although variable, the lowest point of the transverse colon is at about the level of the umbilicus. The transverse colon is the longest and most mobile segment of the colon, extending between the right and left colic flexures. The root of the transverse mesocolon is along the inferior border of the pancreas. The phrenicocolic ligament anchors the splenic flexure to the diaphragm; this left colonic flexure is less mobile than its counterpart on the right [12]. The kidney is retroperitoneal and is covered by other structures like pararenal fat, Gerota's fascia (renal fascia), the renal capsule and the adipose capsule (perirenal fat).

13. D With regard to the contents of the abdominal cavity, the inferior vena cava provides significant physical support to the liver. The ligaments of the liver constitute important sources of support to the liver. The inferior vena cava and the ligaments of the liver do not allow any significant movement of the liver within the abdominal cavity. The major ligaments of the liver are the falciform ligament (attaches the liver to the anterior abdominal wall), coronary ligament (attaches the liver to the diaphragm), triangular ligament (also attaches the liver to the diaphragm), and lesser omentum (which links the liver to the stomach and the duodenum). The ligamentum teres hepatis, a remnant of the umbilical vein, is within the falciform ligament [13]. In patients with portal hypertension, the clinical features are caput medusae, hemorrhoids, and varicosity of the esophageal veins. In portal hypertension, there is venous congestion where there are portocaval anastomoses [13]. The main anatomical sites of portocaval anastomosis are the lower esophagus, umbilicus, and rectum.

Obstruction of major portal veins should be a consideration when there are varices, jaundice, and ascites in a patient with portal hypertension. The patient should be assessed by imaging using ultrasonography or magnetic resonance imaging for the likelihood of Budd–Chiari syndrome or right heart failure; in Budd–Chiari syndrome, there is evidence of hypercoagulability in addition to portal hypertension [14]. Hypercoagulable states in relation to surgery may be found in major trauma, major surgical operations, and cancers like lung and ovarian cancers. The duodenum is retroperitoneal. The jejunum and ileum have mesentery and so can move using the mesentery as their base. The ascending and descending colon are fixed.

14. B Statement A "The large intestine is always wider than the small intestine" is incorrect in cases of small intestinal obstruction; fluid (liquid and gaseous) distension from the pathological process in small bowel obstruction may make the portion of the small intestine above the level of obstruction wider than the colon. When the *small bowel* diameter exceeds 6 cm, the small bowel *obstruction may* be severe enough to compromise the viability of the affected small bowel segment [15].

The longitudinal muscle layer forms a continuous layer round the jejunum and ileum; this is the outer smooth muscle layer of the small intestines. This longitudinal layer contains smooth muscle cells like the circular inner layer at this level of the intestinal tract. The longitudinal layer is not as thick as the inner circular layer. While the outer layer contracts to shorten the length of the intestines, the inner layer contracts to compress the contents of the gut; working together, the two layers propel the contents of the intestines toward the colon. The arrangement of the muscle layers of the colon (excluding the appendix and rectum) is different; in these parts of the colon, the outer longitudinal muscle layer is not continuous but is broken into three strips or bands that are like ribbons. The three thickened muscular bands are the epiploic taenia, libera taenia, and mesocolic taenia; together, they are called taeniae coli (the name is because these three bands are reminiscent of "worms"). The taeniae coli shorten the colon during smooth muscle contraction and, in conjunction with the inner circular layer, move colonic contents toward the rectum. The taeniae coli are responsible for the sacculation (haustra, haustrations) of the portion of the colon where they are found. It is worthy of noting that the absence of taeniae coli at the appendix is due to their merging at this narrow anatomical structure. These readily visually identifiable taeniae coli create an important anatomical landmark during abdominal surgery, whether involving the gut or not. The appendix can be located by following a teniae (taenia) coli down to the cecal tip. [16]. A method that allows automatic teniae coli detection during the non-invasive imaging investigation, computed tomographic colonography (CTC), is a desirable addition for the examination of selected patients with suspected proximal colonic lesions like cancerous lesions in the colon and large polyps [17].

Appendices epiploicae are numerous fatty appendages on the serosal surface of the colon, and they are related to the taeniae coli. While these small fat tags are absent over the cecum, appendix, and rectum, they are plentiful on the distal portion of the descending colon and on the rectum [16].

15. A Pain arising from the stomach is referred to the epigastrium. Pain due to acute appendicitis may involve the whole abdomen, though it is initially umbilical and later right iliac pain. Pain due to cholecystitis may be referred to the right shoulder. The phrenic nerve (subserves the diaphragm) arises from the roots of three cranial nerves (C3, C4, and C5). The nerve that supplies the tip of the shoulder is the supraclavicular nerve; the supraclavicular nerve arises from similar nerve roots as the phrenic nerve, making the pain from the gallbladder (in cholecystitis and cholelithiasis) closely related to the diaphragm, being occasionally referred to the tip of the right shoulder or scapula [18]. This is Collins' sign but it is not pathognomonic of gallbladder disease, as not all patients with the indicated conditions demonstrate it.

Pain arising from the parietal peritoneum is subserved by the anterior rami of the last six thoracic and first lumbar nerves. The T7, T8, and T9 spinal nerves supply sensation to the upper abdomen, and T10 nerve fibers supply the periumbilical area; T11 and T12 nerves cover the lower abdomen, and L1 spinal nerve provides the innervation for the skin over the pelvic girdle and the inguinal area. The iliohypogastric and ilioinguinal nerves arise from the ventral root of the L1 spinal nerve. The ilioinguinal nerve

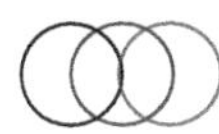

supplies the skin over the medial aspect of the thigh and the inguinal ligament. The ilioinguinal nerve innervates the mons pubis and labia majora in females and the scrotum and root of the penis in males. The ilioinguinal nerve also contributes to the motor innervation of the inferior portions of the transverse and two oblique abdominal wall muscles [19].

Dysfunction of any of the nerves that supply the anterior and lateral walls of the abdomen may eventuate in abdominal wall weakness, hernias, loss of sensation, sexual dysfunction, limitation in range of mobility, chronic pain, and even a reduction in quality of life. Each of these factors can reduce the quality of life of an individual [19]. Pain arising from the visceral peritoneum is not well localized.

16. B It is the superior mesenteric vein that is enclosed by small intestinal mesentery; other contents of small intestinal mesentery are adipose tissue, nerve fibers, and lymph nodes. The small intestinal mesentery also encloses the superior mesenteric artery.

17. A The gastrointestinal tract has four layers. From outside in, these are the serosa, muscular layer, submucosa, and mucosa. Of the layers of the gastrointestinal tract, the innermost (mucosa) has lamina propria. The mucosa has three layers: epithelium, lamina propria, and muscularis mucosae. The lamina propria consists of loose connective tissue. The lamina propria of the mucosal layer of the gut is, therefore, the middle of the innermost layer of the gastrointestinal tract wall [20]. The muscular layer is responsible for the movements of the gut. The muscular layer comprises two coats of smooth muscle tissue—the outer coat, which is longitudinal, and the inner coat, which is circular.

18. D The esophagus is the tubular part of the gastrointestinal tract that transports food from the pharynx to the stomach. Anatomically, the esophagus has three segments: cervical esophagus, thoracic esophagus, and abdominal esophagus. The cervical esophagus spans the distance between the cricopharyngeus and the suprasternal notch. The esophagus runs posterior to the trachea in the thorax. The esophagus exits the thorax at the esophageal hiatus in the diaphragm. The esophagus has an upper sphincter and a lower sphincter; these two esophageal sphincters are functional sphincters [21]. The upper esophageal sphincter (UES) is a high-pressure zone at the boundary of the changeover from the pharynx to the cervical (topmost/uppermost portion of the) esophagus. This sphincter is also referred to as the pharyngo-esophageal sphincter. A similar high-pressure zone exists at the lower part of the esophagus, the junction between the lower esophagus and the stomach. The lower esophagus tends to be at more risk than the upper esophagus principally because of the characteristic acidic milieu of the stomach, unlike the boundary between the pharynx and the cervical esophagus. The lower esophageal sphincter (synonym for cardiac sphincter) is at the level of the esophageal hiatus [22]. The lower esophageal sphincter has two components—extrinsic and intrinsic; the extrinsic component has the crura of the diaphragm and the ligament that links the diaphragm with the lower esophagus (the phreno-esophageal ligament), which anatomically supports the lower esophageal sphincter. The intrinsic component of this sphincter consists of fibers of the muscles of the esophagus [22]. A normally functioning lower esophageal sphincter (or cardiac sphincter) prevents regurgitation of stomach contents [22].

As indicated, the lower esophageal sphincter is made up of two parts: an intrinsic and an extrinsic part. When either the intrinsic component or the extrinsic component becomes dysfunctional, the individual is prone to developing gastroesophageal reflux disease (GERD). GERD may be complicated by Barrett's esophagus, which is the result of mucosal changes in the esophagus from the normal squamous epithelium to columnar epithelium; it is a premalignant condition [23].

19. D The four parts of the stomach are the cardia, fundus, body, and pylorus. The stomach has two valves. The valve between it and the small intestine is the pyloric sphincter. Gastric glands produce secretions, which also contain intrinsic factor; other secretions are pepsin, lipase, and hydrochloric acid.

20. A The stomach is J-shaped when it is "empty" and viewed in the vertical orientation; the J shape is formed by the organ's greater and lesser curvatures, which make the stomach highly asymmetric structurally. The stomach has rugae; rugae consist of folds of mucosa and submucosa, which allow increases in the surface area of the stomach. They allow the stomach to distend according to the amount of contents that it receives [21]. When the stomach distends, the rugae progressively flatten out, and the "full" stomach is able to assume and accommodate a higher volume than when the stomach is in its "empty" state. The stomach is involved in the initial act of digesting proteins; the enzyme, pepsin, is involved in this biochemical process, while the rhythmic contractions churn and mix gastric contents by gastric muscular activity—this is an enabling mechanical action for the initial digestion of food [24].

The stomach has three layers of smooth muscle—the external (outer) longitudinal, middle circular, and inner oblique layers. This third layer of smooth muscle is unique to the stomach and is particularly prominent close to the esophageal opening; it is also present at the body of the stomach. The rhythmic muscular contractions followed by relaxation result in the formation of chyme. The gastric glands that play a major role in the biochemical breakdown of food are the parietal cells, chief cells, G-cells, mucous neck cells, and foveolar cells [25].

21. A The gastric fundus is sometimes filled with air, which shows in plain radiographs of the abdomen; the presence of fundic gas shadow is occasionally useful in reading and interpreting radiographs. This shadow is located just inferior to the left dome of the diaphragm. Fundic gas is mainly carbon dioxide; this gas is formed by gastric acid (containing hydrochloric acid) action on digestive secretions that gastric glands produce and on bicarbonate (in the mucosal layer of the stomach as protection for the stomach). Not only is carbon dioxide produced, but also water [26]. Regarding the pylorus, the correct order is that the pyloric antrum becomes the pyloric canal prior to the small intestine. The pylorus is the fourth part of the stomach; the three proximal parts are the cardia, followed by the fundus and body. Mucous (goblet) cells are located close to the pits, at the neck (the cardia, which is where the esophagus meets the stomach). Chief (peptic) cells and parietal (oxyntic) cells are located deeper, with the chief cells at the base. Gastric (oxyntic) glands open into gastric pits.

22. D The pancreatic duct and the common bile duct join at/form the ampulla of Vater before they empty their contents into the second part of the duodenum. The common bile duct carries the secretions of the liver, which are stored and concentrated in the gallbladder prior to their eventual release into the common bile duct; the pancreatic duct transports the exocrine secretions of the pancreas. The hepatopancreatic ampulla (ampulla of Vater) opening is identifiable at the posteromedial aspect of the mucosal surface of the second part of the duodenum as the major duodenal papilla. The ampulla is a channel surrounded by the smooth muscles of the sphincter of Oddi. The sphincter of Oddi controls the release of the combined secretions in the ampulla

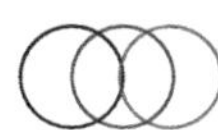

of Vater into the duodenum; the secretions are essential in the digestion of contents received from the stomach. The pancreas is both an endocrine and exocrine gland; the endocrine portion produces insulin, while the exocrine component produces pancreatic juice. The pancreas is retroperitoneal; it lies horizontally between the duodenum and the spleen. The head of the pancreas lies in the duodenal curve, and the tail is related to the spleen. Although the exocrine secretions by the pancreatic acini are released into an elaborate network of ducts, they are eventually transported mainly by the main pancreatic duct.

The main pancreatic duct is the duct of Wirsung; it spans the length of the pancreas and usually joins the distal end of the common bile duct to form the ampulla of Vater. The duct of Santorini is the accessory pancreatic duct; it similarly opens into the second part of the duodenum but about 2 cm proximal to the major duodenal papilla at a location called the minor duodenal papilla [27].

23. D The falciform ligament divides the liver into its major lobes. The liver is the largest internal organ. A normal-sized liver normally extends from the fifth intercostal space superiorly to the subcostal margin inferiorly, with the measurement taken in the right-midclavicular line. The right lobe is larger than the left. The relationships of the other two lobes are as follows: Quadrate, gallbladder; caudate lobe, inferior vena cava. Regarding the caudate lobe of the liver, there is a close relationship with the ligament of the inferior vena cava. This close association may result in leakage of bile or hemorrhage during manipulation of the two structures if adequate care is not observed [28].

24. C The liver is linked with the diaphragm by the coronary ligaments. The coronary ligaments consist of a fold of visceral peritoneum; they are formed as a reflection of visceral peritoneum from the bare area of the liver to connect with the inferior surface of the diaphragm. A hepatic lobule of cells is arranged radially about a central vein. The hepatic portal vein transports blood from the digestive tracts in vascular channels, the hepatic sinusoids.

25. B The liver is partially surrounded by the lower ribs antero-laterally. The liver allows the mixture of nutrient-rich blood and oxygen-rich blood in its sinusoids. The liver has sinusoids, which separate plates of cells of functional liver units from one another. Kupffer cells are in the sinusoidal endothelium. Canaliculi coalesce to form hepatic ducts.

26. C The gallbladder is located in a depression on the inferior surface of the liver. The gallbladder is pear-shaped. It is lined with columnar epithelial cells. It is connected to and continues as the cystic duct. The duct of the gallbladder (cystic duct) and the duct from the liver (hepatic duct) join to form the common bile duct.

The biliary tract has extrahepatic and intrahepatic parts. Drainage of bile within the liver (the intrahepatic biliary drainage system) follows the supply by the portal vein and the hepatic artery. The pattern of branching of the biliary tract in the liver functionally creates right and left lobes and segments. The umbilical fissure is where the round ligament is located; the fissure divides the left lobe of the liver into medial and lateral sectors, i.e., left lateral and left medial. The lateral sector of the left lobe (left lateral) has two sections called the superior and inferior segments; the superior is designated segment II, while the inferior is segment III. Inside the liver substance there is a merger of the ducts of segment II and segment III posterior to the umbilical component of the left portal vein to form the left hepatic duct. The left hepatic duct receives the duct from segment IV. Segment IV of the liver is the medial portion of the right lobe (the quadrate lobe). The right lobe of the liver is divided into anterior and posterior sectors, each of which is further divided into superior and inferior segments [29].

27. A The capacity of the gallbladder is 30–50 milliliters. Regarding the gallbladder, its strong muscular wall contracts in response to stimulus by cholecystokinin. The hepatopancreatic sphincter (sphincter of Oddi) is normally closed because the sphincter muscle is normally contracted. Release of bile into the duodenum is a result of hepatopancreatic sphincter relaxation. Gallstones in the bile duct may block bile flow and cause obstructive jaundice.

28. D The small intestine is about 25 cm at its first part. It is not of the same length in a living adult compared with the dead; it is considerably shorter in the living because of normal intestinal muscle tone that is lost in the cadaver. The small intestine consists of three parts—the duodenum, jejunum, and ileum. It is C-shaped at the level of the duodenum.

29. B The duodenum is anterior to the first three lumbar vertebrae and the right kidney. The duodenum is the part of the small intestine that contains Brunner's glands. Brunner's glands secrete an alkaline fluid that reduces the concentration of acid in the chyme that enters this first part of the small gut before it traverses the rest of the small intestines. A relatively alkaline environment in the small intestine is a requirement for small intestinal enzymes to act on their contents. The ileum is longer than the jejunum. The jejunum is intraperitoneal. The duodenum is retroperitoneal.

30. B The jejunum and ileum hang from the mesentery, while the duodenum is retroperitoneal. The crypts of Lieberkühn are intestinal glands. The mesentery is a double layer of visceral peritoneal fold. Intestinal villi increase mucosal surface area as well as increase absorption. Villi are complex in their structure and genetic, cellular, and non-cellular characteristics. When exposed to various influences, small intestinal villi may be modified to abnormal forms, leading to abnormal function. Since villi play a significant role in the handling or processing of food, there may be health challenges from derangements in the structure and other characteristics of villi. In individuals who are genetically predisposed to hypersensitivity response to ingestion of gluten, there is a marked change in the morphology of villi [30, 31]. Heavy intestinal loads of bacteria like *Klebsiella pneumoniae, Escherichia coli,* and *Enterobacter cloacae* cause tropical enteropathies akin to sprue, and parasites like *Giardia lamblia* (giardiasis), *Entamoeba histolytica* (amebiasis), *Strongyloides stercoralis* (strongyloidiasis), *Cystoisospora belli* (cystoisosporiasis), and *Cryptosporidium parvum* (cryptosporidiosis) may also result in marked alteration of the architecture of small intestines with a malabsorption syndrome [31, 32].

31. C Peristalsis is the movement that propels chyme through the small intestine. Mixing movements are periodical ring-like contractions; this is segmentation. Parasympathetic impulses are what enhance both mixing and propulsive movements. The ileocecal sphincter normally stays closed.

32. D The large intestine is about 1.5 meters (150 cm) long. It commences at the right side of the abdominal cavity. It is wider than the duodenum. The large intestine is devoid of villi. From the beginning to the end, the large intestine consists of the cecum (to which the appendix is attached), colon, rectum, and anal canal.

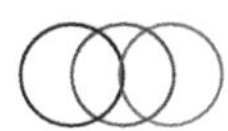

33. B The colon has four parts: Ascending, transverse, descending, and sigmoid colon. The hepatic flexure is the right colic flexure of the ascending colon. The transverse colon is the longest and most mobile part of the large intestine. The rectum is rigidly attached to the anterior part of the sacrum by peritoneum. The rectum commences at the end of the sigmoid colon at the level of the third sacral vertebra. It is approximately 15 cm in length. In its entirety, the posterior surface of the rectum is not covered by peritoneum; its posterior surface is therefore retroperitoneal or extraperitoneal. This surface of the rectum abuts the retroperitoneal space. The rectum is devoid of taeniae coli, appendices epiploicae, and sacculations (haustra) which are present in the earlier portions of the colon except the appendix. There are six to ten or slightly more longitudinal columns or folds of mucosa in the anal canal superior to the pectineal line (dentate line); these are anal columns (columns of Morgagni) and they contain the terminal branches of the superior rectal blood vessels [33].

34. C The rectum commences at the recto-sigmoid junction (S2 or S3 level), where it tends to be narrower than the rest of the large intestine; it continues below the tip of the coccyx and ends about 2 to 3 cm anterior and slightly inferior to the coccygeal tip (i.e., at the anorectal junction); at this junction, the rectum makes a sharp turn posteriorly (anorectal flexure, or perineal flexure) and becomes the anal canal. The transverse colon runs obliquely (*not* transversely) from right to left. The sigmoid colon is S-shaped. The ascending colon links the cecum with the right colic flexure. Only the external anal sphincter muscles are made up of skeletal muscle fibers; the internal sphincter consists of smooth muscles.

35. C Gastric mucosa is lined by simple columnar glandular epithelium. The greater curvature and lesser curvature of the stomach extend between the esophagus proximally and the duodenum distally. The greater curvature forms the lateral and inferior margin of the stomach; the lesser curvature forms the superior and medial aspect of the stomach. The stomach in tall individuals assumes a vertical orientation, while in short people it is relatively horizontal. Gastric rugae are evident in an emptying or empty stomach; rugae are longitudinal folds of mucosal and submucosal layers. In the stomach, the muscularis externa consists of three layers: the outer layer is longitudinal, the middle layer is circular, and the inner layer is oblique.

36. C In the stomach, mucous neck cells produce mucus that protects mucosa from not only hydrochloric acid (HCl) but also enzymes. Chief cells produce gastric lipase during infancy, which enables infants' stomachs to digest fats; secretion of this enzyme does not extend into adulthood. Enteroendocrine cells stimulate gastric motility by producing serotonin; they also produce histamine, but histamine stimulates production of hydrochloric acid. Parietal cell intrinsic factor enhances vitamin B_{12} absorption; this action takes place in the small intestine (distal ileum), not in the stomach where the intrinsic factor is secreted.

37. A Opening the upper abdomen either during surgery or at dissection and viewing the liver anteriorly shows the left lobe of the liver and the falciform ligament. The other parts of the liver are the right lobe (which is larger than the left) and the ligamentum teres. The falciform ligament is a sheet of mesentery that separates the right lobe of the liver from the left lobe; this ligament suspends the liver and runs between the diaphragm and the anterior abdominal wall [13]. At the inferior part of the liver is the ligamentum teres (round ligament); this is the remnant of the fetal umbilical vein that links the placenta with the fetal liver in intrauterine life. The ligamentum teres, not the quadrate lobe, may be seen anteriorly; the quadrate lobe is visible from an inferior view. The caudate lobe is posterior to the quadrate lobe; the gallbladder is visible from the inferior view. The bare area is at the superior surface of the liver.

38. C The hepatic triad consists of a bile ductule and two blood vessels. The blood vessels are small branches of the hepatic artery and small branches of the hepatic portal vein; the blood supply to hepatic sinusoids is therefore dual: well-oxygenated blood from the celiac trunk via the hepatic artery and nutrient-rich blood from the gastrointestinal tract via the hepatic portal vein. In normal conditions, without any pathological activity, the intrasinusoidal pressures in the portal vein and the hepatic artery are equalized. Nutrients and oxygen derived from the systemic circulation get to hepatic parenchymal cells and are distinctively delivered throughout hepatic acini. In these normal conditions, proteins (like albumin, lipoproteins, and coagulation factors) from the liver are also supplied to the systemic circulation [34].

It is the right lobe of the liver that occupies the right hypochondrium. Each hepatic lobule has a central vein surrounded by hepatocytes, which are cuboidal cells. The liver secretes bile directly into bile canaliculi. The bile then passes into bile ductules (cholangioles) and, thereafter, into the right and left hepatic ducts.

39. D The hepatopancreatic ampulla (ampulla of Vater) is a short channel that terminates in the fold of tissue called the major duodenal papilla; this is in the wall of the duodenum, and its opening is visible in the mucosal surface of the middle part of the duodenum [27]. The major duodenal papilla contains the hepatopancreatic sphincter (sphincter of Oddi). This sphincter of smooth muscle surrounds the ampulla of Vater and regulates the passage of both bile and pancreatic juice into the duodenum. The right and left hepatic ducts form the common hepatic duct on the inferior surface of the liver. The cystic duct is the continuation of the neck of the gallbladder. The hepatopancreatic ampulla is formed by the union of the bile duct with the pancreatic duct close to the duodenum—*not* as the bile duct enters the pancreas.

40. B The interior of the gallbladder is lined by simple columnar epithelium. The biliary tree is a continuation of the gallbladder at the neck (cervix), *not* the body (fundus), of the gallbladder. The fundus of the gallbladder sometimes projects below the lower edge of the liver. The length of a normal gallbladder is about 10 cm, while its width and depth are about 4 cm [35].

41. C The accessory pancreatic duct (duct of Santorini) branches off the pancreatic duct; it opens into the duodenum at the minor duodenal papilla proximal to the major pancreatic papilla. This arrangement makes it possible for the accessory pancreatic duct to bypass the sphincter of Oddi and deliver pancreatic secretions into the duodenum when the sphincter of Oddi is closed in-between meals [27]. The duodenum virtually encircles the head of the pancreas. Secretory acini open into small ducts, which unite and eventually enter the pancreatic duct along its length. The pancreas is a retroperitoneal gland.

42. C During surgery, the ileum is identified among intestinal loops in the right lower abdominal cavity. The first part of the small intestine, the duodenum, is about 25 cm in length; the duodenum commences at the pyloric valve. The ileum is still longer than the jejunum in the cadaver, just as in a living person; in the adult cadaver, the ileum is about

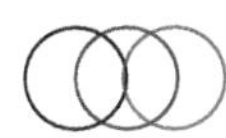

3.6 meters and the jejunum approximately 2.5 meters. During surgery, the jejunum is identifiable in the left upper abdominal cavity.

43. A The dorsal pancreatic artery is a branch of the splenic artery. Although the dorsal pancreatic artery (DPA) commonly arises from the splenic artery, the alternative origins of this artery, in reducing frequency, are the superior mesenteric artery, the common hepatic artery, the celiac trunk, the replaced right hepatic artery, and the inferior pancreaticoduodenal artery. Knowing and keeping this fact in mind is essential for ensuring safety when performing pancreatic resection [36].

The ileocecal artery, jejunal artery, and ileal artery are branches of the superior mesenteric artery. The arteries that arise from the superior mesenteric artery include the inferior pancreaticoduodenal artery, the middle colic artery, the right colic artery, and the ileocolic artery. The inferior pancreaticoduodenal artery arises as a common artery, which divides into the posterior and anterior branches of the inferior pancreaticoduodenal arteries.

44. C A point 1/3 the distance along the spino-umbilical line marks the appendix. This point is the McBurney's point; clinically it is one of the pointers to an inflamed appendix. It was in 1891 that Charles McBurney described a point of maximal tenderness on palpation of the abdomen in patients with acute appendicitis, reflecting inflammation that had involved the parietal peritoneum in patients with a classically located appendix. This point, McBurney's point, has been an important anatomic point of reference before and during surgery for appendicitis, which involves the open approach. The open approach in the surgical management of appendicitis is still used, although the laparoscopic option is widely in use [37].

Obstruction of the lumen of the appendix, culminating in inflammation, is the primary pathology of appendicitis. There are a variety of factors for appendiceal obstruction, and they include appendicoliths, intestinal parasites, hypertrophic lymphatic tissues, and appendiceal tumors [38].

The artery that supplies the appendix, the appendicular artery, runs in the mesoappendix. The appendix is rich in lymphoid tissue and thus plays a positive role in immunity. The rectus abdominis is outside the operative area for appendectomy; the muscles that are encountered are the external oblique, internal oblique, and the transversus abdominis before gaining access into the abdominal cavity via the peritoneum.

45. B The greater omentum arises from the stomach just as the lesser omentum does; while the greater omentum arises and hangs from the greater curvature of the stomach and covers the transverse colon, jejunum, and ileum, the lesser omentum arises from the lesser curvature of the stomach and attaches both the stomach and the duodenum to the inferior surface of the liver. Omentum is a fibro-fatty structure made up of a double layer of visceral peritoneal reflections from the stomach.

The omentum is also a source of resident inflammatory and stem cells. These cells are involved in controlling local infection, and when there is tissue injury, the omentum participates in wound healing and regeneration of affected tissues. The omentum is intricately linked with systemic blood vessels. The omentum is also in communication with the central nervous system and the hypothalamic–pituitary–adrenal axis [39]. Omentum is structurally similar to mesentery because it is a double layer of peritoneum (in this case attaching the small intestines to the posterior abdominal wall) and encapsulates blood vessels, nerves, fatty tissue, and lymphatic tissue.

The lymphoid aggregates in the omentum are called milky spots, which contain macrophages and lymphocytes; milky spots play a role in immunity of the peritoneal cavity because they enable the omentum to gather not only pathogens from the peritoneal cavity but also antigens and particulates which are all processed to counter infection [40]. In the presence of intraperitoneal sepsis, the size and number of milky spots in the omentum increase markedly. Milky spots additionally support innate-like B1 cell responses and local immunoglobulin M synthesis in the peritoneal cavity [41]. The B1 cell is a unique B cell subset that has an innate capability to immunologically respond rapidly to infection and act as a phagocyte—similar to macrophages [42]. B1 cells are different from B2 cells, and they are able to respond rapidly to infective threats without and before T cell activity [43].

46. B The blood supply of the ascending colon is by the right colic artery, which is a branch of the superior mesenteric artery. The ascending colon commences at the ileo-cecal valve opening into the cecum. The ascending colon is retroperitoneal. It terminates at the right colic (hepatic) flexure, which is close to the right lobe of the liver.

47. B The ileocolic artery is a branch of the superior mesenteric artery; from the ileocolic artery the appendicular artery arises. The appendix has both sympathetic and parasympathetic innervation from the superior mesenteric nerve plexus. The sympathetic afferent fibers are from the spinal cord at the T10 spinal level; this explains the central location of visceral pain attributable to an inflamed appendix. The autonomic innervation of the appendix is the autonomic nerve supply to the midgut—the midgut is the embryological origin of the appendix; the specific autonomic innervation originates from the superior mesenteric plexus. In acute appendicitis, the incoming (afferent) sympathetic sensory fibers from the inflamed appendix run in the sympathetic nerve fibers and enter the spinal cord at the T10 spinal level. This level corresponds to the umbilical dermatome. Remember that the appendix is innervated by the autonomic nervous supply to the midgut. Inflammation in the appendix activates afferent sympathetic fibers, which enter the spinal cord at T10, resulting in pain being referred to the periumbilical area as colicky pain [44]. Lymphatic drainage of the appendix is into lymph nodes in the mesoappendix and then to the ileocolic lymph nodes, which surround the ileocolic artery. As just indicated, the appendix is derived from the embryologic midgut; with respect to the gastrointestinal tract, the embryologic hindgut is between the distal (left) 1/3 of the transverse colon and the superior part of the anal canal. The hindgut ends in the cloaca, which is the common origin of the rectum and upper anal canal (in the gastrointestinal tract) and the urinary bladder and the urethra (in the urogenital tract).

48. D The blood supply of the descending colon is by the left colic artery, which is the first branch of the inferior mesenteric artery. The descending colon terminates at the beginning of the sigmoid colon. Being retroperitoneal, the descending colon is not readily mobile. In its length it is related to the left loin.

49. C The arteries to the sigmoid colon run in the sigmoid mesocolon. After their origin from the inferior mesenteric artery, sigmoid arteries run in the sigmoid mesocolon and eventually supply the sigmoid colon via their numerous straight branches (arteriae rectae). Tenia coli are found in the cecum, ascending colon, transverse colon, descending colon, and sigmoid colon. They are three longitudinal strips of the muscularis externa of the colon. It is the muscle tone of the tinea coli that creates haustra in the parts of the colon mentioned. The

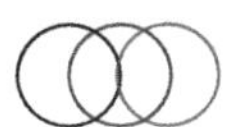

descending colon makes an infero-medial turn to form the sigmoid colon; this takes place at the pelvic inlet, which is not as wide as the abdominal cavity. Sigmoid veins enter the inferior mesenteric vein independent of the left colic veins.

50. C The rectum is one of the sites of porta-caval anastomoses. The other sites of porta-caval anastomoses are the esophagus, periumbilical area, and the retroperitoneum; the venous anastomoses are, respectively, esophageal, periumbilical, and retroperitoneal. In the rectum, the anastomoses occasionally result in hemorrhoids when there is incompetence of the valvular integrity of the veins. The longitudinal layer of rectal muscularis externa forms a complete layer, resulting in the absence of tinea coli in the rectum. In the rectum, projections of the inner (circular) muscle layer form three folds; these folds function as valves and prevent passage of stool when an individual passes flatus. The folds are called the superior rectal valve, middle rectal valve, and inferior rectal valve. Epiploic appendages (appendices epiploicae) are present in the transverse and sigmoid parts of the colon.

Defects that occur during embryogenesis of the gastrointestinal tract may result in conditions like atresia, stenosis, dysfunctional peristalsis, malrotation, or various degrees of patency of a tubular structure that should have become closed before birth [45]. Examples include esophageal, duodenal, jejunal, and ileal atresia (atresias); hypertrophic pyloric stenosis (stenosis); Hirschsprung's disease, which is the result of aganglionosis at the Meissner's plexus (submucosa) and Auerbach's plexus (muscularis) of the terminal rectum and slightly proximally (dysfunctional peristalsis); gastroschisis and vitelline fistula (fistulas or other degrees of non-closure); volvulus, Ladd's bands, and omphalocele (from malrotation of the gut). The Auerbach's plexus is located between the circular smooth muscle layer and the longitudinal smooth muscle layer.

The types of midgut malrotation are as follows: non-rotation, incomplete rotation, reverse rotation, and anomalous fixation of the mesentery [45]. The differential diagnoses of midgut malrotation include the following: bowel obstruction in the newborn with failure to pass meconium within 48 hours after birth and pediatric gastroesophageal reflux, intussusception in older infants may lie in a derivative of the embryologic midgut or hindgut such as duodenal atresia, annular pancreas, jejunoileal atresia, meconium ileus, Hirschsprung's disease, small left colon syndrome; neonatal sepsis; intestinal volvulus; and congenital bands [45].

Ladd's bands are congenital bands that constrict the duodenum; Ladd's bands are thick fibrous peritoneal bands that stretch from the cecum to the right upper quadrant of the abdomen and to the duodenum. They may be asymptomatic; Ladd's bands could cause acute intestinal obstruction from a volvulus in pediatrics, but the acute condition could occur much later in adulthood. Intestinal malrotation results from an incomplete or total failure of 270° counterclockwise rotation of the midgut around the superior mesenteric vessels during fetal development [46].

51. D Above the pectinate (dentate) line, i.e., the superior 2/3 of the anal canal, only the superior rectal vein provides drainage; it eventually drains into the hepatic portal vein. Below the dentate line, i.e., the inferior 1/3 of the anal canal, two veins are responsible for venous drainage; the veins are the middle rectal vein and inferior rectal vein, both of which drain into the inferior vena cava. Thus, venous blood from the upper 2/3 of the anal canal drains into the portal circulation, while from the lower 1/3, drainage is into the systemic circulation.

The anal canal spans the short distance between the anorectal junction and the anus. The dentate line, the line of demarcation, divides the anal canal into two unequal parts—the proximal (superior) 2/3 and the distal (inferior) 1/3. While the external anal sphincter consists of skeletal muscle fibers, the internal anal sphincter consists of smooth muscle.

Regarding the mucous layer (mucosal lining) of the anal canal, it consists of three parts—the colorectal zone, the transitional zone, and the anoderm. The colorectal zone is the uppermost part; it consists of simple columnar epithelium just like rectal mucosa. Just below it is the transitional zone, which is between the colorectal zone and the anoderm; this transitional zone is made of simple columnar epithelium and stratified columnar epithelium. The anoderm, the most inferior zone of the mucosal lining of the anal canal, consists of non-keratinized stratified squamous epithelium.

On the other hand, the cutaneous zone of the anal canal, is the lowermost part of the external part of the perianal skin; this part (which is not a part of the mucosal lining, but skin lining) consists of keratinized stratified squamous epithelium—it is like skin in other parts of the body and is subject to pain, sweating, and hair growth (since the skin is non-glabrous). This provides the explanation of internal hemorrhoids causing no pain, but external hemorrhoids and anal fissures cause patients pain.

Summary: The anoderm is the mucosal lining of the anal canal starting from the pectinate (dentate) line superiorly to the anal verge inferiorly. The colorectal zone (also referred to as the columnar zone) and the transitional zone (which is synonymous with the intermediate zone), in combination, cover/line the upper 2/3 of the length of the anal canal, which starts from the beginning of the anal canal and ends at the pectinate line. The anoderm forms the lower 1/3 of the anatomical extent of the anal canal. The skin-like part of the anal canal, the cutaneous zone (also referred to as the squamous zone or perianal zone) of the anal canal, has features of non-glabrous skin.

52. B The muscles that form the levator ani are puborectalis, pubococcygeus, and iliococcygeus. The puborectalis arises from the pubic rami, goes posterior to the rectum, and forms a sling. The puborectalis is responsible for (creates and maintains) the sharp posterior angulation of the rectum (anorectal flexure) at the anorectal junction [47]. The pubococcygeus arises lateral to the origin of the puborectalis; posteriorly it inserts at the coccyx. Though it is part of the pelvic diaphragm, the piriformis is more posterior and is not part of the three-muscle levator ani.

53. B Injury to the spleen is expected from a bullet entry wound at the left 9th rib. The splenic artery arises from the celiac trunk. The spleen is dorsolateral (posterolateral) to the stomach and inferior to the left dome of the diaphragm. The white pulp contains lymphocytes and macrophages; red pulp contains erythrocytes [48].

The Retroperitoneum

54. D Kidneys are bean-shaped but have a smooth surface. Normal dimensions of the kidney are 12 × 6 × 3 cm. A kidney is retroperitoneal and lies lateral to the vertebral column. Kidneys are held in place by renal fascia and surrounding renal fat [49].

55. A The upper poles of the kidneys are slightly posteromedially disposed. The left kidney is about 1.5–2.0 cm higher than the right. The medial surface of a kidney is concave, while the lateral surface is convex. The renal pelvis is the funnel-shaped part of the upper ureter and is within the kidney. The tunica fibrosa renis is the fibrous capsule or renal capsule; it encloses the kidney.

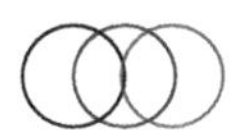

56. C Though kidneys are 1% of body weight, 25% of the cardiac output supplies them via renal arteries. The urinary bladder is inferior to the parietal peritoneum. From inside to outside, the bladder wall has a first layer (mucosa or mucous coat), a second layer (submucosa, or submucous coat), a third layer (muscularis, or muscular coat), and a fourth layer (serosa or serous coat) that consists of parietal peritoneum. The renal vein drains into the inferior vena cava.

57. D The kidneys are retroperitoneal; the same applies to the adrenals, ureters, and bladder. The normal dimensions of the kidney are $12 \times 5 \times 2.5$ cm in length, width, and thickness, respectively. The lateral surface of the kidney is convex; the medial surface is concave. The right kidney is slightly lower than the left due to the presence of the liver.

58. B Structures in the hilum at the medial surface of each kidney are the renal blood vessels, lymphatics, renal nerves, and ureter.

59. C The renal cortex and medulla, the minor and major calyces, the renal columns and pyramids, and the pelvis are identifiable macroscopically [50]. Nephrons are histologically identifiable.

60. C The fibrous renal fascia is the first, attaching the kidney to the posterior abdominal wall. The middle layer is the adipose capsule that provides cushioning to the kidney. The renal capsule is the innermost. It is the left kidney that has the left adrenal on its superior pole; the right adrenal gland rests superomedially between the superior pole and the hilum. A kidney of normal size usually lies between the twelfth thoracic vertebra and the third lumbar vertebra.

CHAPTER 10

ANSWERS AND NOTES FOR MCQs ON THORAX

1. C The thin sheets of tissue that encompass or cover the body, body cavities, and organs within the cavities of the body are referred to as membranes. Membranes are basically divided into two types: epithelial membranes and connective tissue membranes.

Epithelial membranes are further divided into two—serous membranes and mucous membranes. Serous membranes provide lining for body cavities that do not communicate directly with the exterior; such cavities are in the abdomen (abdominal cavity, called peritoneal cavity) and in the thorax (thoracic cavity, called pleural cavity and pericardial cavity). A serous membrane is simple squamous epithelium. Serous fluid is what the epithelial cells of serous membranes produce; it is thin. The cells that line the epithelium of serous membranes produce fluid that lubricates their surfaces and therefore helps in reducing friction between the structures that they line (cover) and surrounding structures. In the thorax, pleural fluid reduces friction between the visceral pleura, which covers the outer (external) surface of the lungs, and parietal pleura, which covers the inner wall of the thoracic cage. There is movement during inspiration and expiration, and this movement is smooth and seamless when the amount and quality of pleural fluid are normal; when there is inflammation, like in pleuritis, pneumonia, or pleural effusion, the patient experiences pain due to friction and other products of inflammation [1]. In pleuritic pain, there is sharp chest pain that is localized to the part of the pleurae that rub against one another; the pain is aggravated by inspiration and further worsens when the patient attempts to engage in deep breathing. Other activities that precipitate or accentuate the pain of pleurisy are sneezing, coughing, or laughing. Although it may appear to be idiopathic, pleurisy usually points to an underlying pathological process like viral infections by agents like influenza virus, respiratory syncytial virus, and coxsackieviruses. Depending on the clinical presentation associated with pleuritic pain, other conditions that should be ruled out include pulmonary embolism, myocardial infarction, pneumothorax, pericarditis, and aortic dissection [1]. The digestive tract in its entirety and portions of the urinary tract, respiratory tract, excretory tract, and reproductive tract, which have openings to the outside of the body, are lined with mucous membranes. There is variability in the organization of the protective mucus system across the digestive tract. The structures in the mouth, stomach and duodenum, and colon, are not the same. For example, the same mucin, MUC2, behaves differently in the small intestine and colon [2].

Connective tissue membranes are the second category of membranes. Connective tissue membranes comprise connective tissue solely. Examples of connective tissue membranes are synovial membranes and meninges. Synovial membranes line the surfaces of freely moveable joints like the joints at the shoulder and elbow in the upper limb and hip and knee in the lower limb. Synovial membranes are similar to serous membranes in the sense that they line surfaces that do not directly communicate with the exterior. However, they are different from serous membranes by lacking a layer of epithelium; what they have are synoviocytes, which line the inner surface of the joint capsule and synthesize synovial fluid to lubricate the cartilaginous articular surfaces of the apposing bones in synovial joints; these cells basically have the same function as epithelial membrane cells [3]. Synovial fluid is thick and viscid [4]. The lubrication

DOI: 10.1201/9781003783961-12

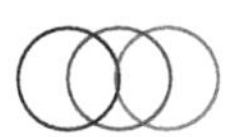

that synovial fluid affords these freely moveable joints allows them smooth function. In patients with synovitis (inflammation of the synovium), there is pain, swelling, and tenderness worsened by movements about the affected joint. Synovitis is a characteristic of rheumatoid arthritis, osteoarthritis, gouty arthritis, psoriatic arthritis, and joint involvement in systemic lupus erythematosus [5].

2. C The angle of Louis is at the level of the disk between the 4th and 5th thoracic vertebrae (T4 and T5). The position of the male nipple corresponds with the level of the 4th intercostal space. The 10th rib forms the lowest part of the costal margin.

3. A The second thoracic vertebral spine (and not the seventh) is at the same level as the superior angle of the scapula. The root of the scapular spine is at the level of the third thoracic vertebral spine. When it is at the anterior axillary line, the apex beat indicates lateral displacement of the apex, which is a feature of left ventricular enlargement. However, regarding enlargement caused by left ventricular dilatation, the size of the apex beat seems to be a more reliable diagnostic sign than its location [6].

4. A The internal thoracic vessels are also known as internal mammary vessels. Bilaterally, the internal thoracic vessels are about 2 cm lateral to the sternum. The internal thoracic arteries provide arterial blood to the sternum, anterior chest wall, breasts, pericardium, and thymus. Each internal thoracic artery originates from the proximal part of the subclavian artery and runs a vertical and downward course along the posterior (inner) surface of the anterior chest wall. In its descent, it lies in between muscles and cartilages. Anterior to each artery are the internal intercostal muscles and costal cartilages; posterior to these arteries is the transversus thoracis muscle. Prior to their bifurcation, they supply each intercostal space with branches called anterior intercostal arteries; they also yield perforating branches. These arteries each terminate at the level of the sixth or seventh costal cartilage by bifurcating and becoming two arteries (the superior epigastric artery and musculophrenic artery) [7].

There is danger to the intercostal vessels when inserting a needle into the pleural cavity through the lower border of a rib because the intercostal vessels lie in the costal groove just posterior to the lower portion of ribs 2 to 11; that is why in procedures like thoracentesis, the needle must be inserted directly above the superior surface of the rib [8]. A similar risk occurs during supracostal percutaneous nephrostolithotomy [9]. An upward tilt of the needle may injure the vessels, and this must equally be avoided. Rib fractures do endanger the intercostal vessels because of the close relationship with the lower rib margin.

5. B The left intercostobrachial nerve is associated with referred pain of myocardial ischemia; this is because visceral sensation from the heart shares the same roots in the spinal cord (T1 to T5). In myocardial ischemia, the pain is not well localized, and therefore it is referred to the patient's left arm and neck (the dermatomes that correspond with T1 to T5), which are served by the intercostobrachial nerve. The intercostobrachial nerve is unique in being the only nerve that supplies the upper limb but does not pass through the brachial plexus. It is the lateral cutaneous branch of T2—the second intercostal nerve. This nerve provides peripheral sensory innervation of the medial aspect of the upper arm up to the elbow. Clinically, damage to the intercostobrachial nerve during mastectomy may result in postmastectomy pain—a neuropathic pain that presents as axillary and upper arm pain. The patient also experiences altered sensation in the same areas that are supplied by this nerve (the axilla and skin over the arm medially) [10].

Fractures of lower ribs endanger the liver and spleen as they encage these organs. There is a significant relationship between rib fractures involving the middle zone of the thoracic cage and abdominal solid organ injury. Injuries to intra-abdominal organs are not limited to the ones due to fractures of the lower ribs; it is therefore imperative to bear in mind the possibility of such injuries when attending to patients with blunt trauma with concomitant rib fractures [11].

Pain from inflammation at the central portion of the diaphragmatic parietal pleura is referred to the shoulder. This is because the innervation of the parietal pleura that lines the central part of the diaphragm is by nerve fibers that travel with the phrenic nerves. Embryologically, the diaphragm arises from the cervical region and migrates downward to its definitive thoracic location. The phrenic nerve similarly arises from the C3, C4, and C5 spinal cord segments, which serve sensory innervation of the neck and shoulders [12]. Mediation of chest pain may be by somatosensory nerves or autonomic nerves; when it is by somatosensory nerves, the pain is well localized, but when it is by autonomic nerves, it tends to be poorly defined and tends to radiate (be referred) [12].

6. D Since the intercostal nerve is the most inferior of the neurovascular structures in the costal groove located in the lower portion of a rib, accessing the nerve is best achieved by injecting the local anesthetic agent just below the inferior margin of the rib, the nerve of which is of interest. A long-acting agent (e.g., ropivacaine 0.2% or bupivacaine 0.25%) is preferred. The patient may be in the lateral, sitting, or prone position—the prone position being the best option for an inexperienced professional [13]. Complications can be avoided by performing an intercostal nerve block under ultrasound guidance and aseptic conditions. Ultrasound guidance ensures that the anesthetic agent is delivered optimally and is neither injected into the nerve nor a blood vessel; ensuring aseptic conditions minimizes the risk of infection. It is also preferable to perform this procedure on a patient who is awake rather than one who is under deep sedation or general anesthesia; this is because the patient's reaction in pneumothorax or intraneural injection of the local anesthetic agent would alert the person performing the procedure. It is essential for the doctor performing this procedure to be cognizant of seizures, alteration in mental status, blood pressure abnormalities, cardiac arrhythmias, and even cardiac arrest, all of which are presentations of local anesthetic systemic toxicity (LAST) [13]. Apart from the standard requirements for this sterile procedure, the equipment required are a marking pen, ultrasound scanner, EKG/ECG monitor, blood pressure monitor, and pulse oximeter [13]. Liposomal bupivacaine has been suggested as a treatment option for severe acute post-thoracotomy pain in patients for whom other treatment options are contraindicated or have proved ineffective [14].

Mediastinal shift is demonstrable clinically by lateral deviation of the trachea in the suprasternal notch. An infero-lateral displacement of the apex beat indicates enlargement of the heart. A pulsatile swelling at the suprasternal notch may indicate aortic aneurysm.

7. D The last five pairs of ribs are false ribs, as they are not attached to the sternum. The last two pairs of ribs are floating ribs; they are also called vertebral ribs. Vertebrochondral ribs are the 8th, 9th, and 10th pairs of ribs; they are the ones usually referred to as false ribs. False ribs are ribs that are not attached to the sternum, but while ribs 8 to 10 are attached to the cartilages of the rib above each of them, ribs 11 and 12 are not attached to either the sternum or any cartilage—they are "floating." Floating ribs are also known as vertebral ribs. The hyaline cartilage of rib 7 to which rib 8 is attached (and the next two are attached indirectly) is what links these three ribs to the sternum. This indirect attachment anteriorly permits chest wall expansion during breathing (particularly inspiration). True ribs are attached to the sternum anteriorly by their cartilages; they are the first seven ribs.

8. C The sternum is a flat bone with a thin outer layer of compact bone; the inner part of the sternum is the core and it consists of spongy bone. The sternum has three parts: the manubrium, body, and xiphoid process [15].

The manubrium is also referred to as the manubrium sterni; this component of the sternum is quadrangular. This part of the sternum has an upper segment called the suprasternal notch or the jugular notch. Laterally, the manubrium has clavicular notches that articulate with the medial end of each clavicle, therefore forming the right and left sternoclavicular joints. By their cartilages, rib 1 on both sides articulates with the manubrium sterni.

The body is the next part of the sternum; it is the longest portion. The body of the sternum is also called the mesosternum. The ridges at its lateral ends are points of articulation of the costal ends of the right and left second ribs. The sternal angle (angle of Louis) corresponds with the level of the intervertebral disk between the fourth and fifth thoracic vertebrae (T4/T5). Moreover, the angle of Louis is also significant because an imaginary horizontal plane traversing this angle from front to back to meet the T4/T5 intervertebral disk passes through the inferior border of the superior mediastinum. The structures in the superior mediastinum are the aortic arch, brachiocephalic veins, superior vena cava, thymus, vagus nerve, phrenic nerve, esophagus, and trachea. It is also at this anatomical landmark that the trachea terminates by bifurcating into the right and left bronchi; it also represents the level of the aortic arch and the pulmonary trunk [16]. The sternal angle is, consequently, an important reference point for performing thoracic surgery and procedures. It is also important for regular outpatient and inpatient clinical care; this is because correctly identifying the sternal angle in a patient is helpful in the clinical examination of a patient by a clinical-year medical student or a practicing physician—palpating the sternal angle is valuable for locating the 2nd rib and proceeding to pinpoint the intercostal spaces during auscultation of the chest and when placing the chest leads for electrocardiography. However, this identification often proves difficult and uncertain in individuals who are obese, particularly those who are morbidly obese. The aortic valve is auscultated at the second intercostal space on the right, while the pulmonic valve is at the equivalent space on the left side. The site for auscultating the tricuspid valve is usually between the fourth and fifth intercostal spaces; for auscultating the mitral valve, the ideal location is the fifth intercostal space.

Xiphoid process: The synonym for the xiphoid process is the xiphisternum or xiphoid; this most inferior component of the sternum is triangular. The entire sternum protects structures in the mediastinum [16]. The sternum may be punctured to obtain bone marrow aspirate for hematological analysis; although it is one of the easiest sites, great caution must be applied during this procedure to avoid injury to nearby vital organs. Imaging of the thorax using computed tomography (CT) scans and magnetic resonance imaging (MRI) are valuable tools in safely evaluating and confidently handling surgical conditions of the structures in the thorax [17].

9. B The bronchial tree starts from the end of the trachea. The origin of the primary (main stem) bronchi corresponds with the level of the fifth thoracic vertebra. The right main bronchus is shorter, wider, and more vertical than the left. There are three right and two left lobar bronchi. The bronchial tree extends to the alveoli, where it terminates.

10. B The right lung is larger than the left lung. The lung reflection is at the hilus. Large blood vessels and the bronchus suspend each lung in the thorax.

11. B Mediolaterally, firm female breasts are between the sternum and axillae; supero-inferiorly they lie between the 2nd and 6th ribs. The areola is the pigmented circular skin area within which lies the nipple. The nipple of a firm breast is at about the level of the fourth intercostal space. Mammary glands—accessory organs of the female reproductive system—are specialized to secrete milk.

12. D In males and females, mammary glands are similar up to puberty. Mammary glands are in subcutaneous tissue. This gland has 15 to 20 irregularly shaped lobes. Mammary glands have lobes separated by adipose tissue and dense connective tissue.

13. C The bronchial tree terminates at the alveoli. The right main bronchus is wider than the left; it is also more vertically disposed than the left. Bronchoconstriction plays an important role in bronchial asthma, not in emphysema.

14. A The anatomical characteristics of the right main bronchus predispose an unconscious patient to aspiration via the right primary bronchus. Risk factors for aspiration include cognitive neurologic impairment in patients who have strokes, seizures, or intoxication from alcohol or drugs of abuse. Other risk factors are the use of a nasogastric tube, tracheostomy tube, or a gastrostomy feeding tube; aspiration could also occur in patients who undergo upper endoscopy (esophagogastroduodenoscopy [EGD]) or bronchoscopy [18]. Features that the clinician should look out for in a patient suspected to have aspirated include cough, tachypnea, rhonchi and rales on lung auscultation, a low peripheral capillary blood oxygen saturation (SpO_2), and absence of breath sounds when there is obstruction of the airway. Since in some patients aspiration may be an ongoing process, it is safe to reevaluate the patient closely and regularly when there is any doubt [18]. It is the right main bronchus that divides into three lobar (secondary) bronchi; it is shorter than its left counterpart, which divides into two lobar bronchi.

15. D The cardiac impression diminishes the size of the left lung. The indentation in the left lung provides accommodation for the heart. The apex of each lung projects above the corresponding clavicle. The hilum of the lung—at the mediastinal surface—consists of the lobar bronchus, blood vessels, nerves, and lymphatic vessels. The mediastinal surface is concave and smaller than the costal surface of each lung.

16. C A pulmonary lobule is a part of the lung that is supplied by one bronchiole. Bronchioles do not have cartilage; the trachea has cartilage that is arranged as rings, but the cartilage in lobar and tertiary bronchi does not form rings, rather overlapping plates. A bronchopulmonary segment is supplied by a tertiary bronchus. Terminal bronchioles are formed by a bronchiole dividing into 50 to 80 units.

17. C Although terminal bronchioles have ciliated cells like the parts of the respiratory tract that are proximal to them, the ciliated cells in these tiniest conducting part of the respiratory tract are sparse and consist of simple ciliated cuboidal epithelium. The majority of the epithelial cells in the terminal bronchioles are club cells that have a non-ciliated epithelium. The conducting portion of the respiratory tree consists of the nasal cavity, pharynx, trachea, bronchi, and bronchioles; it terminates at the terminal bronchioles, which are branches of bronchioles. Terminal bronchioles divide into respiratory

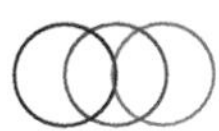

bronchioles. The respiratory bronchioles are the starting points of the respiratory portion (division, zone) of the respiratory tract where gas exchange occurs. The conducting part is a conduit that conditions (moisturizes and warms) inspired air prior to its accessing the lungs and, by its mucociliary escalator, moves inhaled particles proximally to prevent them from entering the lung substance. These functions of the conducting division of the respiratory tract are achieved by specialized cells in the respiratory epithelium, which is essentially ciliated pseudostratified columnar epithelium. There are five types of cells, namely, ciliated cells, goblet cells, basal cells, brush cells, and neuroendocrine cells [19]. Ciliated cells perform a regulatory function on the mucociliary escalator which is a primary defense mechanism by removing particulate debris [20]. Goblet cells produce mucin granules, which trap inhaled particulate matter [20]. Brush cells, also called type III pneumocyte cells, are columnar or flask-shaped. Brush cells have an apical layer that is covered by short microvilli, mimicking a brush. Brush cells are associated with unmyelinated nerve endings [21]. Synonyms for neuroendocrine cells are small granule cells and Kulchitsky cells. Their cells possess neurosecretory-type granules. Their secretions include serotonin, calcitonin, and gastrin-releasing factors [22].

18. B Regarding the 32-year-old patient who, within the past 10 days, had fever, cough, and malaise with leukocytosis and marked neutrophilia, the recent development of sharp right-sided chest pain (pleuritic pain) and shortness of breath of 2 days most likely points to right pleural effusion. The pathology would be in the right costo-phrenic angle.

19. A The medical student manifests features of bronchial asthma, and the site of the pathology is the bronchi. Patients with bronchial asthma have a presentation like: "A medical student in the middle of the professional examination in the final year develops a runny nose, dry cough, breathlessness that has become worse in the past 8 hours and which is preventing her from making complete sentences without a break. She had a similar but significantly milder episode 2 years earlier."

20. B Serratus anterior and pectoralis minor are involved in protraction; protraction is the principal movement that effects the desire of the boxer to give an opponent a knockout punch, as indicated in the question. In conjunction with the trapezius, the serratus anterior enables an individual to lift an object over their head [23]. Rhomboid(eus) major and rhomboid(eus) minor are involved in elevation, medial rotation, and retraction of the scapula. The result of dysfunction or loss of innervation of the rhomboids is winging of the medial border of the scapula and inferior scapular angle rotation [24, 25].

21. D Ribs 1–7 are the true ribs; they are so called because each of them has hyaline cartilage that links their distal end (i.e., the anterior end) to the sternum—this cartilage is called costal cartilage. False ribs have either no link with the sternum or link with the sternum indirectly; the false ribs are ribs 8 to 12. There are three false ribs that link with the sternum indirectly, i.e., by being attached via their costal cartilages to the costal cartilage of rib 7; these are ribs 8, 9, and 10. The remaining ribs (the last two), i.e., ribs 11 and 12, are floating ribs; they are so designated because they are not attached to the sternum or other ribs but are embedded in muscles of the thoracic wall.

22. C The central tendon of the diaphragm is a fibrous structure formed by the convergence of the fascicles of the diaphragm. It does not pass through any of the anatomic openings of the diaphragm. The openings are for the inferior vena cava, aorta, and the esophagus [26].

23. C The internal intercostals are not needed in quiet expiration; however, during activities that require forced expiration, they are required and are utilized. When the internal intercostal muscles contract, they pull the ribs posteroinferiorly; this downward and inward movement of the thoracic cage when forcefully expelling air from the lungs reduces the volume of the thoracic cavity [27]. The intercostal nerves supply both the internal intercostals and external intercostals; paralysis of the intercostal nerves would affect both sets of muscles. The diaphragm is innervated by the phrenic nerve. The external intercostal muscle fibers are disposed at about 90° to the fibers of the internal intercostal muscles.

24. B The lower esophageal sphincter is physiological rather than anatomical. In normal cases the sphincter prevents reflux of gastric contents into the esophagus; the constriction by mainly the diaphragm on the inferior end of the esophagus, with contribution from the tonus of the muscle at the sphincter, provides the sphincter effect [28]. The length of the esophagus between its exit from the mediastinum at the hiatus and entry into the stomach at the cardia is usually 3 to 4 cm. The muscularis externa consists fully of skeletal muscle only in the proximal 1/3 of the esophagus; the middle 1/3 is a combination of skeletal muscle fibers and smooth muscle fibers; the lower 1/3 of the esophagus consists of just smooth muscle fibers. The mucosa of the esophagus consists of nonkeratinized stratified squamous epithelium. The submucosa of the esophagus contains esophageal glands, nerves, blood vessels, lymphatics, and connective tissue.

25. B The axillary artery has three divisions. The artery arises at the lateral margin of the 1st rib; it is a continuation of the subclavian artery. The ulnar artery is a relatively small artery located in the forearm. Direct branches of the axillary artery include the **s**uperior thoracic artery, **t**horacoacromial artery, **l**ateral thoracic artery, **s**ubscapular artery, **an**terior humeral circumflex artery, and **p**osterior humeral circumflex artery [29]. The superior thoracic artery is the first branch of the axillary artery; this small artery arises as the only branch of the first division of the axillary artery. Clinically, the superior thoracic artery is palpable two fingerbreadths inferior to the clavicle in the midclavicular line [29].

26. D The heart is a cone-shaped organ whose primary function is a muscular pump. The heart is situated in the mediastinum (central portion of the chest behind the sternum). The heart has four chambers—two upper and two lower; the upper chambers are the right and left atria, while the lower chambers are the right and left ventricles. The right atrium and ventricle constitute the right heart, and the left atrium and left ventricle function as the left heart [30].

Regarding the blood supply to the heart, it is important to remember that a constant and optimal supply of oxygen and nutrients is essential to satisfy the energy demands of cardiac muscle to achieve continuous contraction and relaxation [31]. The myocardium is the thick middle layer of the walls of the heart.

The coronary arteries, the first branches of the aortic root (i.e., ascending aorta), provide arterial supply to the heart, while venous drainage by the cardiac veins via the coronary sinus accesses the right atrium. There are left and right coronary arteries. The right coronary artery takes its origin from the right aortic sinus and provides arterial blood to the right ventricle and the bundle of His [31]. In the majority of individuals, the posterior descending artery—a branch of the right coronary artery—is responsible for providing the blood supply to the atrioventricular node, the posterior portion of

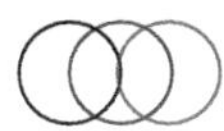

the interventricular septum, the posteromedial papillary muscle, and the ventricles [31]. The origin of the left main coronary artery is the left aortic sinus. The left main coronary artery gives off the left circumflex coronary artery and the left anterior descending artery. The left circumflex coronary artery provides arterial supply to the lateral and posterior walls of the left ventricle, sinoatrial node, atrioventricular node, and the anterolateral portion of the papillary muscle. The left anterior descending artery supplies the anterior surface of the left ventricle and the anterior portion of the interventricular septum [31].

The pericardium consists of two parts—fibrous pericardium and serous pericardium. The serous pericardium has two components—the outer parietal layer and the inner visceral layer. While the outer parietal layer lines the inner part of the fibrous pericardium, the inner visceral layer (synonymous with epicardium) lines the outer surface of the heart. The pericardium, therefore, covers the heart and the proximal portion of its associated great vessels. The pericardial cavity lies between the visceral and parietal layers of the serous pericardium—within the cavity is serous fluid (pericardial fluid). The fibrous pericardium, the outermost of the layers of the pericardium, is attached to the sternum anteriorly.

27. C The lungs are lateral to the heart. The 2nd rib defines the base of the heart, while the fifth intercostal space defines the apex of a normal-sized heart.

28. B The endocardium is continuous with the endothelium of the great vessels that arise from the heart. Purkinje fibers are found in the endocardium. The endocardium contains blood vessels. The epicardium contains nerve fibers and lymph capillaries. The middle of the three layers of the heart is the myocardium. There are, therefore, three walls of the heart—the epicardium, myocardium, and endocardium. Note that the sac that covers the heart (pericardium) also has three parts—the outermost, tough, fibrous pericardium, the parietal layer of serous pericardium, and the visceral layer of serous pericardium.

29. A The pulmonary circulation shunts deoxygenated blood from the heart to the lungs to be re-saturated with oxygen prior to being distributed into the systemic circulation. The inferior vena cava conveys deoxygenated blood from the inferior half of the body to the heart. Similarly, deoxygenated blood from the upper body is transported to the heart by the superior vena cava. The two vena cavae discharge venous blood into the right atrium. From the tricuspid valve, blood flows into the right ventricle and thence into the pulmonary artery via the pulmonic valve prior to being emptied into the lungs. Within the lungs, blood is distributed into pulmonary capillaries. Carbon dioxide is released by the capillaries, which take up oxygen. Blood that is maximally saturated with oxygen is transported by the pulmonary vein into the left atrium. The left atrium contracts and transmits blood through the mitral valve and into the left ventricle. The contraction of the atria is not as strong as that of the ventricles; the left ventricle sends blood that is saturated with oxygen to the systemic circulation via the aortic valve and the aortic arch [32].

30. D The mitral valve is synonymous with the bicuspid valve. The mitral valve allows blood flow from the left atrium to the left ventricle. The pulmonary valve is semilunar and has three cusps. Contraction of the right ventricle leads to tricuspid valve closure. Relaxation of the right ventricle leads to closure of the pulmonary valve.

31. D The left atrium is related to oxygenated blood and four pulmonary veins. The aortic valve has three cusps and is at the base of the ascending aorta. Left ventricular contraction leads to closure of the mitral valve. Left ventricular relaxation coincides with closure of the aortic valve; closure of the aortic valve is the first event when the heart is in diastole [33].

32. A The skeleton of the heart consists of rings of dense fibrous connective tissue at atrioventricular orifices and bases of the aorta and pulmonary trunk. The interventricular septum is part of the skeleton of the heart. Blood from the coronary sinus into the right atrium is of low oxygen concentration and high in carbon dioxide. The pulmonary trunk has two branches. Blood supply to the myocardium is via the coronary arteries.

33. C When the atria contract, the ventricles relax—and vice versa. The main parts of the electrical conduction system of the heart are the sinoatrial (S-A) node, Bachmann's bundle, atrioventricular (A-V) node, the bundle of His, Tawara branches, and Purkinje fibers [34]. The location of the S-A node is in the upper right atrium; it is the primary pacemaker of the heart and generates electrical impulses automatically [34]. Transmission of impulses between the S-A node and Purkinje fibers is slow between the S-A and A-V nodes and fast along the A-V bundle and Purkinje fibers. Pressure goes up and down cyclically. Vibrations from valve movements are responsible for heart sounds. Closure of the aortic and pulmonary valves is responsible for the second heart sound [35]. The first heart sound is the result of the closure of A-V valves. The cardiac cycle comprises **diastole** (a period of cardiac muscle relaxation) and **systole** (a period of contraction). **Ventricular systole** refers to contraction of the ventricles.

34. D Ventricular repolarization occurs after ventricular depolarization. Particularly, the cardiac action potentials of the pacemaker cells possess an inherent automaticity [36]. The pacemaker action potential has just three phases, which are referred to as phases zero, three, and four—skipping phases one and two. As indicated, ventricular repolarization occurs after ventricular depolarization has taken place. Phase zero of pacemaker action is the phase of depolarization; it commences with attainment of membrane potential of minus 40 mV. –40 mV is the threshold potential for pacemaker cells. Attainment of a membrane potential of –40 mV results in the opening of voltage-gated calcium ion (Ca^{2+}) channels; open calcium ion channels allow an influx of Ca^{2+} ions, and the influx of these cations creates an upstroke in membrane potential from a negative 40 mV to a positive value (–40 mV to +10 mV) [36].

Since phases one and two are absent, they are skipped, and the immediately following phase in pacemaker cells is phase three, which is repolarization. Repolarization entails closure of the calcium ion (Ca^{2+}) channels; this closure blocks the flow of Ca^{2+} ions. Closure of calcium ion channels allows voltage-gated potassium ion (K^+) channels to open; opening of these channels permits an efflux of potassium ions (K^+). This cation efflux is a contributory factor to an expeditious reduction in the membrane potential; the change is from a positive to negative value (+10 mV to –60mV) [36].

The electrocardiogram records the electrical changes in the myocardium during a cardiac cycle. The QRS complex represents ventricular depolarization. The T wave is a normal wave. The P wave represents atrial depolarization.

35. A Regarding capillaries, they link arterioles with venules. Basically, capillaries are thin-walled blood vessels and comprise a single layer of simple squamous epithelium, tunica intima (a basement membrane), and pericytes (scattered connective tissue cells); the capillary wall forms a semi-permeable membrane [37]. There is a tight arrangement

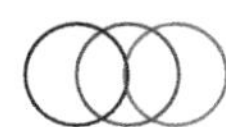

of endothelial cells in brain capillaries; this forms the blood–brain barrier. Arterioles arise from arteries; when arterioles contract, there is a decrease in blood flow to the capillary bed that the arterioles branch off to form. When they undergo dilation, arterioles increase the rate of blood flow into the capillary bed. Arterioles can cause a bypass (shunt) of blood from the capillary bed using metarterioles, by which they access post-capillary venules directly [38]. This is what happens in cold weather when a combination of vasoconstriction and the shunting just described takes place in skin arterioles; the result is a significant reduction in heat loss and diversion of blood supply to the vital organs—heart, brain, and lungs [39].

The flow of blood into capillaries is essentially under the control of precapillary sphincters, which are smooth muscle bands that encompass or surround metarterioles [40]. A subtype of capillaries in the human body is referred to as continuous non-fenestrated capillaries, which are found in the blood–brain barrier, skin, and lungs. They are linked via cellular junctions, have a basement membrane, but are characteristically devoid of fenestrations in the plasma membrane, thus their name. Another subtype of capillaries is called continuous, fenestrated capillaries; this type of capillary is present in intestinal villi and endocrine glands; structurally, they are similar to continuous non-fenestrated capillaries, but their membranes have diaphragmed fenestra. The capillaries in the liver are different because the gaps are wide and the basement membrane is incomplete [41]. In summary, the capillary has a unique anatomical relationship with arterioles and venules that ultimately governs its vascular function.

The higher the metabolic rate, the more capillaries there are. Parts of the body that are rich in capillaries are the heart, lungs, eyes, gut, skeletal muscles, and skin; in the skin, they play a role in sweating or not sweating, and temperature regulation. Capillaries do not link the arterioles with venules in all cases; in certain cases, capillaries are bypassed via metarterioles. Kidneys lack metarterioles and precapillary sphincters. Low oxygen and nutrients make precapillary sphincters open, increasing blood flow [42, 43].

The structure of the capillary system in an organ dictates how permeable that organ is to solutes; it also determines the degree of gas and nutrient exchange that can take place in that organ. Because arterioles branch into capillary beds on arriving at a tissue in an organ, they also play a significant role in controlling capillary exchange by regulating the flow of blood to the tissues of specific organs [37].

36. D Walls of veins contain less muscle and elastic tissue than arterial walls do. The wall of a vein is thinner than the wall of a corresponding artery. Veins are a merger of venules. The muscle layer in arterial walls is of smooth muscle. Arteries have the intrinsic capacity to withstand the pressure of blood from the heart.

37. B The right coronary artery (RCA) normally arises from the right aortic sinus, which is also referred to as the right sinus of Valsalva; this sinus is a part of the ascending aorta. From this origin, the RCA initially courses anteriorly and to the right, prior to assuming a descending course in the groove between the right atrium and the right ventricle (atrioventricular groove) to provide arterial blood supply to the right side of the heart [44]. The left common carotid artery normally originates directly from the aortic arch. It is both the second and longest branch of the aortic arch. This artery arises in the superior mediastinum from the zenith of the aortic arch and takes an ascending course into the neck. In the neck, it runs lateral to the esophagus and the trachea [45]. Its counterpart on the right does not arise from the aortic arch but from the brachiocephalic trunk. While in the neck, the two common carotid arteries lie posterior and medial to the internal jugular veins. The left and right common iliac arteries arise from the abdominal aorta.

A good understanding of the variants in anatomical branching of arteries from the aortic arch is essential because, although these variants are rare, the surgeon, radiologist, or interventional cardiologist working in the superior mediastinum may encounter such vascular deviations from the normal anatomy. Ignorance of variations or assumptions regarding always encountering the normal may result in surgical complications during procedures carried out in the base of the neck or superior mediastinum. Other serious complications include brain damage and severe hemorrhage that may be fatal [45].

An example of an anomalous branching pattern of the aortic arch that may alter the cerebral hemodynamics, with clinical symptoms, is the "subclavian steal syndrome." This syndrome is characterized by a subclavian artery stenosis sited proximal to the origin of the vertebral artery. The subclavian artery steals reverse-flow blood from the vertebrobasilar artery circulation to supply the arm during exertion, resulting in vertebrobasilar insufficiency. However, because the vertebrobasilar arterial system supplies the peripheral and central auditory and vestibular systems, this syndrome results in neurotological symptoms from the vertebrobasilar insufficiency. Patients who have subclavian steal syndrome have tinnitus, recurrent vertigo, dizziness, and hearing loss. In two of the three documented cases, a positional nystagmus was detected, which was vertical in two [46]. The aortic arch also has left subclavian and brachiocephalic arteries as branches. Subclavian and common carotid arteries provide arterial supply to the head and neck.

38. A Ventricular contraction is responsible for systolic blood pressure. An increase in blood volume to the heart leads to an increase in contraction, an increase in stroke volume, and an increase in cardiac output. The cardiac center is in the medulla oblongata. Central venous pressure is the pressure in the right atrium.

39. B The jugular vein does not gain direct entry into the heart. The great vessels are the arteries that exit the heart and veins that enter the heart directly. They are the aorta, pulmonary trunk, superior vena cava, inferior vena cava, and pulmonary veins.

40. C The circulatory system consists of the heart (which can rightly be considered its pump) and the conduit (which is made up of the complex of vessels of various sizes that transport blood). The conduit of arteries, veins, and their numerous branches forms an efficient reticulation that ends in capillaries that link the arterial system and venous system at the microscopic level. The lymphatic vessels belong to the lymphatic system.

41. D The great vessels arise from the base of the heart and not the anterior surface. The superior part of the heart is its base. In a normal adult heart, the shortest dimension is the distance between the anterior and posterior surfaces, while the longest distance is between the apex and the base.

42. A The pulmonary trunk gives rise to the right and left pulmonary arteries. The pulmonary arteries supply the lungs with oxygen-poor blood, which the lungs enrich with oxygen and send off to the left atrium via the pulmonary veins. The inferior vena cava drains the body inferior to the diaphragm.

43. C The aortic arch, via its branches, supplies the head, neck, and both upper limbs. The blood supply of the diaphragm does not come from the aortic arch but from several

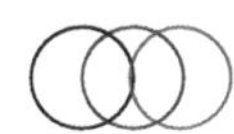

arteries, one of which arises from the thoracic aorta. The superior phrenic arteries arise from the thoracic aorta. Other arteries that supply the diaphragm are the inferior phrenic arteries, musculophrenic arteries, pericardiophrenic arteries, and lower internal intercostal arteries [47]. The superior phrenic artery provides arterial blood supply to the superior and posterior surfaces of the diaphragm; the inferior phrenic artery provides the major arterial blood supply to the diaphragm, the bare area of the liver, and the adrenal glands [48].

44. B The epicardium is the same as the visceral pericardium. The myocardium is the thickest of the three layers of the wall of the heart. The endocardium, composed of endothelial cells, forms the lining of the inner surface of the chambers of the heart and the valves; it extends into the great blood vessels as their endothelium. A fibrous skeleton is present at the origin of the great blood vessels.

45. A The mitral valve is synonymous with the bicuspid valve; it is the left atrioventricular valve. The right atrioventricular valve is the tricuspid valve. Control of blood flow from the right ventricle into the pulmonary trunk is by the pulmonary valve. The aortic valve is one of the semilunar valves; the other is the pulmonary valve. With regard to the heart valves, only the mitral valve has two cusps (bicuspid).

46. B A flask-shaped fibroserous sac with two layers—the fibrous pericardium and the serous pericardium. The pericardium encompasses the heart and the proximal portions of the great vessels that arise from and enter the heart. The serous pericardium itself has two layers; these two layers of the serous pericardium create a potential space, meaning that they are essentially apposed and the space between them is not obvious. These two layers of serous pericardium are the visceral pericardium and the parietal pericardium [1, 49]. The outermost layer of the pericardium is the thick, fibrous pericardium; this layer continues with the diaphragm on which the heart "sits" and superiorly with the great vessels from which the heart "hangs." This same outer, fibrous component of the coat is connected anteriorly to the inner surface of the sternum by sternopericardial ligaments. The lungs are laterally related to the heart on both sides of the heart; the parietal pericardium is associated with the parietal pleura of the two lungs. Posteriorly (to its back), the heart is in a close relationship with not only its descending thoracic aorta but also the esophagus and the bronchi [49].

Relative to the fibrous pericardium, the serous pericardium is thin. Its various attachments maintain the position of the heart in the thorax. The fibrous pericardium helps define middle mediastinal relationships. The epicardium is the visceral component of the serous pericardium—it forms the external (outer) covering of the heart [49, 50].

47. A The serous pericardium has two layers; this part of the pericardium is thin and comprises the parietal layer and a visceral layer—the synonym for the visceral layer of serous pericardium is the epicardium. The parietal layer of serous pericardium lines and forms the inner surface of the fibrous pericardium; the epicardium adheres to the heart and encloses this vital organ [50]. Fluid collection in the pericardial cavity stays within the two leaves of serous pericardium that form a potential space surrounding a normal heart; when there is significant inflammation, e.g., in infections, the cells of the serous membranous lining of the pericardium secrete pericardial fluid in various amounts depending on the gravity of the condition. In severe cases, the patient may develop cardiac tamponade that makes the patient present with distension of the jugular veins, muffled heart sounds, and hypotension (Beck's triad) [51].

48. B There is fat collection (epicardial adipose tissue [EAT]) situated between the myocardium and epicardium. The amount of epicardial fat is variable, but the greatest amounts are in three sites: the interventricular groove, the acute angle of the right ventricle, and the atrioventricular groove [50]. This is visceral fat; it embeds the coronary blood vessels, nerves, and lymphatic vessels. In the pericardial cavity, the small amount of secretion in a normally functioning heart lubricates the serosal surfaces and thus allows unimpeded and painless movement of the heart. This space also contains fat, which is epicardial fat or pericardial fat [50, 52, 53].

49. C The transverse pericardial sinus is posterior to the ascending aorta and the pulmonary trunk; it is also superior to the left atrium and anterior to the superior vena cava. On the right side, the transverse pericardial sinus extends superiorly to form the superior aortic recess; this recess lies between the ascending aorta and the superior vena cava [49, 54]. The zone of serous pericardial reflection that envelops the pulmonary veins takes an inverted "U." The cul-de-sac it forms with the "U" is posterior to the left atrium and is referred to as the oblique pericardial sinus. This sinus is directly adjacent to the tracheal carina and the esophagus posteriorly. The pericardial reflections make not only the anterior and lateral surfaces of the ventricles accessible, but also the apical surface of the ventricles [54].

50. D The parietal pericardium comprises an innermost serosal layer with mesothelial cells that are loosely packed; these cells have a basement membrane on which sit microvilli. Microvilli are essential in the process of synthesizing and resorbing pericardial fluid [55]. Deep to the basement membrane of mesothelial cells is a layer of dense collagen with elastic fibers that assume imprecise directions; this cell layer is the fibrosa. This middle layer, by virtue of containing elastic fibers and the orientation of the fibers, is the layer that allows a degree of distensibility, not the inner layer. After the fibrosa is a third layer, which is the outermost of the layers; it is closest to the mediastinum and, therefore, closest to the fibrous coat of the pericardium. This third layer contains blood vessels, neural structures, and adipose tissue, and it consists of even more elastic fibers than the innermost layer [49, 56].

Requirements for pericardiocentesis are characteristically confirmation of a large pericardial effusion or a cardiac tamponade. Cardiac tamponade is both a clinical instability and demonstrable hemodynamic instability. The main techniques for pericardiocentesis are fluoroscopy-guided pericardiocentesis and echocardiography-guided pericardiocentesis. Fluoroscopy-guided pericardiocentesis entails pointing the needle between 30° and 45° to the patient's skin and directing the needle toward their left shoulder [57]. This accesses the dependent part of the prone patient with massive pericardial effusion or cardiac tamponade. The point of entry at the skin is just inferior to the xiphoid process (sub-xiphoid approach). Regarding echocardiography-guided pericardiocentesis, the advantages are the high degree of access that ultrasound provides and real-time visualization; the latter gives the operator options from which to select the best site to access the fluid on the basis of the distribution of fluid in the index patient [58]. The notorious infection (pulmonary tuberculosis) is a dominant cause of massive pericardial effusion in developing countries [59]. In developed countries, the more likely causes include cancers, connective tissue diseases, and iatrogenic causes, but sometimes the cause is idiopathic [60].

CHAPTER 11

ANSWERS AND NOTES FOR MCQs ON BACK

1. D Keratinocytes are the key features of the deeper layer of cells [1]. The stratum basale receives nourishment from dermal blood vessels. The cells of the outermost layer of the epidermis are dead. The epidermis does not have blood vessels; epithelial cells obtain nourishment from the upper portion of the dermal blood vessels by diffusion [2]. The cells of the outermost layer of the skin form the stratum corneum. Stratum basale cells can reproduce.

The epidermis is the outermost layer of the skin. It comprises layers (strata), and each stratum is composed of cells. From the topmost (outermost) layer down, the layers of the epidermis are stratum **c**orneum, stratum **l**ucidum, stratum **g**ranulosum, stratum **s**pinosum, and stratum **b**asale. The deepest layer (stratum basale) is synonymous with stratum germinativum. Immediately deep to the epidermis is the dermis. The boundary structure that separates the deepest layer of the epidermis from the dermis is the basement membrane, which is also called the basal lamina. The stratum basale is attached to the basal lamina by hemidesmosomes. Stratum basale stem cells are mitotically active, producing keratinocytes and melanocytes. The epidermal layer just before the stratum basale is the stratum spinosum, also called the prickle cell layer. This layer has eight to ten layers of cells. The cells of the stratum spinosum are polyhedral. This layer may also contain dendritic cells [3, 4].

2. C Aggregation and cross-linkage are features of precursors in the cells in the stratum granulosum of the epidermis; the cells that contain these precursors have organelles called keratohyalin granules and the keratohyalin granules contain keratin precursors; when the precursors aggregate and form cross-linkages, they form bundles of keratin. Stratum granulosum has between three and five layers of cells; the cells are diamond-shaped. The cells in stratum granulosum have both keratohyalin granules, and lamellar granules. Lamellar granules are organelles in the cells of this stratum; the organelles produce bonding material (glycolipids); the glycolipids they secrete are released to cell surfaces, and they act as adhesives to ensure cohesion of the cells and serve the purpose of making skin waterproof [5].

3. A With regard to the epithelium of the skin, defensins are products of living keratinocytes in the stratum granulosum (the second of the four layers in thin skin) and the one below it (stratum spinosum). Defensins are released by the lamellar bodies of the stratum granulosum layer of the epidermis [6]. Human β-defensin-2 (HBD-2) is an antimicrobial peptide that possesses a broad spectrum of activity against pathogenic microbes, with the exception of *Staphylococcus aureus*. HBD-2 is produced as a preprodefensin; this preformed material contains a typical signal sequence for targeting to the endoplasmic reticulum [6]. Preprodefensin is a precursor that is a much larger molecule than defensin, the ultimate product. Preprodefensin consists of a "pro," which is a signal peptide and a pre-sequence; during processing, both are cleaved off, leaving a much smaller active peptide (defensin) [7]. The stratum corneum consists of corneocytes (anucleate squamous cells), which do not have nuclei and are really flattened dead keratinocytes [6]. These dead cells are filled with keratin—a

DOI: 10.1201/9781003783961-13

proteinous material. Corneocytes therefore retain just *keratin* filaments embedded in the filaggrin matrix [8].

Keratinocytes produce keratohyalin granules [9]. Stratum lucidum is an extra layer of skin found only on thick glabrous skin like the palms and soles [1]. The stratum corneum is made up of flattened anucleate cells.

4. A Sweating allows heat loss from the body through sweat glands in non-glabrous skin; this heat loss is by evaporation. In human beings, it results in maintaining a stable normal body temperature of about 98.6°F or 37°C. This mechanism helps in regulating the body temperature regardless of the high temperature in the environment or in conditions where the human body generates and dissipates a loss of energy, like in rigorous exercise. In sweating, water escapes the liquid phase into the gaseous phase using evaporation—a principle of physics [10]. The transition of water in sweat from the liquid phase to the gaseous phase utilizes latent heat of vaporization obtained from the surface of the human skin. When high-energy water molecules on the skin escape, the remaining sweat cools, and lowers the body temperature. Maintenance of an increased blood flow to the skin brings more heated blood from within the body, and the process continues. The conditions in the person's environment, like degree of airflow, level of humidity, and the type of clothes the individual wears, have an impact on the evaporated molecules staying in the vapor phase. Sweat contains electrolytes; these diminish vapor pressure to a slight degree by causing a slight alteration to the bonding structure of water [10]. *Sweating is the most powerful autonomic thermoeffector.* Sweat that is eventually released onto the skin surface is hypotonic fluid. Sweating increases proportionally with the intensity of the heat challenge as the body works toward achieving heat balance and sustaining a stable internal body temperature. Sweating regulation is modifiable; factors that can modify control of sweating are heat acclimation, dehydration, biophysical factors, and non-thermal factors [11].

Summary: Radiation is the primary means of heat loss when an individual is in a room with still air or there are cold surfaces, with the energy transfer being via infrared electromagnetic waves; in these cases, the individual may lose heat by radiation to the environment or object(s), with the person consequently getting cold. Radiation is not of equal magnitude with convection in terms of efficiency in human body temperature regulation in this kind of still, comfortable, cool environment. Regarding the individual who lies down on a cool floor, this direct heat loss by contact is due to conduction. In convection, cool air replaces warm air, which is less dense and has moved away from the surface of the skin. Since cool air currents enhance heat loss from the surface of the skin, a person who uses a fan or is in an outdoor environment in windy conditions loses fluid by convection with a resultant feeling of cold. When submerged in water that is not heated, there is also loss of heat by convection—water, which forms the person's environment in this circumstance, extracts heat efficiently from their skin because water has a higher thermal conductivity. This is part of the explanation for a person who is submerged in cold water being more prone to becoming hypothermic than a person surrounded by air of the same temperature as the cold water.

5. C This network of skin blood vessels, the rete cutaneum, is located between the dermis and the subcutaneous layer [12]. It assists in conserving body heat because of the insulating property of adipose tissue.

6. B Meissner's corpuscles, receptors for perception of light touch, are present in the dermal papillae of glabrous (hairless) skin; this type of skin is found in the fingertips, palms,

 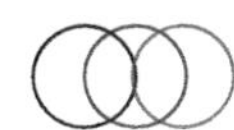

and soles [13]. Visceroceptive sense (appreciation of information from the viscera—also called interoceptive sense) is a component of the somatosensory system [14]. Every Meissner's corpuscle is comprised of three primary components: elongated Schwann cells, a connective tissue capsule, and a central axon. In Meissner's corpuscles, changes occur in aging and central or peripheral nervous system injury. In disease, these structures are of interest to pathologists regarding the diagnosis of some peripheral neuropathies and neurodegenerative diseases [15]. Relaxation of muscles stimulates muscle spindles; the reflex to contract the muscle is thus initiated. Golgi tendon organs are stimulated by a reduction in muscle tension.

7. A Thermoreceptors are free nerve endings that detect changes in temperature. Mechanoreceptors are related to the Golgi tendon organ. Muscle spindles detect changes in muscle length; changes in muscle tension are appreciated by the Golgi tendon organ. Pacinian corpuscles are related to deep pressure. Pacinian corpuscles go by two synonyms—Vater-Pacini corpuscles and lamellar corpuscles; they subserve vibration and deep pressure and are necessary for a person to appreciate proprioception (joint position sense), which allows a person to appreciate their spatial position without utilizing their vision; spatial position is the position of a person in physical space (a place) in relation to other objects. Pacinian corpuscles are distributed in every part of the body but are most highly concentrated in the hands and feet [16, 17]. Capsules and ligaments are where the presence of Pacinian corpuscles enables a person to know joint position [18]. Meissner's corpuscles transmit the sensations of vibration and fine, discriminative touch.

8. D Only the first of the seven costo-sternal joints is a synchondrosis (an almost immovable articulation); the second to the seventh ribs form synovial joints with the sternum. A symphysis is an amphiarthrotic joint (amphiarthrosis) because it allows slight movements. The articulations between vertebrae are amphiarthroses [19]. The connection between the epiphysis and diaphysis in a growing long bone is a synchondrosis.

9. D In a typical vertebra, weight-bearing action and cushioning effects are achieved by the vertebral bodies and intervertebral disks, respectively [20]. An intervertebral disk is composed of a central nuclear zone of collagen and hydrated proteoglycans, which are enveloped by concentric lamellae of collagen fibers. The intervertebral disks constitute about 30% the length of the human vertebral spinal column. In a typical vertebra, the involved vertebral body surfaces are roughened. The vertebral body is the anterior part of the vertebra. Intervertebral foramina are formed by the notches on the inferior surfaces of the vertebral pedicles.

10. D Articulation between an upper vertebra and a lower one involves the vertebral body indirectly, through an intervening intervertebral disk. A disk sits between the lower surface of an upper vertebral body and the upper surface of a lower vertebral body. Viewed from its anterior surface vertically, the anterior part of a typical vertebra bears the semblance of part of a drum; the anterior part of a typical vertebra is where the padding for articulation between the adjoining vertebrae sits. In the human body, there are 25 disks; this is short of the number of vertebrae. The sacrum has just one disk, although it has five segments; there is fusion of the segments in adult life [20]. Intervertebral disks provide the expected degree of flexibility of the spine in individuals with normal spines, provide a shock-absorbing function, and prevent friction in such individuals. An intervertebral disk consists of three parts:

nucleus pulposus (an inner part), annulus fibrosus (an outer part), and cartilaginous endplates; there are two endplates on the surfaces of each intervertebral disk by which they anchor a disc to adjacent superior and inferior vertebrae [21]. The two parts of an endplate are the bony endplate and cartilaginous endplate. A bony endplate attaches to the bony surface of an upper or lower vertebra; it is a layer of porous cortical bone. A cartilaginous endplate is a layer of hyaline cartilage that connects directly with the intervertebral disk [21].

11. A All thoracic vertebrae articulate with ribs at the articulating facets on the sides of their bodies. The spinal cord passes through the vertebral foramen of a vertebra. The openings in a vertebra through which a spinal nerve pair passes are intervertebral foramina. The bony tissue in a cervical vertebra is denser than in a lumbar vertebra [22]. A study of the cervical, thoracic, and lumbar vertebrae using Hounsfield units (HUs) showed that bone density values generally decreased with age; this occurred in all spinal segments. Significantly, however, the reduction was gross in male and female adults aged >50 years [22]. The relevance of the findings from this study have implications for preoperative evaluation of patients with surgical conditions that affect the spine; it also provides biomedical engineering companies with insight that could help them come up with devices that can adapt to the variations in the demands of various spinal regions and various age strata of the patients [22].

12. B Transverse foramina are for the passage of arteries. The atlas has almost no body. The most common justification for naming the first cervical vertebra "atlas" is that the vertebra sustains the globe of the cranium the way the mythological ancient Greek god Atlas holds up the globe of the heavens [23]. This name was the name that the Romans originally assigned to C7, the seventh cervical vertebra. Prior to the name change, the original name given to C1 was "astragalus," which is also the original name for the talus. There are seven vertebrae (C1 to C7) in the cervical spine. In the cervical spine, there are two segments. With the occiput, the two most cephalad vertebrae, i.e., the atlas (C1) and the axis (C2), form the craniocervical junction. The lower (caudad) five cervical vertebrae, C3 to C7, form the sub-axial spine. The cervical spine bears the weight of the cranium, and its constituent bones are pivotal in making motions of the head and neck [24]. Although the atlas (C1) has transverse foramina, these foramina are for the vertebral artery, vertebral vein, and sympathetic nerves to traverse, but not for spinal nerves to pass through. Spinal nerves exit the spinal cord through the intervertebral foramina; these foramina are located between vertebrae which, by design, leave a foramen on each side to accommodate the exiting spinal nerves on the left and right sides. The atlas lacks a body. It takes the shape of a ring; this bone consists of an anterior arch, a posterior arch, and two lateral masses; the lateral masses bear the transverse processes. The name "vertebra prominens" refers to the seventh cervical vertebra.

13. D The axis enables turning of the head from side to side; the axis is the second cervical vertebra. It has a bifid spinous process, like the third, fourth, and fifth cervical vertebrae. The dens is on the body of the axis. Dens is synonymous with odontoid process. The dens of the axis provides a pivot for the atlas for the turning movement. The axis has muscular attachment at its spinous process. The axis is a typical cervical vertebra in the sense that it has a bifid (Y-shaped) spinous process. The third, fourth, fifth, and sixth cervical vertebrae (C3–C6) share this characteristic with C2, making the number of typical cervical vertebrae in the human body five. The posteriorly

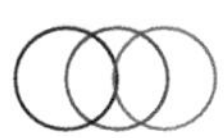

disposed cleft shape ensures that there is an increased surface area; this design makes provision for the attachment of the *ligamentum nuchae* and the muscles in the cervical region [24]. The axis articulates superiorly with the atlas by a special bony structure, the dens or odontoid process. The dens projects superiorly from the body of the second cervical vertebra to achieve the articulation with the first cervical vertebra. It is the dens that allows the pivoting motion, which provides an increased range of lateral rotation of the head [25].

14. B The clavicle and the scapula are the bony components of the pectoral girdle, which attaches an upper limb to the axial skeleton; the clavicle, therefore, belongs to the appendicular skeleton—not the axial skeleton. The specific part of the axial skeleton that the clavicle links the appendicular skeleton to is the sternum at the sternoclavicular joint, a synovial joint [26]. The axial skeletal system consists of the skull, 12 pairs of ribs, sternum, and the 33 vertebrae.

15. C The characteristic articulations in the spine allow rotation and bending movements. The spinal canal is a central lumen; the body of every vertebra features in (contributes to) this canal; the spinal canal harbors the spinal cord. Spinal nerves exit from the spinal cord via the intervertebral foramina at each vertebral level; the spinal nerves form the sympathetic trunk and splanchnic nerves. The diameter of the spinal canal is variable, depending on the segments of the vertebral column; while the diameter is smaller in the thoracic region, it is wider in the cervical region and lumbar regions. Weight bearing is one of the primary functions of the spinal column [27]. There would be no point in having this core component of the musculoskeletal system and nervous system if it could not support the skull and its contents, accommodate the weight of the rest of the body, and distribute the weight to the feet of humans; severe spinal injuries and diseases are a testament to the primacy of the spine to the efficient functioning of every human being.

16. B Posterior intercostal arteries supply the spine; they originate from the thoracic aorta. Vertebral arteries do not arise from the axillary artery but from the subclavian artery. Vertebral arteries branch, with each giving off one anterior spinal artery and two posterior spinal arteries. An anterior spinal artery supplies the anterior part of the spinal cord, while the two posterior spinal arteries supply the posterior portion of the spinal cord. The ascending cervical arteries of the spine also arise from the subclavian artery. Lumbar arteries arise from the abdominal aorta. In the pelvis, the lateral sacral arteries branch from the internal iliac arteries [27]. Every artery that supplies the spine divides into an anterior branch and a posterior branch. While the anterior branch serves the body of a vertebra, the posterior branch provides the blood supply of the vertebral arch. The vertebral arch forms the middle portion of the posterior aspect of the vertebra, and from it arises the spinous process of the vertebra. Radicular arteries take a course along the middle and supply mainly the roots of the spinal nerves and respective dura mater, and to some degree the interior of the vertebral canal and vertebral column [27].

17. A Blood from the internal and external vertebral veins and blood from the smaller veins of the spinal cord enter radicular veins. It is blood from radicular veins that empty into segmental and intervertebral veins. Hierarchically, segmental and intervertebral veins are larger than radicular veins, and larger veins receive venous blood from the smaller ones, just like larger arteries supply blood to the smaller arteries. The spine is drained by a venous system that consists of a network of valveless veins [28]. Venous drainage of the cervical spine is carried out by the superior vena cava. The inferior vena cava primarily drains the lumbar and sacral spine. Venous blood from the thoracic area of the spine enters the azygos and hemiazygos veins [27].

18. B Spinal nerves, cranial nerves, and their ganglia constitute the peripheral nervous system [27]. The spinal cord and spinal column are not synonymous; the spinal cord is the principal nervous tissue that occupies the spinal canal created by the bony structure called the spinal column. Meningeal nerves are branches of spinal nerves; these branches provide the innervation of the vertebrae.

19. D The filum terminale is a delicate lengthening or addendum of the spinal cord from the conus medullaris; the filum terminale becomes attached to the dorsum of the coccyx. The number of spinal nerves that leave the spinal cord and pass through intervertebral foramina to innervate the periphery is 31 pairs [27]. The spinal cord commences from the base of the brain and terminates at the conus medullaris, which extends spinal cord neural tissue to the filum terminale. Beyond this true end of the spinal cord is the cauda equina, which consists of spinal nerve roots. It is essential to remember that while the conus medullaris (the cone-shaped tapered inferior limit of the spinal cord) usually has its inferior limit at L1–L2 in adults, it is known to be further down to the L3–L4 level as a variant. This means that even when accessing the spinal column in a frequently performed procedure like lumbar puncture (using the L3/L4 intervertebral space as a reference point for safety), caution should still be applied, as the variation from L1, L2 to even L4 may be the case with the index patient.

20. A Serratus posterior inferior is not a superficial muscle. The superficial extrinsic back muscle group consists of the trapezius, levator scapulae, latissimus dorsi, rhomboideus major, and rhomboideus minor; the rhomboids are also called rhomboid major and rhomboid minor. The superficial extrinsic muscles participate in movements of the upper limbs, like movements of the proximate bones, scapula, and humerus.

21. A The extrinsic muscles also comprise an intermediate group of muscles, which are the serratus posterior superior and serratus posterior inferior. The intermediate extrinsic muscles help in carrying out rib movement and thus participate in respiration [27].

22. D The intrinsic muscles of the back muscles are in three layers: superficial, intermediate, and deep. The superficial layer comprises the splenius cervicis and splenius capitis. Splenius cervicis and splenius capitis are put into action during flexion, rotation, and extension of the neck. The paraspinal (erector spinae) muscles—the iliocostalis, longissimus, and spinalis—mostly constitute the intermediate layer of intrinsic muscles. These muscles are therefore essential for sustaining the central curvature of the spine; they are required for achieving movements of the spine and maintaining chosen postures involving the back [27].

23. C The deep layer of intrinsic muscles of the back is synonymous with the paravertebral muscles. The deep layer of the intrinsic back muscles comprises muscles that lie between the transverse processes and spinous processes of vertebrae. The muscles are in three groups. The semispinalis is the most superficial of these muscles, followed by the multifidus. The semispinalis is prominent in the cervical and thoracic regions. The multifidus is most prominent in the lumbar region. The deepest of the three muscles

 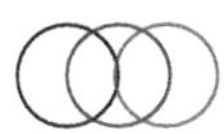

that constitute the deep layer of intrinsic muscles is formed by the rotatores muscles; these muscles are most prominent in the thoracic region [27].

24. C The muscles that make up the suboccipital triangle are the rectus capitis posterior major, obliquus capitis superior, and obliquus capitis inferior.

25. B By their attachment to the skull, the suboccipital muscles form an important anatomical landmark—the suboccipital triangle. This vital anatomical landmark contains the vertebral artery and the suboccipital nerve that, respectively, provide arterial blood supply and innervation to the posterior part of the head and upper part of the neck. There are four suboccipital muscles, namely, the rectus capitis posterior major, rectus capitis posterior minor, obliquus capitis superior, and obliquus capitis inferior. The muscles cause extension of the head. In the suboccipital triangle, the vertebral artery makes a loop from the transverse foramen of the atlas and accesses the foramen magnum. The vertebral artery provides the arterial supply of the brainstem (midbrain, pons, and medulla oblongata).

26. D By stimulating the overlying ectoderm to form neuroectoderm, the notochord forms the neural plate, which gives rise to the neural tube. The rostral and caudal parts of the neural tube respectively become the adult brain and spinal cord [29]. Formation of the notochordal process commences at about day 17. Notochordal plate arises from the floor of the notochordal processes; this occurs after the fusion of the roof of the yolk sac. After this event, an inward fold of the notochordal plate results in the notochord. The notochord plays a crucial role because it is involved in sustaining the structure of the embryo and is the site where the vertebral column develops [30].

27. B Sclerotome in the mesodermal somites grows around the notochord and neural tube; this event results in the formation of vertebral arches, vertebral bodies, annulus fibrosus, and ribs. Gastrulation of the embryo commences at about 3 weeks. Formation of a vertebral body is by the process of segmentation, which entails fusion of the cranial and caudal halves of a sclerotome. It is in week 6 of embryogenesis when cartilage formation first occurs. By week 8, cartilage is replaced by bone in the growing embryo.

28. C Gibbus is an acquired condition of the vertebrae (usually in the thoracic vertebrae) due to tuberculosis of the spine. The other conditions are congenital, and they are fused vertebrae, misshapen vertebrae, and missing or extra vertebrae [30]. Congenital anomalies that present with associated vertebral defects include **A**nal atresia, **C**ardiac defects, **T**racheo-**E**sophageal fistula, **R**enal anomalies, and **L**imb anomalies; with the V for Vertebral defects, the acronym VACTERL is apt.

29. D Arnold–Chiari malformation is usually associated with myelomeningocele. In spina bifida there is a neural tube defect, which is the result of incomplete closure of the vertebral column and meninges. Three types are recognized, with spina bifida occulta as the mildest form and myelomeningocele as the most severe. In degree of severity, meningocele sits in-between spina bifida occulta and myelomeningocele [31].

30. B Regarding kyphosis, there is exaggeration of the anterior *concavity* of the thoracic spinal level. Kyphosis may result from osteoporosis. Another predisposing condition is poor posture due to chronically assuming a slouching posture; this may lead to kyphosis even in children who engage in this habit [32]. Older people are prone to developing kyphosis. In kyphosis, there is an anterior curvature of the thoracic portion of the vertebral column. Severe accidents like vehicular accidents with vertebral fractures may lead to kyphosis. In adolescents with Scheuermann's disease, the irregularly shaped intervertebral disks and vertebrae may cause kyphosis [33]. The person with kyphosis is said to have humpback or hunchback.

31. C In a patient with abnormal lordosis, there is an increase in the anterior *convexity* of the affected vertebral bodies. The lumbar spine is a common site for this condition. Straightening of the normal curvature of the affected portion of the spine is usually due to spasm of the spinal muscles [34]. Obesity is sometimes associated with abnormal lordosis. An increase in lumbar lordosis is usual during pregnancy since it is a physiological adaptation for maintaining balance and stability; this compensatory mechanism in response to the anterior shift in the center of gravity by the uterus growing in size and weight as pregnancy progresses is more in the third trimester of pregnancy [35].

In the case of patients who develop neck pain and the pain is assessed by plain digital radiography or magnetic resonance imaging, the finding of loss of cervical lordosis could still raise issues as to the propriety of reassuring the index patient or carrying out further investigations, depending on the symptomatology and the overall clinical presentation of some other patients; modalities of treatment and prognosis would depend on the precise findings [36]. In patients with pain that leads to loss of lumbar lordosis or cervical lordosis, strong muscle contractions produce spasms, which constitute a protective mechanism to minimize injury or prevent instability to that part of the spine—at least in the initial phase of the pain.

32. A There is abnormal lateral deviation and curvature of the spine in individuals with scoliosis. Weakness of vertebral muscles, absence of a component of a vertebra, or malrotation of a vertebra may be the cause of scoliosis. Although there may be a genetic predilection, scoliosis may be idiopathic or secondary to trauma. Disk herniation is not a cause but one of the likely results of scoliosis; another result is compression of neural tissue, like the exiting nerves. The condition usually occurs in females in the teenage years [37]. Patients with kyphoscoliosis have a combination of the features of kyphosis and scoliosis.

33. C Pott's disease is from osteomyelitis of vertebral bodies and intervertebral diskitis; the patient with Pott's disease has advanced tuberculosis of the spine, which must have been left undiagnosed, or diagnosed but not treated, or not treated with the appropriate drugs for an acceptable duration. There is usually destruction of vertebral body/bodies with a wedge collapse that results in a gibbus; the patient is likely to develop compression of the cord with motor weakness in the lower limbs (paraparesis) and, in severe cases, paraplegia. Patients who have severe osteoporosis also stand an increased risk of developing a vertebral compression fracture [38].

Pathology of the spine from spinal cord injury at the level of the C3 vertebra would result in tetraplegia if there were transection of the cord at that level. When there is a tear of the annulus fibrosus with involvement of the nucleus pulposus, the tear is likely from disk herniation; there is a decrease in reflexes because this is a lower motor neuron injury from compression of exiting spinal nerve roots [39]. Patients with annular fissures are usually without symptoms; however, in patients who develop chronic pain due to annular fissures, the pain may be the result of granulation tissue formation or growth of nerve endings into the area of disruption, close to the dorsal root ganglion—this is apart from the possibility of nucleus pulposus of the disk herniating [40]. Other presentations are paresis, paresthesia, and pain.

In spondylolisthesis, there is an anterior (forward) displacement of an upper vertebra over a lower vertebra. There are various degrees of spondylolisthesis; in type 1 the displacement is less than 25%, and in type 5 it is 100% or more. The symptomatology and full clinical presentation depend on the degree, which may be back pain or weakness or paralysis below the site of the combined bony and cord displacement; the treatment of spondylolisthesis may be surgical or non-surgical [41].

34. A Spinal canal stenosis is the most likely pathology in a patient who suffers from back pain that is relieved by bending forward. In canal stenosis, there is narrowing of the central spinal canal. Other clinical features in this condition are paresthesia and paresis of the upper or lower limbs, depending on the site of the stenosis. Relief of back pain in patients with spinal canal stenosis (canal stenosis) when there is flexion of the affected spine is due to the posture increasing the space in the spinal canal and reducing spinal nerve root compression. There is also relaxation of the ligaments—these combine to ameliorate the pain [42]. A patient with canal stenosis may already have a history of severe trauma involving the vertebral column; other preceding and causative conditions include osteoarthritis, rheumatoid arthritis, or Paget disease of the bone.

Neurogenic claudication is one of the features of spinal canal stenosis. A main characteristic of neurogenic claudication is pain increasing when the back is extended (bent backward) and pain becoming less when the patient flexes the lower back (i.e., bends the back forward). There is, therefore, pain relief when a patient sits, squats, leans forward, or lies/lays down. For many patients, inactivity makes them asymptomatic [42]. In simian stance, the erect posture of the patient with spinal stenosis is flexing/bending the lower back at the hip and stooping the trunk forward, reminiscent of the way lower primates stand and walk [43]. Simian stance ameliorates the pain in spinal canal stenosis. Treatment may be surgical or non-surgical; surgical, by open surgery or minimally invasive surgery, aims at decompression—this generally provides early results of pain relief and reduction or prevention of the risk of falling [44].

35. C Seronegative spondyloarthropathy consists of chronic inflammatory rheumatic diseases that principally target the axial skeleton. This condition, which characteristically affects the sacroiliac joint, is considered a hallmark for diagnosis of seronegative spondyloarthropathy and manifests in this joint first [45]. Seronegative spondyloarthropathies include psoriatic arthritis, reactive arthritis, ankylosing spondylitis, juvenile spondylitis, inflammatory bowel disease-associated spondylitis, and idiopathic arthritis. In seronegative spondyloarthropathy, a disease that affects the vertebral column, there is an absence of the serum marker antinuclear antibodies and an increased incidence of the human leukocyte antigen-B27 (HLA-B27).

36. A With respect to the sacrum, the bone is a fusion of five vertebrae. Components fuse in the age range 18–30 years. The sacrum has dorsal foramina through which both nerves and blood vessels emerge. The five sacral vertebrae are fused to form a triangular unit. The sacrum forms the posterosuperior portion of the bony pelvis. The sacrum has a curve that creates a concavity anteriorly and a convexity posteriorly. The sacrum is wider at its proximal end; the bone is tapered progressively toward its distal end. The superior (upper) end is the base, and the inferior (lower) end is the apex. Four paired foramina are present in the sacrum. The foramina are narrower anteriorly than they are posteriorly. The anterior surface of the sacrum is relatively smooth when compared with the posterior surface from which the median sacral crest (equivalent of a vertebral spinous process) arises; the median sacral crest is, however, short in comparison with the spinous processes of lumbar vertebrae, which are immediately proximal to the sacrum [46].

Anterior inferior view of the pelvic (anterior) surface of the sacrum: At the superior end of the anterior surface of the sacrum is the sacral promontory in the midline. There are five basically transverse linear elevations on the anterior surface of the sacrum. The most proximal (superior) of them is bilateral—one on either side of the sacral promontory; these elevated areas (linea terminalis), in conjunction with the sacral promontory, form the sacral part of the pelvic brim. The contributions to the ring called the pelvic brim are the anterior projection of the body of the first sacral segment (S1), which is the largest of the five sacral segments, plus the ilium and, anteriorly, the pubic bone (pubis). Each linea terminalis is on the ala (wing) of the sacrum, and on both sides they form alae (wings). Just inferior to (below) the linea terminalis is the first of the four pairs of sacral foramina; these are the anterior sacral foramina. There are four anatomical transverse ridges of the sacrum, and they are slight linear elevations in the midline; each transverse ridge represents the point of fusion of two sacral vertebrae—and it runs between the corresponding pair of foramina [47, 48].

Posterior superior view of the dorsal (posterior) surface of the sacrum: In the midline is a prominent longitudinal crest—this is the median sacral crest. There are two other crests that lie lateral to the median sacral crest and are smaller and less prominent than their median equivalent. These are the intermediate sacral crest and the lateral sacral crest—unlike the median crest, which is single, they are bilateral. The posterior sacral foramina are located between the median sacral crest and the lateral sacral crest. Lateral to each lateral sacral crest is the sacral tuberosity. At the superior end of the sacrum are two superior articular processes—one on each side; each posteriorly disposed articular process has a facet. Each of the superior articular processes articulates with lumbar vertebra 5 (L5) via its articular facet for the sacrum. At the inferior end of the sacrum is the sacral hiatus, bounded superiorly by the terminal part of the median sacral crest and an inferiorly facing sacral cornu on each side. The sacral hiatus is the inferior end of the sacral canal. At the inferior end, the sacrum articulates with the coccyx.

Multiple muscles are attached to the sacrum on its anterior and posterior surfaces. The muscles that are attached to the anterior surface of the sacrum are the iliacus, piriformis, and coccygeus. On the posterior surface of the sacrum are attached the following three muscles: gluteus maximus, erector spinae, and multifidus lumborum [46].

The sacral promontory and the rest of the body of S1 articulate superiorly with the body of the fifth lumbar vertebra (L5), forming the lumbosacral joint; this is the joint that the iliolumbar and lumbosacral ligaments strengthen. The auricular surface of the sacrum is on the upper part of each lateral end (alae) of the sacrum. The auricular surface is covered with hyaline cartilage and is the site of the sacroiliac joint—a major synovial joint in the pelvis. The alae (wings) of the sacrum, therefore, articulate with the iliac bones on each side, forming the sacroiliac joints. The articulation between the axial skeleton (the vertebral column) and the appendicular skeleton (lower limbs) is essential in achieving the transfer of forces from the lower extremities to the vertebral column. The anterior sacroiliac ligament, the posterior sacroiliac ligament (with two components—the long posterior sacroiliac ligament and short posterior sacroiliac ligament), and the interosseous sacroiliac ligament all contribute to the stabilization of the sacroiliac joint [49]. The interosseous sacroiliac ligament is a rather short but strong ligament that directly links the ends of the ilium (iliac bone) with the sacrum—its

 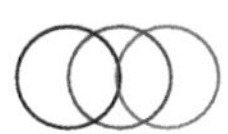

attachment on the sacrum is to the sacral tuberosity, which is close to the auricular surface of the sacrum. Two other ligaments associated with the sacrum are accessory ligaments that connect the sacrum to the ischium at the ischial spines (sacrospinous ligament) and at the ischial tuberosities (sacrotuberous ligament) [50].

Axial low back pain may originate from the sacroiliac joint. Sacroiliac joint pain may result from trauma, sports, pregnancy, repetitive stress, and surgical operations on the spine. The following are some causes to consider and rule out when a patient presents with low back pain. If the history does not say anything about injuries, emphasis should be directed at finding the cause among the following: Spondyloarthropathy, osteoarthritis, infection, discrepancy in leg length, scoliosis, and pregnancy. If, however, history indicates trauma, the physician should consider occupational or domestic injury from a sudden or repetitive lifting of heavy objects or awkward position during lifting, which may cause pain from strain or torsional effects. If these recent and easy-to-remember incidents are ruled out, the list of likely causes should include indirect injury from motor vehicle collision, soft tissue injury from a fall onto the buttock, and fractures to the pelvic ring (sacrum, ilium, ischium, pubis) [51].

37. A With regard to lumbar vertebrae, the spinous processes are almost horizontally disposed; these spinous processes are also short and thick. The cervical and thoracic vertebral bodies are not as big or strong as those of the lumbar vertebrae. Transitional vertebrae at any junction in the vertebral column are characterized by features that are retained from two adjacent regions. The thoracolumbar transitional vertebrae are vertebrae that arise from an overlap or shift of thoracic and lumbar somites at the junction between thoracic vertebrae and lumbar vertebrae. Biomechanically, the thoracolumbar junction is a weak structure; the majority of spine fractures are related to the thoracolumbar region. At the thoracolumbar junction, it is worthwhile to differentiate between the transitional vertebrae and the typical thoracic or lumbar vertebrae. The study by Du Plessis et al. found that the general overlapping characteristics consisted of aplasia or hypoplasia of the transverse process, irregular orientation of the superior articular process, and atypia of the mammillary bodies [52].

This structural weakness often leads to spinal instability that results in injuries, such as spine fractures and thoracolumbar junction syndrome. The feature of thoracolumbar junction syndrome is referred pain, which may originate at the thoracolumbar junction. The thoracolumbar junction spans the twelfth thoracic vertebra to the second lumbar vertebra from functional abnormalities. Clinical features of thoracolumbar junction syndrome are back pain, pseudo-visceral pain, and pseudo-pain on the posterior aspect of the iliac crest; it also features irritable bowel symptoms. During clinical examination, there is tenderness on deep palpation of the facet joints or lateral to the spinous processes [53].

38. D The longissimus cervicis extends the cervical vertebral column, like the iliocostalis cervicis. The iliocostalis cervicis and iliocostalis lumborum respectively extend the cervical and lumbar regions of the vertebral column. The iliocostalis thoracis helps keep the spine erect. The spinalis muscles form the medial group of muscles of the vertebral column.

39. C Wedge collapse of bodies of the lower thoracic and/or upper lumbar vertebral bodies results in sharp angulation of the spine in the affected area. Compression fractures usually involve the anterior column of vertebral bodies, with a resultant wedge-shaped deformity [54]. This is gibbus and is seen in conditions such as tuberculosis of the spine, i.e., Pott's disease, or in osteoporosis and severe trauma that involves the vertebrae in the indicated sites [55, 56]. Kyphosis is an exaggeration of the normal thoracic curvature. Scoliosis is an abnormal lateral deviation of the spine. Lordosis is an exaggerated curvature of the lumbar part of the spine.

40. C Regarding the relationship between spinal nerve roots and vertebrae, there are eight cervical spinal nerves. Although there are seven cervical vertebrae, there are eight cervical spinal nerves; the first cervical spinal nerve exits above the first cervical vertebra, while the remaining seven cervical spinal nerves pass below vertebrae starting from the second cervical spinal nerve, which exits below the C1 vertebra. The C8 cervical spinal nerve consequently exits below C7 (i.e., between the C7 and T1 vertebrae). The cervical enlargement serves all the cervical spinal nerves. Cauda equina does not arise from the lumbar enlargement but are nerve roots that arise from the conus medullaris, which is just inferior to the lumbar enlargement within the spinal canal. The cauda equina consists of the nerve roots from L2 to coccygeal nerve via L2, L3, L4, L5, S1, S2, S3, S4, S5, and the single coccygeal nerve. It is pertinent to note that chiropractic manipulations may lead to this uncommon but inconvenient condition [57]. Patients with cauda equina syndrome and conus medullaris syndrome may present with back pain and sciatica and any (or a combination) of the following conditions: bladder dysfunction, paraparesis or lower limb paresthesia, saddle anesthesia that comprises reduced perineal sensation, fecal retention or fecal incontinence and, in men, sexual dysfunction, i.e., impotence [57].

41. A Regarding the posterior triangle of the neck, semispinalis capitis and splenius capitis form the floor; semispinalis capitis belongs to a deep muscle layer, and so the splenius capitis is superficial to the semispinalis capitis. The trapezius forms the posterior border of the posterior triangle; the anterior boundary of the triangle is formed by the sternocleidomastoid. The great auricular nerve lies anterior and inferior to the lesser occipital nerve. These two nerves share the same nerve root, C2, but the great auricular nerve is also from C3 (C2, C3), while the lesser occipital nerve arises from only the C2 nerve root. Both nerves emerge from the posterior border of the sternocleidomastoid muscle. The origin of the cervical plexus is the ventral rami of the first to the fourth cranial nerves (C1–C4). The cervical plexus forms connections with the facial nerve (CN VII), vagus nerve (CN X), spinal accessory nerve (CN XI), hypoglossal nerve (CN XII), and the sympathetic trunk. This network of nerves is situated anterior and medial to the scalene muscles and deep to the sternocleidomastoid muscle. From the cervical plexus of nerves arise branches that are both sensory and motor [58]. Regarding branches of the cervical plexus that have the skin as their destination (cutaneous branches), they transmit sensory information from the skin of the neck, superior thorax, and scalp; these are the nerves that emerge from the posterior aspect of the sternocleidomastoid muscle [58].

42. A Regarding the vertebral ligaments in the lumbosacral region, the anterior longitudinal ligament attaches to the anterior surface of the sacrum. The posterior and lateral sacrococcygeal ligaments attach to the sacrum and the coccyx. The posterior longitudinal ligament runs along the concave (posterior) surface of vertebral bodies. Supraspinous and interspinous ligaments extend to the coccygeal cornu [50].

Three ligaments are essential to spine stability; the posterior longitudinal ligament is one of the ligaments. The posterior longitudinal ligament extends superiorly from the body of the axis to the sacrum; the ligament runs along the posterior aspect of

 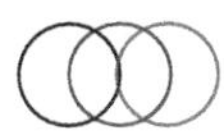

the vertebral body inside the vertebral canal [59]. The posterior longitudinal ligament (PLL) has longitudinal fibers that are denser than the anterior longitudinal ligament. There are two layers of PLL fibers—superficial and deep. The superficial layer of fibers continues from the tectorial membrane at the axis, while the deep layer is the extension of the cruciform (cruciate, cross-shaped) ligament at the atlas. The superficial layer of fibers extends to between three and four vertebrae; the deep layer of fibers connects just adjacent vertebrae—this makes the deeper layer of fibers of PLL less effective than the superficial fibers in preventing excessive flexion of the spine. When compared to the PLL, the anterior longitudinal ligament (ALL) is thicker, broader, and, overall, more robust than the PLL; the ALL resists excessive extension of the spine. Due to the posterior longitudinal ligament being much thinner than the anterior longitudinal ligament, disk herniations have a predilection for occurring posterolaterally [59].

43. A Regarding the sacrum and the coccyx, the apex of the sacrum is its inferior (distal) part; this part is the tapered, lower end of the bone. The base of the sacrum is its upper (superior, proximal) end; the body of the last (fifth) lumbar vertebra sits, via the lumbosacral disk, on the superior surface of the body of the first segment of the sacrum—this is the most robust of the sacral vertebrae. The last lumbar vertebra forms the lumbosacral joint via the articulation of the transverse processes of L5 and the posteriorly directed facets on the superior articular processes of the sacrum—ligaments and capsules are also involved. The sacral promontory on the anterior surface of the base of the sacrum marks the sacral part of the beginning of the true pelvis. The anterior sacral foramina are synonymous with pelvic sacral foramina—there are four pairs. The median sacral crest is the equivalent of a spinous process in other vertebrae. The sacral hiatus is the inferior limit of the sacral canal.

44. B The multifidus is a deep muscle group that starts from the axis (C2) and terminates at the sacrum. It is topographically divided into three portions, namely, the superior, which is the cervical part and consists of multifidus cervicis (multifidus colli); the middle, which is in the thorax (multifidus thoracis), and the inferior, which is in the lower back and is called multifidus lumborum. Multifidus lumborum is the most developed and thickest of these deep-seated muscles [27].

The main action of multifidus is stabilization of the spine. The proximal attachment (origin) of multifidus is multiple and, from top to bottom, consists of the cervical spine (**A**rticular processes of C4–C7), thoracic spine (**T**ransverse processes of T1–T12 [i.e., all]), lumbar spine (**M**amillary bodies), ilium (posterior superior iliac spine), and sacrum (posterior [dorsal] surface). The distal attachment (insertion) of multifidus is made up of the spinous processes of vertebrae two to five levels above its origin; it is different in the atlas (C1), which lacks the usual spinous process. The blood supply of the cervical portion of the multifidus is by deep cervical arteries, occipital arteries, and vertebral arteries. The thoracic portion of this muscle receives arterial blood supply from the dorsal branches of the posterior intercostal arteries, the subcostal and lumbar arteries. Its lowest portion, the sacral portion, obtains arterial blood from dorsal branches of the lateral sacral arteries [27].

Shahidi et al., in their research titled "Lumbar Multifidus Muscle Degenerates in Individuals with Chronic Degenerative Lumbar Spine Pathology," concluded that multifidus muscles in individuals with lumbar spine pathology show extreme muscle loss; the mechanism was multiple and entailed reduced blood supply to multifidus lumborum, an imbalance between degeneration and regeneration, and an increase in inflammation. Consequently, treatments for reversing simple atrophy/muscle overload may be inapplicable. It is a finding in clinical management of patients with this disorder that despite postoperative improvements in pain and rehabilitation efforts, there is a pattern of unresolved "atrophy" [60].

45. C Multifidus lumborum or erector spinae is the most likely muscle that was injured. Multifidus extends and rotates the vertebral column. The semispinalis thoracis is one of the deep muscles in the thoracic region, but in this area, the rotatores are the deepest and most developed muscles among the transversospinales muscles [27]. The origin (proximal attachment) of quadratus lumborum is the inner lip of the iliac crest and the iliolumbar ligament; its insertion (distal attachment) is the internal surface of rib 12 and the transverse processes of the lumbar bodies of the lumbar vertebrae except the last (i.e., L1 to L4). Quadratus lumborum is the major deep muscle of the posterior abdominal region [61]. When the left and right quadratus lumborum contract, they contribute to the stabilization of the lower back; contraction of each quadratus lumborum (a rectangular muscle) flexes the ipsilateral lower back. The serratus posterior moves the ribs.

CHAPTER 12

ANSWERS AND NOTES FOR MCQs ON PELVIS AND PERINEUM

1. D The reproductive tract has mucous membranes. The epithelium of the female reproductive organ differs according to the function of the specific part. The endometrium consists of simple columnar epithelium—during the secretory phase, the glands are coiled but are long tubules in the proliferative phase. The inner layer of the cervix (endocervix) is lined with simple columnar epithelium. The ectocervix is characterized by nonkeratinized stratified squamous epithelium. Between the ectocervix and endocervix (i.e., the transformation zone where scrapings are obtained for cytological examination in a Papanicolaou test), the epithelium is squamocolumnar. Like the ectocervix, the vagina is lined by characterized nonkeratinized stratified squamous epithelium. The lining of the vulva is formed by stratified squamous epithelium. The external surface of the ovary is lined by simple cuboidal epithelium, and the interior of the fallopian tube has ciliated simple columnar epithelium [1]. The mucus in the female reproductive tract has properties that include its ability to flow or undergo deformation; this viscoelasticity depends on the part of the reproductive tract and the stage in the menstrual cycle [2]. Soulsbury and Humphries state that, "viscosity is a fundamental driver in changing spermatozoon structure and, in turn, plays a vital role in shaping the biomechanical movement of the sperm" [3, 4]. In the female genital tract, mucus provides lubrication.

The lining of the nasal cavity similarly has mucous membrane. The oral cavity is lined by stratified squamous epithelium. The small intestine is lined with simple columnar epithelium. Pseudostratified columnar epithelium is the lining of part of the nasal cavity.

2. A The synovial membrane is vascular. The synovial membrane encloses the synovial cavity and has projections that increase its surface area. Synovial fluid is clear and viscous. The inner layer of a synovial joint capsule consists of loose connective tissue. In the pelvis, the hip joints and the sacroiliac joints are the two that are synovial joints.

3. C Regarding the bony framework of the pelvis in thin people, both the anterior superior iliac spines and posterior superior iliac spines can be identified relatively easily; the former is palpable, and the latter creates two dimples on the skin of the lower back above the glutei [5, 6]. The posterolateral surface of the ilium is "roundish" and provides attachments to gluteal muscles—gluteus maximus, gluteus medius, and gluteus minimus. The anteromedial surface is slightly concave and smooth and is occupied by the iliacus. The ilium is the largest of the pelvic bones. The others are the ischium, pubis, sacrum, and coccyx. The ilium, ischium, and pubis constitute the os coxae [7]. The bony pelvis protects the internal pelvic organs. The bony pelvis provides the required support for body weight, stability for the upper trunk, and coordination for efficient movements with the legs. Several ligaments, muscles, neurovascular components, foramina, and various joints allow the axial skeleton and appendicular skeleton, and all contents and attached and communicating structures, to function seamlessly in health—and they contribute significantly to disease when they dysfunction.

DOI: 10.1201/9781003783961-14

4. B The pubic arch in adult females has an angle that is more than 90° compared to adult males, where it is 90° or less [8]. The false (greater) pelvis in females is shallower than in males. The adult female pelvis is more moveable. The pelvic inlet in the adult female (gynecoid pelvis) is ovoid or roundish, with a transverse diameter that is slightly more than the anteroposterior diameter [9]. The pelvic outlet in the adult female is larger than in the male. It is in the adult male that the pelvic inlet is heart shaped.

5. B With respect to the pelvis, the sacral promontory, ileo-pectineal lines, symphysis pubis are boundaries of the true pelvis [9]. The transverse diameter is the widest (about 13.5 cm) at the female pelvic inlet [9]. The broad ligament of the uterus consists of two layers of the peritoneum that link the lateral walls of the uterus with the lateral pelvic walls [10]. The mesometrium forms the most extensive portion of the broad ligament; the mesosalpinx is the portion that contains the fallopian tubes; and the mesovarium forms the connection between the ovaries and the broad ligament. The broad ligament contains the following: Uterine arteries, ovaries, ovarian arteries, ovarian ligaments, fallopian tubes, suspensory ligaments (or infundibulopelvic ligaments), round ligaments, nerves, and lymphatics [11].

The right ureter is expected anterior to the bifurcation of the right common iliac artery; still on the ureters, they lie beneath the broad ligament, and the respective uterine arteries cross them. The ureters are thin tubular structures that are 3 to 4 mm in diameter; they have smooth muscles that contract to direct the flow of urine from the renal pelvis to the urinary bladder [12].

The upper limit of the rectum is at the third piece of the sacrum; the rectum is 18 to 20 cm long, and S3 marks both its commencement and the termination of the sigmoid colon [13].

6. B Regarding the bony framework of the pelvis, the part of the iliac crest that is not listed is the tuberculum; the other parts of this important portion of the ilium are the outer lip, intermediate zone, and inner lip. Other parts of the ilium are the iliac tuberosity, its contribution to the sacroiliac joint, the ala (wing) of the ilium, the greater sciatic notch, and the arcuate lines. The arcuate line is a smooth, narrow ridge on the medial (inner) surface of the ilium that starts posteriorly from the auricular surface of the ilium and extends anteriorly to terminate at the iliopubic eminence [14]. The continuous ring of smooth bony ridge starts from the sacral promontory and sweeps bilaterally across the left and right arcuate lines, then the pectineal lines to the pubic symphysis form the pelvic brim [9].

7. D With regard to measurements of the adult female pelvis, the transverse (intertuberous [between the two ischial tuberosities]) diameter of the pelvic ***outlet*** is narrower than the anteroposterior diameter (from the pubic symphysis to the sacrococcygeal joint) [9]. The plane of the pelvic outlet joins the inferior margin of the pubic symphysis and the tip of the coccyx; this is the anteroposterior diameter of the pelvic outlet. The diagonal conjugate is the distance between the inferior margin of the pubic symphysis and the sacral promontory (which, anatomically, is at a higher level than the tip of the coccyx, which is the lowest point of the vertebral column). The plane of the pelvic inlet is the true conjugate diameter of the pelvic inlet; it joins the superior surface of the pubic symphysis and the sacral promontory. Regarding the pelvic inlet, the true conjugate is shorter than the diagonal diameter by about 1.5 cm.

Summary: The transverse diameter is the widest diameter at the pelvic inlet, but the anteroposterior diameter is the widest diameter at the pelvic outlet. The true conjugate of the pelvic inlet and outlet have the same reference point posteriorly (sacral promontory),

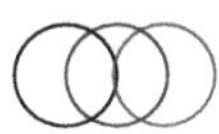

but anteriorly, it is the superior surface of the pubis for the pelvic inlet and the inferior surface of the pubis for the pelvic outlet.

If during clinical pelvimetry (infrequently done) or, more frequently, imaging pelvimetry, the distance between the pubis and the sacral promontory is inadequate, the pregnant woman is advised not to go into labor. In males, the diameters are shorter than in females of comparable body size [9]. In women, the pelvic outlet measurements increase during labor, enhancing delivery of the fetus and the entire pelvic outlet architecture supports and guides the fetus as it exits the birth canal [15, 16].

8. A The ischial spine does not contribute to the outline of the pelvic inlet; the ischial spine is at a lower level. The parts that are involved in the outline of the pelvic inlet are, from anterior to posterior, the superior surface of the pubic symphysis, the pecten pubis (pectineal line), the arcuate line, a portion of the sacroiliac joint, a part of the ala of the sacrum, and the sacral promontory.

9. C It is the ischium and pubis that contribute to the obturator foramen. Regarding the pelvic bones, the other three statements are correct: The sacrum has five segments and four foramina. The ilium and pubis contribute to the anatomy and surgery of inguinal hernias—this is via the reference points formed by the inguinal ligament using the anterior superior iliac spine and the pubic tubercle. The inguinal ligament is a thickened inferior portion of the external oblique aponeurosis; this ligament forms the floor of the canal. The inguinal canal (natural canal with orifices) comprises an anterior wall, a posterior wall, a roof, and a floor. In inguinal hernia, a weakness of the walls and an accompanying widening permit certain structures that are normally within the confines of the abdominal cavity access to the extra-abdominal space [17].

The anterior superior iliac spine is also a reference point for clinically assessing a patient with symptoms suggestive of acute appendicitis. During abdominal examination of a patient with suggestive symptoms, tenderness, guarding, and rebound tenderness following application of pressure by palpation or percussion over McBurney's point are the most reliable *clinical* indicators of *acute appendicitis* [18]. The lesser sciatic notch is closely related to the ischial spine.

10. D The transverse process of the fifth lumbar vertebra (L5) indirectly articulates with the iliac tuberosity via the robust iliolumbar ligament. The iliolumbar ligament arises from the tip and inferior portion of the anterior aspect of the transverse process of L5 and spreads out laterally in two (anterior and posterior) bands that attach distally (anteriorly) to the inner lip of the iliac crest and the anterior portion of the iliac tuberosity [19]. This strong ligament plays a role in supporting the frame of the body and in distributing weight from the spine to the legs through the pelvis [20]. The anterior band of the iliolumbar ligament may consist of just one band, but there may be up to six bands; the posterior band is more consistent, as it is usually just one band [20]. In 70% to 80% of cases, the anterior and posterior bands of the iliolumbar ligament arise from the transverse process of the fifth lumbar vertebra (L5) [20]. The ischial spine separates the greater sciatic notch from the lesser sciatic notch. The pubic arch is formed by the inferior pubic rami linked by the inferior pubic ligament. Using the bony pelvis, the subpubic angle helps forensically to identify the sex of a deceased person.

11. A The false pelvis (greater pelvis) is wide and shallow and is considered to be a part of the abdominal cavity. Regarding the false pelvis, the lower limit is the linea terminalis (also referred to as the innominate line or pelvic brim), while the iliac crests form its upper border. The iliac crest and arcuate line are parts of the ilium. The greater sciatic notch is between the posterior inferior iliac spine and the ischial spine; the posterior inferior iliac spine lies superiorly while the ischial spine is inferior. The lesser sciatic notch is bordered superiorly by the ischial spine and inferiorly by the ischial tuberosity; with attached ligaments, the lesser sciatic notch forms the lesser sciatic foramen. Structures that pass through the lesser sciatic foramen are the tendon of the obturator internus, the nerve to the obturator internus, the internal pudendal artery and vein, and the pudendal nerve. The lesser sciatic foramen links structures between the gluteal region and the perineum.

The anterior gluteal line is on the posterolateral (gluteal) surface of the ilium. The ilio-pubic eminence (formed at the meeting point of the ilium and pubis) is a part of the bony ridge that separates the false pelvis from the true pelvis—it is, therefore, a part of the pelvic brim. The pelvic brim is also called the pelvic inlet, superior pelvic aperture, and upper pelvic narrow [9].

12. C The obturator canal does not pierce the obturator membrane; it is a natural ovoid opening formed between the inferior border of the superior pubic ramus and the superior border of the obturator membrane. The greater sciatic foramen is posterosuperior to the obturator canal. The greater and lesser sciatic foramina are separated by the sacrospinous ligament. The sacrotuberous ligament attaches to the ischial tuberosity inferiorly.

13. C Regarding the bony pelvis, the posterior sacral foramina are lateral to the supraspinous ligament [21]. The supraspinous ligament runs in the midline posteriorly. During pregnancy there is relaxation of the ligaments and cartilages in the pelvis; this is due to hormonal effects; this feature enhances the process of labor and childbirth [22]. Relaxation of the pelvic ligaments is a physical change that commences in the latter part of the first trimester of pregnancy; this physiological change is essential during pregnancy and childbirth. This hormonal change results from relaxin, a peptide hormone secreted by the corpus luteum and placenta in the early stages of pregnancy. The hormone belongs to the insulin-like growth factor family and contributes to remodeling of collagen. Blood levels of relaxin increase during the first trimester, plateau at a high level up to the third trimester, and then taper down. It is only in the first few days in the post-partum period that the hormone is not detectable serologically [23, 24]. It is surmised that relaxin, by achieving alteration of the structure of collagen, enhances pelvic laxity, and makes the pubic symphysis prone to separation [25]. Regarding the pubic symphysis, it is a special joint with two joint articular surfaces formed by the pubic bones; a fibrocartilaginous disk is sandwiched between these joint articular surfaces. The symphysis pubis is able to withstand a variety of forces, including the ones that cause compression, shearing, and tension. The symphysis pubis also allows a slight degree of movement. During pregnancy, increases in mobility and in the width of the pubic symphysis result from the changes that take place in the fibrocartilaginous disk [26].

The ischiopubic ramus is inferior to the superior pubic ramus. The anterior longitudinal ligament extends to the concave surface of only the upper sacral bones.

14. C The transverse acetabular ligament is inferior to the acetabular notch; one of its attachments is the obturator crest. The obturator membrane is not attached to the symphyseal surface of the pubic bone; it is attached to the superior surface of the ischiopubic ramus and the inner surface of the ischium medial to the ischial

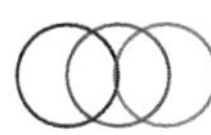

tuberosity. The structure that is attached to the symphyseal surface of the pubic bone is the pubic symphysis. The acetabulum is notched inferiorly. The lunate surface of the acetabulum is crescent-shaped and covered with cartilage; it is the part of the acetabulum with an articular surface that articulates with the head of the femur. The non-articular part of the acetabulum is the acetabular fossa; this part is deeper, and the articular part of the head of femur is not directly in contact with this further recessed part of the acetabular surface [27]. In their study, Shimodaira et al. concluded that although the acetabular fossa has been considered to be located in the center of the acetabulum, the center of the acetabular fossa is positioned anterior to the center of the acetabulum [28].

15. A With regard to the ligaments of the pelvis, the two ligaments on the concavity of the sacrum are not located on the posterior aspect of the pelvic bones; this is because the concave surface of the sacrum is its anterior surface. The two small ligaments are the anterior sacrococcygeal ligaments. Their equivalents on the posterior surface of the coccyx and lower sacrum are the deep posterior sacrococcygeal ligament and the superficial posterior sacrococcygeal ligaments. There are superficial posterior sacrococcygeal ligaments, two on each side, while the deep posterior sacrococcygeal ligament is in the midline posteriorly. Further laterally are the lateral posterior sacrococcygeal ligaments. There are, therefore, anterior and posterior sacrococcygeal ligaments, with the posterior ones being three—deep posterior, superficial posterior, and lateral posterior components [29]. The deep posterior sacrococcygeal ligament corresponds to the posterior longitudinal ligament; the superficial posterior sacrococcygeal ligament acts as the roof for the distal end of the sacral canal and the sacral hiatus. The lateral posterior sacrococcygeal ligaments are similar to the intertransverse ligaments [29].

16. A Regarding the pelvic diaphragm in females, the deep dorsal vein of the clitoris lies between the pubic bone and the urethra. From the posterior to anterior, the correct order of structures is rectum, vagina, and urethra. The tendinous arch of the levator ani muscle links the pubic bone with the ischial spine. The iliococcygeus muscle is anterior to the ischiococcygeus muscle; the ischiococcygeus muscle and coccygeus muscle are synonymous. The levator ani muscle provides support for pelvic viscera and lifts the pelvic floor. Weakness of the pelvic floor may be from obesity, giving birth to many babies, or any condition that causes raised intra-abdominal pressure that is transmitted to the pelvic cavity [30, 31]. Symptomatic pelvic organ prolapse is a bothersome clinical condition that features the descent of pelvic structures. The pathology is from weakness of the structures that support the pelvic floor. The structures that may be involved are various and could be the muscles, ligaments, or fasciae; the organs (or portions of them) that traverse the pelvic floor via the anatomical orifices include the uterus, cervix, vaginal apex, anterior vaginal wall, or posterior vaginal wall [32]. Herniation into the vaginal space causes rectocele, enterocele, cystocele, or uterine prolapse [33]. When it becomes symptomatic, pelvic organ prolapse makes the patient present with symptoms like a feeling of pressure in the pelvis, a sensation of a bulge in the vagina, or a visible bulge in the vagina; other features are difficulty with passing stools or voiding, sexual dysfunction, urinary incontinence, or fecal incontinence [34, 35].

17. D Functionally, the puborectalis is the most anteriorly positioned component of the levator ani muscles; the puborectalis forms a sling posterior to the rectum while it is anchored anteriorly to the pubis. The deep dorsal veins of the penis are anterior to the urethra. The coccygeus muscle lies above (superior to) the sacrospinous ligament and sacrotuberous ligament. The levator ani muscle comprises three muscles: the pubococcygeus, puborectalis, and iliococcygeus muscles.

18. C With regard to the levator ani muscle, arterial blood supply is via the inferior gluteal artery and internal pudendal artery; the internal pudendal artery supplies arterial blood via its perineal and inferior rectal branches. The proximal attachment (origin) of this three-in-one muscle is not only the body of the pubic bone but also the tendinous arch of the obturator fascia and the ischial spine. The six distal attachment (insertion) sites are as follows: (a) the perineal body, (b) the anococcygeal raphe, (c) the coccyx, (d) the prostate wall, (e) the rectal wall, and (f) the wall of the anal canal. Innervation of the levator ani muscle is by the ventral rami of the lower sacral nerves and the perineal nerve.

19. B Regarding the pelvic diaphragm in females, the tendinous arch of the levator ani muscle is not a midline structure; it is located in the lateral aspect of the pelvic diaphragm. The structures that are in the midline include, from anterior to posterior, (a) the inferior (arcuate) pubic ligament, (b) the deep dorsal vein of the clitoris, (c) the transverse perineal ligament, (d) the fascia of the deep perineal muscles, (e) the urethra exiting the hiatus for urethra, (f) the vagina, (g) the interdigitating fibers of the perineum—between the vagina and the rectum, (h) the rectum exiting the anorectal hiatus, and (i) the levator plate of the levator ani muscle, which is synonymous with the median raphe of levator ani muscle. In males, the dorsal veins of the penis replace the deep dorsal vein of the clitoris; there is no vagina.

20. A Regarding pelvic viscera in females, the pouch of Douglas is peritoneal reflection over the uterus; it is the rectouterine pouch. As with other surfaces that have serous membranes, the peritoneal surfaces that create this pouch secrete small amounts of serous fluid. When the secretion is voluminous, it is usually due to an inflammatory process, as may be caused by infections in the surrounding organs, like an infection (salpingitis with pelvic inflammatory disease) in the fallopian tubes. When a pelvic examination is performed on the patient, there may be tenderness from motion of the cervix, which is transmitted to the inflamed fallopian tube(s). This cervical motion tenderness is also referred to as the Chandelier sign [36]. A more common and non-invasive examination is pelvic ultrasound scanning, which shows the presence of more than normal fluid collection [37]. There are many indications for abdominopelvic ultrasound scanning, but regarding abdominal masses and pelvic masses, the following should be noted: Ascites and ovarian malignancy, large subserosal leiomyoma in the broad ligament, multiple uterine leiomyomas (fibroids), ovarian mass, tubo-ovarian mass, adenomyosis that exceeds the size of a uterus with a 12-week-old pregnancy, molar pregnancy, hematometra, pyometra, rudimentary horn ectopic pregnancy, and choriocarcinoma [37].

Sometimes, lower abdominal pain and pelvic pain may be from a dire emergency like a ruptured ectopic pregnancy causing hemorrhage into the pelvic cavity [38]. An ovary lies posterior to the external iliac artery and external iliac vein. The vesicouterine pouch is at a higher level than the rectouterine pouch—the rectouterine pouch is, therefore, the deepest/lowest portion of the pelvic cavity in females.

21. D When viewing the pelvis from the abdominal cavity, the rectouterine folds are at a higher level than the rectouterine pouch (pouch of Douglas). The peritoneal folds

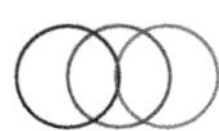

that form ridges on the uterosacral ligament are responsible for the rectouterine folds; the rectouterine folds form the upper ends and sides (lateral walls) of the pouch of Douglas; therefore, the folds must be at a higher level than the fluid-collecting bottom of the pouch of Douglas—the lowest (deepest) point of the female pelvis, especially when the woman is in the erect position. The fundus of the non-pregnant uterus is wholly in the pelvic cavity. The round ligament of the uterus is attached to the lateral wall of the uterus at the uterine cornu just anterior and inferior to the origin of the corresponding fallopian tube, which is the uterotubal junction; it then takes a course anterior to the fallopian tube [16]. The ovary is on the posterior wall of the broad ligament.

22. B Regarding the female reproductive organs, the cardinal ligament is a part of the broad ligament; it is a band of connective tissue located at the base (inferior end) of the broad ligament. The cardinal ligament is synonymous with Mackenrodt's ligament; this ligament is also referred to as the transverse cervical ligament and lateral cervical ligament. In the ligament run the uterine artery and vein on both sides. The uterine artery arises from the internal iliac artery after it branches off from the external iliac artery. The ligament runs transversely bilaterally from the lateral sides of the cervix. The uterine cervix is enveloped by the uterovaginal fascia. There are two sacrouterine ligaments and they arch posteriorly to link the uterus with the sacrum and rectum; these ligaments are also called rectouterine ligaments. Between the cervix and vagina anteriorly and the rectum posteriorly, there are two potential spaces called rectocervical and rectovaginal spaces. The fascial ligaments of the uterus are the cardinal ligament, the uterosacral ligament, the round ligament of the uterus, and the ligament of the ovary. The uterosacral ligament and the cardinal ligament are the ligaments that primarily provide apical support to the upper vagina and the uterus [39].

23. B The uterus is a muscular organ with an internal hollow; it has a cross-section that is pear-shaped and like an inverted triangle with the apex distally. In an adult, non-pregnant female, the dimensions of the uterus are approximately 8 × 5 × 4 cm in length, width, and thickness. It has a capacity of 80 to 200 mL. The normal uterus is both anteverted and anteflexed. Anteversion means that the uterus is flexed forward (anteriorly) at the cervix; anteflexion indicates that it is also flexed forward at the isthmus [40]. Superoinferiorly, the parts of the uterus are the fundus, body, isthmus, and cervix [41]. The cervix uteri commences proximally at the internal os which opens into the uterine cavity; it ends at the external os, which opens into the vagina [40]. The uterine wall consists of three layers. From the exterior inward, the layers are perimetrium, myometrium, and endometrium. The perimetrium is a continuation of the parietal peritoneum of the pelvic cavity. The myometrium is the muscular layer of smooth muscle. The endometrium consists of two parts—a thin stratum basalis and a thick stratum functionalis. It is the stratum functionalis that is involved in monthly shedding in females with normal menstrual cycles [40]. The uterus is completely pelvic in its non-pregnant state. The uterus is linked to the labia by the round ligament. Cord-like, the round ligament of the uterus is made up of fibro-muscular connective tissue. By one of its sides, the round ligament is linked to the superolateral aspect of the uterus at the uterine cornu. The round ligament crosses the pelvis through the deep inguinal ring. The ligament goes through the deep inguinal ring and the superficial inguinal ring of the inguinal canal. After exiting the inguinal canal, the round ligament accesses the labium majus. The mons pubis is the terminal point of each round ligament [16].

24. B An acutely inflamed fallopian tube does not become gangrenous because of its dual arterial blood supply. Each ovarian artery arises from the abdominal aorta and courses in the infundibulopelvic ligament (suspensory ligament of the ovary) [11]. The fallopian tubes are supplied by both ovarian arteries and uterine arteries; this makes it difficult for an acutely inflamed fallopian tube to become gangrenous. Even when it is not an acute condition (like in hydrosalpinx or pyosalpinx), it is still rare even for a patient to have an isolated torsion—torsion of an organ usually precedes gangrene; the twisting of the organ involved in torsion leads to ischemia by compromising the arterial supply to the organ, and sustained compromise of arterial blood supply to the organ leads to gangrene. Torsion in the adnexa is usually related to the ovaries (due to ovarian cysts), but a rare case of torsion of a fallopian tube associated with hydrosalpinx in a 27-year-old pregnant woman during the third trimester has been documented [42]. Awareness and a high index of suspicion by clinicians are imperative to ensure early diagnosis and appropriate intervention to prevent permanent damage to an affected fallopian tube [42]. Due to the presence of extensive collateral circulation in the mesosalpinx, the likelihood of compromise of ovarian function is remote following female sterilization using electrocoagulation, clips, or the older method of ligation with sutures of the fallopian tube bilaterally. The collateral circulation provides a branch to the infundibulopelvic ligament that supplies ovarian circulation from the opposite direction [43].

The fimbriae are at the most lateral portion of the fallopian tubes. The level of the pouch of Douglas is lower than that of the utero-vesical peritoneal reflection in the erect position.

25. D The ovaries are the primary sex organs. The full dimensions of a normal-sized ovary are about 3.5 × 2.0 × 1.0 cm in length, width, and thickness, respectively. Each ovary is ovoid and lies in an ovarian fossa (fossa ovarica) [44]. The outer part of the ovary is the epithelial layer of simple cuboidal epithelium (the germinal epithelium). Deep to this layer is a connective tissue of collagen (the tunica albuginea). Further deeper is the cortex, composed of ovarian follicles. The innermost zone of the ovary is the central zone or the medulla (or hilus); the medulla consists of loose connective tissue with nerves, lymphatic vessels, and large spiral arteries [45]. In a nulliparous adult female, an ovary lies in the ovarian fossa. The external iliac artery and vein are anterior to the fossa, and the internal iliac artery and vein lie posterior to the fossa—the ovarian fossa is, therefore, between the external and internal iliac vessels. The boundaries of the ovarian fossa are as follows. The infundibulum (funnel-shaped portion) of the fallopian tube is superior to the ovary. The medial umbilical ligament is anterior to the ovary; the medial umbilical ligament is the remnant of the obliterated umbilical artery. The internal iliac artery and ureter lie posterior to the ovary. The proper ligament of the ovary and the suspensory ligament of the ovary are the two ligaments of the ovary, while the suspensory ligament bears the ovarian artery, ovarian vein, the sympathetic plexus, and the parasympathetic plexuses. The proper ligament of the ovary is the remnant of the gubernaculum and contains no blood vessel [11]. The "proper ovarian ligament" (ovarian ligament, or utero-ovarian ligament) is the cord-like fibrous tissue in the broad ligament.

26. A The uterus and oviducts are female internal accessory organs. Synonyms of oviducts are uterine tubes and fallopian tubes. The order of the portions of the fallopian tube, starting from the uterus, is as follows: intramural, isthmus, ampulla, and infundibulum. The fimbriae are at the distal end of the infundibular part of the fallopian tube [46]. The fimbriae are closest to the ovary. The luminal diameter of

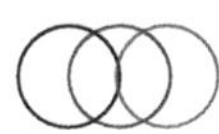

a fallopian tube is less than 1 mm, but the length is between 11 and 12 cm [47]. The vestibule is part of the external reproductive organ; it is the space enclosed by the labia minora. The labium majus is an external reproductive structure; two make up the labia majora, which correspond to the scrotum in the male.

27. B Testes are the primary sex organs. The human testis is ellipsoid in shape. Each of the testes is about 2.5 × 4 cm in diameter. Each testis is enclosed by tunica albuginea, which is a tough, white, active connective tissue capsule. The tunica albuginea provides support to the internal structures of the testis; it is essential in ensuring that the pressure that the testis requires for production of spermatozoa is achieved and maintained. About 370 conical lobules form the testicular parenchyma; the lobules are separated by thin septula testis. Each lobule contains seminiferous tubules and intertubular tissue. It is the intertubular connective tissue that contains groups of Leydig cells [48]. Lobules of highly convoluted glandular tubules make up the testis. The testis contains Leydig cells, Sertoli cells, and germ cells. Leydig cells are in the groups of interstitial cells found in testicular loose connective tissue. Sertoli cells provide support to developing sperm cells; the Sertoli cells are in seminiferous tubules, and they project internally toward the lumen from the basement membrane. The testis also contains germ cells in the periphery of the basement membrane; they develop from spermatogonia through primary spermatocytes, secondary spermatocytes, spermatids, and finally to spermatozoa, which are the mature sperm released into the seminiferous tubule lumen. The maturing cells (spermatocytes), in the process of spermatogenesis, move toward the lumen of the seminiferous tubule [49, 50]. Fetal Leydig cells produce testosterone; the levels become higher in adult Leydig cells; it is also surmised that pharmacological means may be used to increase serum testosterone via Leydig cell stimulation [51].

Tunica albuginea is a tough, white, fibrous capsule that encloses the testes. The testes are the sites for production of both testosterone (endocrine function) and spermatozoa (exocrine) function.

28. B A testicular lobule may have up to four seminiferous tubules. A seminiferous tubule is about 70 cm long. Seminiferous tubules are lined by spermatogenic cells and interstitial cells. The rete testis is in the mediastinum testis. The epididymis is made up of ducts of the rete testis.

29. C The scrotum is an external reproductive organ, just as the penis is. Internal accessory organs of the male reproductive system are the prostate, seminal vesicles, and bulbourethral glands. Bulbourethral glands are synonymous with Cowper's glands.

30. B The embryology, histology, gross anatomy, and physiology of the constituents of the male reproductive system are intertwined. Embryologically, the testis is an abdominal structure. The testis and associated structures get "dragged" down into and, eventually, out of the pelvis. It becomes an external structure after it passes through the internal ring and external ring of the inguinal canal on each side. The two testes find their final "accommodation" in the scrotum.

The testes cannot perform their full function in reproduction if they cannot send their exocrine products (spermatozoa) out of the body. To access the exterior (via the penile urethra, which it is very close to, anatomically, but does not have direct access to), the testis sends spermatozoa through the entire length of the vas deferens (from the testes to the prostatic urethra). This means going back into the pelvis through the inguinal canal [52].

The vas deferens, testicular artery, artery to the vas deferens, pampiniform plexus of veins, ilioinguinal nerve, autonomic nerves, and lymphatic vessels are the constituents of the spermatic cord. The spermatic cord has coverings that reflect the coverings of the anterior abdominal wall; this means that it has cremaster muscle and fascial coverings (external spermatic fascia, cremasteric fascia, and internal spermatic fascia). The structure in the spermatic cord must be protected when performing inguinal hernia operations.

After entering the pelvis, the vas deferens of each side runs on the superolateral surface of the urinary bladder and takes a posterior and inferior course toward the seminal vesicle. The vas deferens becomes enlarged toward its terminal end—this is the ampulla of the ductus deferens. The seminal vesicle is located in the rectovesical space; it also lies immediately posterior to the urinary bladder and anterior to the recto-prostatic (Denonvilliers') fascia; posterior to this fascia is the rectum covered by rectal fascia. The duct of the seminal vesicle and the duct of the vas deferens meet to form an ejaculatory duct; the ejaculatory duct enters the prostate gland. Each ejaculatory duct traverses the prostate from the posterolateral position by taking an inferomedial course toward the prostatic urethra. The prostatic duct joins the ejaculatory duct and they open into the prostatic urethra at an elevation called the verumontanum or seminal colliculus [53].

31. D Regarding the parts of the urinary bladder, the apex points forward (anteriorly), not upward. Vesical fascia lines the external surface of the urinary bladder. The fundus of the bladder is the posterior part of the organ. The bladder neck is just superior to the prostate gland. The body of the bladder lies between the apex and the fundus. The trigone is the part of the bladder where the ureters enter and the urethra commences; the trigone is a smooth-surfaced triangular area of the inner wall at the bladder base/floor. The trigone allows the bladder to receive from the kidneys via the ureteric openings and prevents exit of the urine from the bladder until the person desires to urinate. Mechanoreceptors at the trigone respond to bladder wall distension, allowing the individual to know when to empty a full bladder. The sphincter effect of the detrusor muscles at the proximal (internal) urethral orifice maintains continence. Tiny valves at the ureteric openings allow unidirectional flow of urine into the bladder and prevent backflow. When there is excessive pressure inferior to the valves (or superior to them), the raised pressure may progress to the development of hydroureters or hydronephrosis, which could be unilateral or bilateral, depending on the etiology [54].

32. A The trigone is at the floor of the urinary bladder; it has a smooth surface and has the openings of the two ureters and that of the urethra. A full, normal bladder can accommodate up to 0.8 liters of urine. The bladder fills up superiorly and the superior surface of a distended bladder may be palpable in the suprapubic region. The mucosa of the urinary bladder and the ureters are composed of transitional epithelium [55].

33. C With respect to the prostate, the prostatic venous plexus is superior to the transverse perineal ligament; the transverse perineal ligament is the anterior thickening of the perineal membrane. A penetrating injury from a narrow and sharp-pointed object through an entry point superior to the symphysis pubis is unlikely to involve the prostate but likely to affect the bladder. Anatomically, the prostate has five lobes—anterior lobe, posterior lobe, two lateral lobes, and a median lobe [56]. The prostatic venous plexus is located anterior to the prostate gland. An enlarged median lobe of the prostate gland is most commonly implicated in bladder outlet obstruction; by virtue

 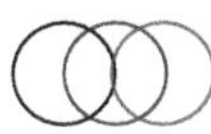

of its growth superiorly into the bladder neck and causing a distortion, the enlarged median lobe creates a ball-valve effect, preventing voiding of urine [57].

34. C The symptomatology of gradual onset of urinary frequency, urgency, terminal dribbling, and spending a longer time than usual to urinate, with no dysuria, hematuria, or weight loss and no increase in volume of urine passed by a 65-year-old man would primarily point to benign prostatic hyperplasia. It is less likely to be an infection (schistosomiasis, prostatitis, or urethritis), cancerous (cancer of the prostate), endocrine (diabetes mellitus), urethral stricture, or primarily a urinary bladder pathology. These are differential diagnoses, and the patient needs to be examined physically and investigations carried out to rule out the mimics or the possibility of comorbidity.

35. A Regarding the rectum, superoinferiorly, the structures anterior to it are rectovesical pouch, seminal vesicle, prostate, and Denonvilliers' fascia; Denonvilliers' fascia is the recto-prostatic fascia [58]. The ampulla is the distal portion of the rectum. From out to in, the wall of the rectum consists of muscularis externa, submucosa, and mucosa. Rectal mucosa comprises epithelium, lamina propria, and muscularis mucosae. The rectum has three distinctive or characteristic folds (transverse rectal folds or valves of Houston) called the superior rectal valve, middle rectal valve, and inferior rectal valve [59]. Each fold is the result of invagination, or in-folding of, from inside to out, the mucous membrane, submucosa, and a portion of the circular inner layer of smooth muscle, which is thickened. The synonym for middle rectal valve is Kohlrausch's valve; it is the most prominent of the usually three valves, with two on the left side and one on the right. On the external surface of the rectum, these valves produce three permanent transverse deepenings or constrictions. On the internal surface of the rectum (its lumen), the valves are transverse protrusions. Vitamin B_{12} absorption takes place in the distal ileum in the presence of intrinsic factor, which is synthesized in the stomach; vitamin B_{12} is attached to the glycoprotein, which enhances absorption of this vitamin.

36. B The functions of the rectum do not include secretion of digestive enzymes. The upper portions of the gut produce the enzymes for digestion of food. Functions of the rectum include storage of contents of the gut delivered by the sigmoid colon, further absorption of water from stored contents leading to an increased solidification of fecal matter, absorption of electrolytes, secretion of mucus to lubricate feces, signaling the commencement of the process of defecation consequent upon distension of its walls by sufficient fecal load, delivery of fecal material to the anal canal, and controlling/determining the timing of fecal expulsion by working in conjunction with the external anal sphincter (which contains striated muscles) [60]. Consumption of a high-fiber diet and much water eases transit of colonic and rectal contents; this enhances relative cleanness and health of the colon and, therefore, lessens diverticular disease risk, maintains healthy colonic flora, and ultimately decreases the risk of diarrhea, constipation, infectious colitis, and abdominal bloating from excessive gas [61].

37. A Digital rectal examination is a painful procedure if the patient has an anal fissure. The examining finger does not reach the colon. It may be done in patients who are suspected to have anorectal neoplasm but should be carried out gently and carefully because it may trigger rectal bleeding, especially when there is an accompanying recent history of bright red rectal bleeding (hematochezia). The details of the procedure are well laid out under "Technique" in the referenced journal article [62].

38. D Gonadal veins are testicular veins in males and ovarian veins in females. The left gonadal vein drains into the left renal vein, while the right gonadal vein drains into the inferior vena cava. Other veins that drain into the inferior vena cava are the lumbar veins, renal veins, and inferior phrenic veins; therefore, the venous drainage of the left kidney is first to the left renal vein, then to the inferior vena cava [63].

39. B The deep circumflex iliac vein is formed by the veins that accompany (venae comitantes of) the deep circumflex iliac artery; the vein courses medially and parallel to the inguinal ligament and empties into the external iliac vein either alongside or in conjunction with the inferior epigastric vein. It provides deep drainage of the muscles of the lower abdominal wall (hypogastric region) just as the inferior epigastric vein does—these are the two large veins that provide deep venous drainage in this area [64]. The deep circumflex iliac vein also drains the iliac area and the major deep muscles in the pelvis [65]. Apart from the deep external iliac vein, superficial epigastric vein, and lateral accessory vein, the veins that form tributaries of the great saphenous vein include the superficial circumflex iliac vein, superficial external iliac vein, superficial external pudendal vein, small saphenous vein, and anterior accessory saphenous vein [66].

40. B The external urethral orifice is located between the vaginal orifice and the clitoris. The female urethra extends from the internal urethral sphincter to the external urethral orifice. When the female external sphincter muscles contract, they constrict not only the urethra but also the vagina [67]. In the adult female, the length of the urethra is short, unlike in the adult male. Its length is short (about 4 cm) in comparison to about 20–22 cm in the adult male [68]. This length does not protect the female urethra from involvement in infections; rather, infections tend to ascend with relative ease toward the bladder. The short length of the female urethra usually makes easier in women than men—if the external orifice is identified before introducing a urethral catheter.

41. A Regarding fasciae and ligaments in the female perineum, the levator ani lies in between the superior fascia of the pelvic diaphragm and the inferior fascia of the pelvic diaphragm [69]. The anococcygeal body (anococcygeal raphe, anococcygeal ligament) lies posterior to the external anal sphincter and the anal canal. The site of the perineal body is between the vagina and the rectum [70]. The perineal body is a point of attachment for several muscles; this structure is involved in providing strength to the pelvic floor. The muscles include the internal anal sphincter, external anal sphincter, external urethral sphincter, levator ani muscle (the puborectalis, pubococcygeus, and iliococcygeus), rectourethralis, bulbospongiosus, deep transverse perineal muscle, compressor urethrae, and longitudinal anal muscle (which lies between the internal anal sphincter and the external anal sphincter) [70]. The perineal membrane forms the superior border of the superficial perineal space, while Colles' fascia forms the inferior border of the superficial perineal space; Colles' fascia is also called superficial perineal fascia [71]. Other structures in the anterior part of the perineum are inferior pubic ligament (arcuate ligament), transverse perineal ligament, suspensory ligament of the clitoris, and sphincter urethrae and sphincter urethrovaginalis muscles.

42. B Regarding the female perineum and external genitalia, Gallaudet's fascia is the deep perineal fascia—also called investing fascia. The bulbospongiosus muscle is the medial wall of the space formed by the ischiocavernosus muscle, superficial transverse

 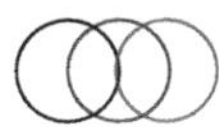

perineal muscle, and bulbospongiosus muscle. While the suspensory ligament of the clitoris is a midline structure, the round ligament is not; round ligaments are medial structures, each of which runs lateral (but close) to the midline. From the anterior to posterior, the structures are the hymenal caruncle, posterior commissure of labia majora, and perineal raphe, which covers the perineal body. Structures in the anterior part of the female external genitalia are the anterior commissure of the labia majora, prepuce of the clitoris, pudendal cleft (which is the groove between the labia majora anteriorly), glans of the clitoris, and frenulum of the clitoris. Between the frenulum of the clitoris and the vaginal orifice is the external urethral orifice; to clearly access the external urethral orifice and safely insert a Foley catheter for urethral catheterization, the clinician should part the lips of each labium minus laterally. Just posterior to the urethral orifice are the orifices of the paraurethral ducts (Skene's ducts) [72].

43. D The terminal part of the urethra is lined by stratified squamous epithelium; this is close to the external urethral orifice. The part close to the urinary bladder is lined by transitional epithelium, just like the bladder. The middle portion of the urethra has pseudostratified columnar epithelium. Control of urine involves coordinated actions of the external urethral sphincter and the internal urethral sphincter (which is a continuation of the detrusor muscle). When detrusor (involuntary muscle) contraction occurs concomitantly with urethral sphincter (skeletal muscle) relaxation, the result is an individual urinating (voiding). Detrusor muscle activity is controlled by the autonomic system. When there is detrusor muscle pathology, a patient may manifest the dysfunction as urinary retention, urinary incontinence, or a combination of the two conditions [54].

The prostatic urethra is the first part of the male urethra and is about 2.5 cm long; this makes the middle region (membranous urethra) the shortest, with a length of just 0.5 cm, as it is the part of the urethra that traverses the not-so-thick muscular pelvic floor. The most distal portion is the penile (spongy) urethra; with a length of 15 cm, it is the longest part of the male urethra. The male urethra is S-shaped [73].

44. D Cowper's glands are embedded within the fibers of the sphincter urethrae (external urethral sphincter). The pea-sized glands are at the level of the membranous urethra. They, however, secrete their alkaline pre-ejaculate fluid into the spongy portion of the urethra to protect spermatozoa in seminal fluid during sexual intercourse [74]. Covered by the perineal membrane, the dorsal nerve of the penis runs lateral to internal pudendal artery; the dorsal nerve of the penis is consequently closer to the ischiopubic ramus than the internal pudendal artery is. The internal pudendal artery gives off the artery of the bulb of the penis, deep artery of the penis, dorsal artery of the penis, and urethral artery [75]. The bulbospongiosus lies in the superficial perineal space; the space is superficial to the perineal membrane. Gallaudet's fascia (deep perineal fascia) is the investing fascia that surrounds the bulbospongiosus—the muscle is, consequently, deep to this fascia [76]. Covered by the perineal membrane, the dorsal nerve of the penis runs lateral to the internal pudendal artery. The internal pudendal artery gives off the artery of the bulb of the penis and dorsal artery of the penis. The bulbospongiosus muscle is external to the corpus spongiosum [75].

45. D A cross-section of the penis shows the intercavernous septum of deep fascia dorsal to the urethra. The lateral superficial vein is lateral to the deep dorsal vein and the dorsal artery. There are two lateral superficial veins. Each lateral superficial vein is also lateral to the dorsal nerve. Mediolaterally, the arrangement from the deep dorsal vein, which is a median structure like its superficial counterpart (the superficial dorsal vein), is the deep dorsal vein, dorsal artery, and dorsal nerve [77]. The dartos fascia of the penis lies between the penile skin and Buck's fascia of the penis; the dartos fascia of the penis is the superficial fascia of the penis, while Buck's fascia of the penis is the deep fascia of the penis. The penile urethra traverses the corpus spongiosum and its tunica albuginea; the corpus spongiosum and its tunica albuginea therefore surround the centrally located penile urethra as it courses through this spongy part of the penile architecture. There are two corpora cavernosa; each corpus cavernosum with its tunica albuginea is penetrated by a deep artery of the penis [78].

CHAPTER 13

ANSWERS AND NOTES FOR MCQs ON UPPER LIMB

1. A Melanocytes lie in the deepest part of the epidermis. By the process of cytocrine secretion, melanin granules may be introduced into non-melanocyte epidermal cells; In cytocrine secretion, keratinocytes phagocytose the tips of melanocyte processes [1]. Melanocytes protect the skin by producing melanin, which absorbs light and consequently protects deeper cells from the deleterious effects of ultraviolet radiation. Melanocytes synthesize melanin, which is a macromolecule. The enzyme tyrosinase catalyzes the first step in melanin synthesis. Tyrosinase converts tyrosine to **d**ihydr**o**xy**p**henyl**a**lanine (DOPA). Albinism results from the lack of tyrosinase. Mammalian and avian melanin is in two forms: eumelanin and phaeomelanin; the former is black or dark brown, while the color of the latter is yellow or red. Melanogenesis produces toxic intermediates. This biosynthesis takes place in melanosomes; melanosomes are unique organelles in that they are modified lysosomes. Melanocytes essentially do not retain melanin although they synthesize it; the melanin granules get transported along microtubules to the tips of dendrites—long cell protrusions; the movement of the granules continues to nearby keratinocytes in the skin and hair of mammals [2]. Calluses are found on palms and soles.

2. C The dermis contains collagenous fibers. Sebaceous glands and sweat glands are in the dermis. Both smooth and striated muscle fibers may be present, depending on the site. Pacinian corpuscles are stimulated by heavy pressure, while Meissner's corpuscles appreciate light touch. Striated muscle fibers are found in the face, while smooth muscle fibers are present in the dartos muscle in the scrotum. There are about 30 muscles on each side of the human face. Facial muscles are striated muscles that connect facial skin to bones of the skull; these striated muscles are involved in executing essential daily actions like chewing and expressing our emotions [3]. The scrotum, a thin external sac in the male perineum, is composed of skin and smooth muscle and is located below the penis [4].

3. B Specialized epithelial cells produce nails. Nails have keratinized cells. They grow most actively at the base of the nail plate. The half-moon-shaped portion is called the lunula. The nail plate overlies the nail bed. The upper and lower extremities are where nails are found. The plate of fingernails and toenails is made by keratinocytes. The nail plate is about 0.5 mm thick and slightly curved. The nail is securely attached to the underlying nail bed. The hyponychium is the skin at the tip of the digit (finger or toe) that connects the proximal part of the free edge to the distal portion of the nail bed; it protects the nail bed. At the tip of the fingers and toes, there is an extension of the nail plate from the nail bed to form the free edge; the length of the protruding nail plate depends on how long the individual desires to keep it [5].

4. C The structural unit of a hair follicle is the pilosebaceous unit, which comprises a hair follicle and associated sebaceous gland and arrector pili [6]. Hair has living and non-living components; the hair shaft, which is above the epidermis, is a thin, flexible cylinder of non-living, keratinized epithelial cells, while the hair follicle is the portion

DOI: 10.1201/9781003783961-15

below the epidermis, is living, and enlarges at its base forming the hair bulb [7]. The hair follicle is the part of the hair from which hair grows; it has an outer sheath and an inner sheath. The portion of a hair follicle where active production of hair takes place is the bulb; the bulb is divided into two parts by the Auber line. In the dermal layer of skin, the bulb encloses dermal papilla. The papilla is the specific part of the bulb of the follicle that is responsible for hair growth, utilizing growth factors like insulin-like growth factor, keratinocyte growth factor, stem cell growth factor, and bone morphogenetic protein. Hair papilla contains capillaries and nerve fibers. The hair shaft determines the color, texture, and strength of the hair; the hair shaft has a cortex, cuticle, and sometimes a medulla [6]. Hair may be readily visible above the skin surface, not readily visible, or absent. Terminal hair is hair that is easily seen principally because it is long, darker, and thicker [7]. Fine hair, also called vellus hair, is the type that is not easy to see; this is because it consists of just medulla and is short. The type of fine hair in a fetus is lanugo hair; it is usually shed into the amniotic fluid. Some babies are born with lanugo hair [8]. Terminal hair and vellus hair may become club hair; club hair is hair that has stopped growing and is bound for shedding. Parts of the body that do not have hair at all are called glabrous skin; examples are in the palms and fingertips, soles, the inner surface and vermillion border of lips, and labia minora [9]. Other parts are eyelids (save the margins where eyelashes grow), glans penis, glans clitoridis (clitoral glans, head of clitoris). Hairlessness makes treatment of genital vitiligo difficult [10].

The arrector pili muscle has smooth muscle cells. Hair follicles are also absent on the lips, palms, and soles. In hair shedding, old hair is pushed out by new ones [11].

In the normal hair cycle, there is scalp hair replacement between 3 and 5 years [3]. The most common cause of diffuse hair loss is telogen effluvium. Other causes of diffuse hair loss include hair shaft abnormalities like unruly hair and breakage of hair, diffuse type of alopecia areata, congenital hypotrichosis, congenital atrichia, anagen effluvium, loose anagen hair syndrome, and trichotillomania [12].

When a patient complains of hair loss, it could be an increase in the number of hairs lost daily or hairlessness in one or more parts of the body; the first is effluvium and the second is alopecia [13]. Effluvium may occur after childbirth; in this case it could be physiological. This condition of excessive loss of hair may be pathological; this occurs in systemic conditions like thyroid dysfunction, iron deficiency, or the effect of medications. Telogen effluvium is the usual cause of diffuse non-scarring alopecia. The feature of telogen effluvium is the sudden onset of diffuse hair loss, which usually occurs 2 to 3 months after exposure to the cause. While acute telogen effluvium is a self-limiting condition that usually resolves within 6 months, chronic telogen effluvium continues even after 6 months [11]. Telogen is the resting or quiescent phase in hair growth cycle, with the hair in readiness to be shed.

Androgenetic alopecia (with diffuse hair thinning) may occur in females over the scalp top; it may also affect males, in which case the patient presents with receding hairlines in the temporal scalp and the parietal region inferior to the vertex. Other conditions with scalp hair loss are alopecia areata, folliculitis decalvans, lichen planopilaris, and Kossard's frontal fibrosing alopecia, which presents as a receding frontal hairline and loss of eyebrows. The description differentiates from a patient with Hansen's disease (leprosy) who has superciliary madarosis without frontal hairline recession [14].

5. D The external part of sweat glands is found on the skin surface and is the pore. Sweat glands are responsible for certain people's hands being moist. Eccrine glands are common on the back, the neck, and the forehead. The type called apocrine glands produces secretions with a scent; they are found in the axillae and groin. Ceruminous glands and female mammary glands are modified apocrine sweat glands.

6. B With respect to long bones, the diaphysis is synonymous with the shaft. The epiphysis is at the ends of the bone. The part of the bone that participates in a joint is covered with hyaline cartilage. The periosteum is vascular. Cortical bones are found in the bone shaft, and cancellous (spongy) bones are in the epiphysis.

7. C In children, vitamin D deficiency leads to rickets. Androgens and estrogens are responsible for significant growth of long bones during puberty. Also, growth hormone encourages growth of long bones at the epiphyseal disks. Vitamin C is required for collagen synthesis in bone. Exercise tends to strengthen bones. Exercise boosts a person's quality of life. There are types of exercise that are designed to increase muscle strength. Muscle strength is one of the determinants of bone strength and a person's ability to maintain balance and coordination. Anyone, particularly those in the age bracket where falls are rife, whose level of coordination and balance is high is less at risk of developing osteoporosis. Although exercise is recognized to be useful in the prevention and treatment of osteoporosis, the number of physicians who know the appropriate exercise regimens to prescribe for various conditions is inadequate [15].

8. D Synovial joints are more complex than cartilaginous joints. Most joints in the human body are synovial joints [16]. Synovial joints are diarthrotic joints; diarthroses allow free movement. Synovial joints have both synovial membrane and articular cartilage. Synovial joints possess a joint capsule.

9. A In a synovial joint, there is an articular cartilage surface, which sits on a subchondral plate of dense cortical bone; cancellous (spongy) bone is deeper and provides support to the subchondral plate [17]. Dense connective tissue is a feature of the outer layer of the joint capsule. Ligaments reinforce the articular capsule. Parts of the synovial joint capsule that are subjected to compression forces during movement become fibrocartilaginous. When it is injured, the synovial capsule becomes lax, constricted, or attached to surrounding structures. Changes in synovial capsule are significant in disease conditions like osteoarthritis, rheumatoid arthritis, and ankylosing spondylitis [18]. Less elasticity occurs on healing.

10. D Elevation is the movement that is performed when shrugging the shoulders; the muscles that are utilized in elevation of the shoulders are the upper fibers of the trapezius, the levator scapulae, the rhomboid major, and the rhomboid minor. Regarding stabilizing the shoulder (glenohumeral) joint, the rotator cuff muscles are used via their tendons; there are four such muscles—the supraspinatus, infraspinatus, subscapularis, and teres minor [18, 19]. The shoulder girdle consists of two bones (the clavicle and the scapula); in addition to the rotator cuff muscles (that help to stabilize and protect the glenohumeral joint by holding the humeral head to the glenoid cavity), the muscles at the shoulder girdle are not limited to pectoralis major, pectoralis minor, deltoid major, deltoid minor, trapezius, and serratus anterior [19].

In their study, which involved dividing the subscapularis into three portions (superior, middle, and inferior), Omi et al. demonstrated that the deltoid, supraspinatus, and subscapularis muscles worked significantly during arm elevation in the scapular plane. The superior one-third of the subscapularis muscle performed significantly more than the inferior two-thirds during the exercise. The performance of the infraspinatus and teres minor muscles was comparatively low. Their findings suggest that the superior one-third of the subscapularis muscle contributes to arm elevation from 0 to 90° in the scapular plane in neutral rotation of the arm. The subjects in the study carried out arm elevation exercises in the scapular plane. The researchers defined the scapular plane as a plane that inclines 30° anteriorly from the coronal plane [20].

Supination is the movement of turning the hand so that the palm faces upward. Eversion results in the sole facing laterally. Lifting the upper limb to a horizontal position and making a 90° angle with the side of the body is abduction. Pushing one's chin forward is an example of protraction.

11. C The elbow joint capsule covers the radioulnar joint. The elbow is a complex joint, not just a hinge joint. There are three articulations in the elbow joint: the ulnohumeral joint, radiohumeral joint, and proximal radioulnar joint [21]. Several muscles are related to the elbow joint, with the result that this joint is the second most frequently injured joint in sports-related activities [21]. When examination of a patient with elbow joint dislocation shows instability of the joint or there are complex dislocations at the joint, surgical intervention may be a necessity. The aftermath of simple elbow dislocations is impressive, justifying the sportsperson returning to engage in their chosen sports with no significant impediment [22]. The knee joint is not only the largest but also the most complex synovial joint. The shoulder joint is a ball-and-socket joint, like the hip joint. The fibrocartilage, acetabular labrum, makes the acetabulum deeper.

12. B The rotator cuff consists of tendons of several muscles that blend with the capsule of the shoulder joint. The rotator cuff is a support for and reinforcement to the shoulder joint. The glenoidal labrum, a fibrocartilaginous tissue, forms a fibrocartilaginous rim that deepens the glenoid cavity. The scapular coracoid and acromion processes protect the articulating surfaces of the glenohumeral joint [23].

13. D Regarding the shoulder joint, the acromioclavicular and coracoclavicular articulations further enhance the range of shoulder movements [24]. The acromioclavicular joint is a diarthrodial (synovial) joint; this joint is formed by the lateral end of the clavicle articulating with the acromion process. The acromioclavicular joint is a plane-type synovial joint; it usually permits just gliding movement. By making the scapula attach to the thorax, an additional range of motion to the scapula is achieved; this joint, therefore, participates in effecting arm movements like flexion and abduction at the shoulder joint. The acromioclavicular joint also allows forces from the upper arm to be transferred to the rest of the body. The articulating surfaces of the acromioclavicular joint are lined with fibrocartilage [24].

The shoulder joint is completely covered by the capsule. The attachments of the capsule of the shoulder joint are the anatomical neck of the humerus and the circumference of the glenoid cavity. However, inferiorly, the capsule of the glenohumeral joint extends to attach to the medial aspect of the surgical neck of the humerus. This inferior part of the capsule does not enjoy the reinforcement caused by the attachment of rotator cuff muscles and associated ligaments and makes it weaker than the anterior, posterior, and superior portions of the capsule. This inferior part of the capsule of the shoulder joint, however, allows additional movement of abduction at the shoulder joint. Falling on an outstretched arm may easily overcome the supporting structures of the joint.

In the glenohumeral joint, there are multiple synovial bursae; they provide a cushioning effect between tendons and thus lessen friction inside the joint. The bursae that are present in the shoulder joint are the subscapular bursa, subacromial (subdeltoid) bursa, and subcoracoid bursa. The function of the subscapular bursa is a reduction in damage to the subscapularis from friction during internal shoulder rotation. Regarding the subacromial bursa, its function is to minimize friction under the deltoid muscle, thus extending the range of motion at the joint. The location of the subcoracoid bursa is between the coracoid process and the subscapularis muscle. Two of these bursae are important to doctors in clinical practice because they are prone to injury—they are subacromial and subscapular bursae [23].

14. D The elbow joint is an articulation between the humerus and both the ulna and radius. It is a hinge joint, which allows flexion and extension movements. The articulation between the humerus (at its capitulum) and the head of the radius (with a slightly concave surface) is a hinge joint. The articulation between the circumferential part of the radius in the annular ring and the radial notch of the proximal ulna is what constitutes a pivot joint; at this joint (the proximal radioulnar joint), pronation and supination take place. The elbow joint, by the ends of the humerus and ulna, allows flexion and extension movements. The main contributors to the hinge joint characterization of the elbow joint are the trochlea of the distal humerus and the trochlear notch of the proximal ulna (the ulnohumeral joint).

15. B Lymphatic organs in humans exclude the skin; this is because although the skin contains a rich network of lymphatic vessels and immunologic cells, it does not contain characteristic features of lymphoid tissue—specialized encapsulated structures and sites where development, maturation, and activation of lymphoid cells occur. The skin is strongly associated with the immune system, but it is not a primary or secondary lymphatic organ; rather, the skin contains "skin-associated lymphoid tissue" (SALT) [25]. The bone marrow and thymus are the primary lymphoid organs; they are where lymphocytes are synthesized and go through the maturation process. Secondary lymphoid organs, on the other hand, are where activation of immune responses takes place; the organs in this group are tonsils, spleen, lymph nodes, and mucosal-associated lymphoid tissues (like Peyer's patches, which are present in gut mucosa). The thymus, spleen, mucous membranes, bone marrow, tonsils, and lymph nodes are lymphatic organs—primary or secondary.

Regarding the thymus, the superior portion of the retrosternal mediastinum is its location. This organ is bilobed; the two lobes converge near the level of the manubrium sterni. The thymus measures 3.0–4.0 cm long and 2.5–3.5 cm wide [26]. A greater part of the thymus is in the anterior and anterosuperior mediastinum. Cervical extensions of the gland may cause the gland to assume a more superior location; it may, therefore, reach the inferior border of the thyroid gland. The connection between the thymus and the thyroid gland is the thyrothymic ligament [27].

Histologically, the thymus consists of cortex and medulla. The gland is made of four types of cells: epithelial, dendritic, mesenchymal, and endothelial cells [28, 29]. In humans, the thymus attains full maturity in utero. It undergoes progressive involution from about puberty. With declining immunological decline, the parenchyma of the thymus is replaced with adipose tissue. The thymus serves as the primary production and maturation site of immune cells, especially small lymphocytes. This organ provides progenitor cells to lymphoid tissues that are located in peripheral parts of the body; the thymus also supports their maturation and functionality [30].

With regard to the thymus gland, the most common indications for resection are myasthenia gravis or thymoma. It may be difficult to differentiate between the thymus and mediastinal fatty tissue; this is because of the consistency and appearance of the thymus gland that is undergoing involution and the replacement of its parenchyma with fatty tissue. It is, therefore, important not only to have a sound understanding of the anatomy and the relationships between the thymus gland and adjoining structures but also to exercise caution during surgical interventions on the thymus or in the area of the gland [31].

16. C Lymph channels are the origin of lymphatic vasculature; they are initially blind-ended capillaries that become small vessels that drain proximally via many lymph nodes. Superficial lymph vessels originate in subcutaneous tissues, and deep lymph vessels arise from deep tissues and accompany deep arteries, not veins. Collecting vessels exit from lymph nodes rather than drain into them; collecting vessels are synonymous with lymphatic trunks. The right lymphatic duct and the thoracic duct are a convergence of lymphatic trunks. The two lymphatic ducts open into their termination at the root of the neck, specifically at the right and left venous angles, respectively. The junction of a subclavian vein and internal jugular vein forms a venous angle.

17. D Regarding the lymph nodes of the upper limb, central nodes are related to the second part of the axillary artery—the part of the artery that lies posterior to the pectoralis minor muscle. Posterior nodes are synonymous with the subscapular nodes; they drain the posterior thoracic wall and the scapular area. Lateral nodes are also referred to as humeral nodes; these nodes that are the primary draining nodes of the upper limb are sited posterior to the axillary vein. Anterior nodes are the same as pectoral nodes; the anterior nodes drain the breast and the anterior wall of the thorax. Apical nodes are located near the first part of the axillary artery and vein. Filtration of lymphatic fluid (lymph) from the central nodes of the axilla takes place in this group of lymph nodes. The subclavian lymphatic trunk arises from the apical group of lymph nodes; the subclavian trunk then drains its contents into the right lymphatic duct. Both superficial and deep lymphatics of the upper extremity ultimately drain into the lymph nodes in the axilla (axillary nodes). Cubital lymph nodes and supratrochlear lymph nodes are also present at the elbow, and there are further lymph nodes (brachial lymph nodes and deltopectoral lymph nodes) that drain lymphatic fluid from the upper limb [32].

In the upper limb, the superficial lymphatic vessels run inside subcutaneous tissue; they do so in close relationship with the main subcutaneous veins. Most upper limb lymphatic vessels flow into one main lymph node in the axillary region (referred to as the sentry lymph node). Some lymphatic vessels course along the posterior aspect of the forearm and bypass the sentry node to access lymph nodes that are smaller than sentry nodes. Sentry nodes are larger than regular lymph nodes [33].

18. C Lymph from the breast goes to the anterior lymph nodes [34]. The axillary lymph nodes are in the axillary pad of fat; the axillary lymph nodes are in five groups. The five groups are the anterior lymph nodes, the posterior lymph nodes, the lateral lymph nodes, the central lymph nodes, and the apical lymph nodes [35]. Pectoral lymph nodes are synonymous with anterior lymph nodes. Lymph from the arm drains into the lateral lymph nodes. Lymph from these anterior lymph nodes drains into the central and apical lymph nodes. Lymph that the pectoral (anterior) lymph nodes receives is from the breasts, the skin and muscles of the anterolateral wall of the body superior to the umbilicus. The anterior lymph nodes are located along the inferior border of the

 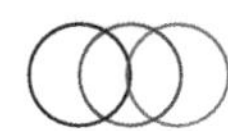

pectoralis minor and in proximity with the lateral thoracic artery and lateral thoracic vein. Lymph from the arm drains into the lateral lymph nodes. Lateral lymph nodes are synonymous with humeral lymph nodes. These lymph nodes are located on the lateral wall of the axilla. The lymph from the lateral lymph nodes continues to the apical lymph nodes, central lymph nodes, and deep cervical nodes.

The apical lymph nodes are the terminal lymph nodes. Their location is deep in the apex of the axilla. These lymph nodes receive lymphatic fluid from all other axillary groups of lymph nodes and from the upper portion of the breast. The convergence of efferent vessels from the apical group forms the subclavian lymphatic trunk which, on the right, drains into the right venous angle via the right lymphatic duct, and on the left, drains directly into the thoracic duct [36].

19. C The latissimus dorsi muscle contributes to the posterior wall of the axilla; other structures that form the posterior wall of the axilla are the subscapularis muscle and the teres major muscle. The serratus anterior and the intercostal muscles with ribs 1, 2, 3, and 4 form the medial wall of the axilla. The structures that form the anterior wall of the axilla are the pectoralis major muscle, pectoralis minor muscle, and clavipectoral fascia. The lateral wall of this important anatomical reference in the upper limb constitutes the short head of the biceps brachii muscle, coracobrachialis muscle, and the intertubercular groove of the humerus. Other borders of the axilla are the apex and the floor (base). Three bony structures create the superior wall (inlet, apex) of the axilla; these are the superior border of the scapula, the lateral border of the first rib, and the posterior surface of the clavicle. Skin and fascia that link the anterior and posterior walls of the axilla form its floor (base) [37].

20. A The bifurcation of the brachial artery occurs in the cubital fossa; this location is not in the axilla but much further distally. Structures that are present in the axilla are the axillary artery, axillary vein, and axillary lymph nodes. The axillary artery is the major artery that supplies arterial blood to the upper limb. The axillary artery starts from (or continues from) the subclavian artery as the subclavian artery appears under the first rib; at this point of entering the axilla, the subclavian artery is "renamed" the axillary artery. Prior to ending as the brachial artery, the axillary artery gives off six branches. The axillary artery is involved in important disease conditions; these include aneurysms, thrombosis, embolism, thoracic outlet syndrome, arteritis, and pseudoaneurysms. This artery and its branches are significant landmarks when specialists carry out surgical procedures like axillary lymph node dissections, shoulder operations, and bypass grafting. In these and related interventions, avoiding damage to the axillary artery is a vital requirement. Failing in the duty of care to the patient puts the patient's function of the rest of the upper limb in jeopardy. The relevant professionals are, therefore, required to be familiar with the anatomy of the axillary artery to minimize morbidity in patients who require interventions on or around the axillary artery [38].

21. C Irrespective of whatever tests that you may choose to request, the test that you must perform on this patient is electrocardiography (ECG, EKG). This is because of the history of a sudden illness, diaphoresis, and no evidence of trauma, yet the patient's principal complaint that draws the flatmate's attention is severe pain in the left arm; this is most likely referred cardiac pain to the left arm. In referred pain from the viscera, the pain is usually not very defined or precise and tends to travel along the same pathway with other nerves. Thus, visceral pain signals from the heart are transmitted by the sympathetic cardiac nerves to the upper thoracic segments (T1–T5) of the spinal cord. In the spinal cord, there is a synapse at the second-order neurons at the T1 to T5 level; the second-order neurons at this same level receive somatosensory input from the skin of the inner (medial) aspect of the left arm (including the upper lateral aspect of the left side of the chest). The intercostobrachial nerve is a lateral cutaneous branch of the second intercostal nerve. The afferent fibers, which subserve somatosensory sensation by the intercostobrachial nerve, enter the spinal cord at the T2 level, just like the afferent sympathetic cardiac nerves. Therefore, at the secondary spinothalamic neurons at the T2 spinal cord level, fibers from the heart and from the skin over the medial (inner) aspect of the arm converge. The patient's brain interprets this pain, which really originates from the heart in acute myocardial infarction from myocardial ischemia, as an unusually severe pain that arises from the inner aspect of the left upper arm. The patient with this referred pain would most likely also complain of pain of various degrees of severity from mild chest pain to stabbing chest pain. The intercostobrachial nerve (ICBN) is a cutaneous nerve that provides sensation to the lateral aspect of the chest, medial aspect of the upper part of the arm, and the axilla [39].

22. D ***Cords*** is the correct word and not "C**h**ord." The purpose of this multiple choice question is to draw the attention of the medical student and clinician to the importance of paying attention to spellings and other apparently small issues in the study and practice of medicine. Trunks, roots, divisions, and branches are the other terms used to describe structures in the brachial plexus [40].

23. D From its proximal to distal portions, the brachial plexus is divided into roots (also called rami), trunks, divisions, cords, and terminal branches. The brachial plexus is a large neurovascular bundle that traverses the axilla to provide innervation to the upper extremities. The anterior primary rami of C5 through T1 form the brachial plexus; the brachial plexus is responsible for the sensory and motor innervation of the upper limb. The trunks of the brachial plexus are present in the posterior triangle of the neck, specifically between the anterior scalene muscles and middle scalene muscles.

24. C In the brachial plexus, trunks have anterior and posterior divisions that form three cords. The anterior divisions of two trunks merge to form one of the cords, while the anterior division of the third trunk continues as another cord. The two anterior divisions of the superior and middle trunks merge to form the lateral cord. The anterior division of the inferior trunk is what continues as the medial cord. The three posterior divisions of the three trunks merge and form the posterior cord. In simple terms, of the six divisions, three merge to form the posterior cord, two merge to form the lateral cord, while one simply continues by changing its name at the transition point/boundary to become the medial cord. The ventral rami of the brachial plexus are from C5 to T1 spinal nerves; they are the five roots of the brachial plexus. The fibers of the rami intermix and form three trunks [40]. The three trunks of the brachial plexus are the superior trunk, middle trunk, and inferior trunk. It is the continuation of the C7 root that forms the middle trunk of the brachial plexus. The three trunks of the brachial plexus are formed in the posterior triangle of the neck. Each of them proceeds into the axilla.

In the supraclavicular fossa (just above the upper surface of the clavicle) of the posterior triangle, the C5 and C6 roots merge to form the superior trunk; in a similar fashion, C8 and T1 roots form the inferior trunk. The middle trunk has just been mentioned as a continuation of the anterior ramus of the C7 spinal nerve.

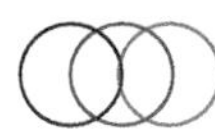

Spinal nerves are mixed nerves; they have a direct interaction with the spinal cord. A spinal nerve subserves motor information (efferent via **e**fferent fibers) and receives sensory information from the external surface of the body via the **a**fferent fibers. Each spinal nerve is derived from nerve fibers (rootlets), which are referred to as fila radicularia. Fila radicularia connect the posterior (dorsal) roots to the spinal cord, while the anterior (ventral) roots of spinal nerves connect the nerves to the anterior column of the spinal cord. The roots connect via interneurons. The formation of a spinal nerve is from the joining of the root fibers inside the intervertebral foramina.

While the ventral root consists of efferent motor axons, the dorsal root comprises afferent sensory axons that transmit visceral and somatic sensations from peripheral receptors and transmit the information to the central nervous system [41]. In the upper limb, the spinal nerves between C5 and T1 carry out these important motor and sensory functions. Cords of the brachial plexus receive their arterial blood supply from the subclavian artery, axillary artery, and subscapular artery [42].

25. D The radial nerve (C5–T1) is the continuation of the posterior cord and provides motor innervation to all muscles in the posterior arm and forearm. In the arm, the muscles include triceps brachii, anconeus, brachioradialis, and extensor carpi radialis longus. The muscles that the radial nerve supplies motor innervation to in the forearm are the supinator and extensor carpi ulnaris, and in the wrist and digits, it provides motor innervation to the abductor pollicis longus and all the extensor muscles, such as the extensor digitorum, and the rest [43]. The median nerve provides motor innervation to the pronator teres; the pronator teres is one of the flexor muscles of the arm. Other muscles that the median nerve supplies are the flexor carpi radialis, flexor digitorum superficialis, and palmaris longus.

26. A The long thoracic nerve innervates the serratus anterior muscle; the long thoracic nerve takes its origin from the rami of C5, C6, and C7. The only other nerve that originates directly from the rami in the brachial plexus is the dorsal scapular nerve, which supplies the levator scapulae muscle; the dorsal scapular nerve arises from the rami of just one spinal nerve—C5. It is because the phrenic nerve obtains some fibers from C5 (C3, C4, C5), which creates irritation of the diaphragm (e.g., from blood in hemoperitoneum in a ruptured ectopic pregnancy), that a patient may experience pain in the shoulder tip, which receives sensory innervation through the suprascapular nerve (C4, C5, C6) and dorsal scapular nerve (C5). The long thoracic nerve courses alongside the lateral thoracic artery. The lateral pectoral nerve arises from the lateral cord, and it is a sole nonterminal branch; being the only nerve that branches off the lateral cord of the brachial plexus means that the lateral pectoral nerve is not among the other nerves that the lateral cord eventually gives off to supply the upper limb. The lateral pectoral nerve innervates the upper part of the pectoralis major muscle.

The three nonterminal branches that the medial cord gives off are the medial pectoral, medial brachial cutaneous, and medial antebrachial cutaneous nerves. The medial antebrachial cutaneous nerve innervates skin over the medial aspect of the forearm and not motor innervation to the pectoralis minor. Motor innervation to both the pectoralis minor muscle and pectoralis major muscle is by the medial pectoral nerve (C8–T1); innervation by another cutaneous nerve—the medial brachial cutaneous nerve—is to the medial aspect of the arm. The middle subscapular nerve (C6–C8) is synonymous with the thoracodorsal nerve; this nerve innervates the large muscle, latissimus dorsi, and the nerve courses alongside the thoracodorsal artery. The teres major muscle derives its innervation from the lower subscapular nerve (C5, C6); the lower subscapular nerve also innervates the subscapular muscle (subscapularis). The upper subscapular nerve innervates the subscapularis. The upper subscapular nerve, middle subscapular nerve, and lower subscapular nerves are the three non-terminal branches of the posterior cord of the brachial plexus. *NB*: The upper and lower subscapular nerves supply the respective portions of the subscapularis, while the middle subscapular nerve (thoracodorsal nerve) supplies the latissimus dorsi. The brachial plexus has five terminal branches: the axillary nerve, musculocutaneous nerve, median nerve, radial nerve, and ulnar nerve. There may be physiological variants of the brachial plexus; one that is relatively common is when there are contributions from C4 and T2 to the brachial plexus [44].

Two conditions of clinical significance pertaining to the brachial plexus are Erb's palsy and thoracic outlet syndromes. Erb's palsy results from obstetric trauma during childbirth; the injury is to the C5 and C6 roots of the brachial plexus in 40%–50% of cases. The clinical presentation of Erb's palsy is medial rotation at the shoulder, pronation of the forearm, and flexion at the wrist. Spontaneous recovery occurs in 90% of the patients [45]. Thoracic outlet syndromes are outcomes of compression of the brachial plexus in the thoracic outlet. The patient presents with pain in the neck, shoulder, arm, chest, and over the trapezius muscle [46].

Injuries to the brachial plexus or the peripheral nerves related to it characteristically pose significant impairment to the patient; the impairment is to the ipsilateral upper limb. If there is avulsion of a cervical nerve root, the incidence of neuropathic pain, from somatic nerve fiber and sensory nerve fiber damage, may reach 95% [45]. Treatment of the severe pain by a multidisciplinary approach may be required and could involve pharmacological, occupational therapy, psychological, and transcutaneous electrical nerve stimulation (TENS). In patients with extreme and refractory cases, neurosurgical interventions are available options [47].

27. A The trapezius enables a person to carry out multiple actions at the shoulder joint: elevation, lateral rotation, depression, and retraction. Elevation is achieved by its upper fibers, and depression is through its lower fibers.

28. C While the surgical neck, greater tubercle, intertubercular sulcus, anatomical neck, and the head of the humerus are in the proximal portion of the humerus, the deltoid tuberosity—for distal attachment of the deltoid muscle—is on the lateral aspect of the shaft of the humerus. Action at this point enables the deltoid muscle to achieve movement of the arm away from the body (abduction).

29. D The median cubital vein is relatively superficial and is large enough in most individuals to enable venipuncture. The four pulmonary veins return oxygenated blood to the left atrium. A brachiocephalic vein is formed by a subclavian vein and an internal jugular vein uniting—there are two brachiocephalic veins: the right and the left. The two brachiocephalic veins join to form the superior vena cava at the inferior border of the first right costal cartilage. Major veins maintain a path parallel to the corresponding main arteries. Blood from the liver travels to the inferior vena cava through hepatic veins.

30. B The basilic vein is a superficial vein that, at the wrist, takes its origin from the venous network of veins on the dorsum of the hand. It runs on the medial aspect of the forearm and, with the brachial veins, forms the axillary vein. While the basilic vein is a superficial vein, the brachial veins are paired deep veins; they are also called venae

 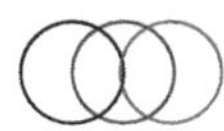

comitantes. These deep veins course in the arm in the company of the brachial artery. The brachial veins join with the basilic vein at the inferior border of the teres major to form the axillary vein. The unification of the radial vein and ulnar vein at the cubital fossa creates the brachial vein.

31. B The deltoid convexity is reduced or obliterated in shoulder dislocation. The convexity of the shoulder is principally due to a proper seating of the head of the humerus in the glenoid fossa of the scapula; in this normal situation, the overlying deltoid muscle with the skin covering creates a rounded contour. The acromion process is the flattened projection of the scapula, which lies posterior to the hook-shaped coracoid process, which is anteriorly disposed. In shoulder dislocation, there is disruption of the relationship between the humeral head and the glenoid fossa, with the head of the humerus taking a new position inferior to the glenoid cavity and assuming a forward (anterior) tilt. There is distortion or loss of the natural convexity at the shoulder from a combination of an emptiness or void posteriorly and a flattening inferior to the position of the acromion process. The displaced head of the humerus may be palpated in its new anterior location, where it lies inferior to the coracoid process.

The sternocleidomastoid causes elevation of the medial portion of a fractured clavicle. It is the third part of the axillary artery that is palpable in the axilla. The axillary and radial nerves may be damaged in patients who use crutches. The brachial artery is palpable in the medial part of the arm.

32. C Involvement of the radial nerve in fracture of the humeral shaft results in wrist drop. For efficiency of grip, the ideal position of the wrist is a slight dorsiflexion (extension occurring at the wrist) of about 20 degrees and a slight ulnar deviation of about 10 degrees. It is in this position that the extrinsic finger flexor tendons can produce maximal force; this is difficult or impossible in wrist drop. In wrist drop, the hand and fingers are forced by the unopposed functional flexor muscles of the wrist and digits to assume a flexed or dropped position; this position is due to paralysis of the extensor muscles that ought to have maintained the wrist in an optimal position for the balance of forces between the flexors and extensors to allow desired grip. The clavicle is the most frequently fractured bone of the shoulder girdle and one of the most frequently fractured bones in the entire body. The proximal part of the humerus is abducted when the humeral fracture line is below the insertion of the deltoid muscle; this is because the deltoid, by its three distal attachments at the same location (deltoid tuberosity), is able to pull the proximal part laterally away from the distal part of the humerus. The posterior border of the ulna is palpable throughout its length. The "anatomical snuffbox" is distal to the radial styloid process.

33. D Injury to the median nerve proximal to the flexor retinaculum makes thumb opposition impossible; this is because of damage to the median nerve proximal to (before) the origin of the motor branch, which supplies the opponens pollicis that performs opposition of the thumb. Damage to the deep branch of the radial nerve (posterior interosseous nerve) does not cause total wrist drop, which presents with flaccidity; this is because extensors of the carpus or the brachioradialis may not have been involved in the injury to the nerve. Injuries to the ulnar nerve are likely in fractures of the humeral medial epicondyle because of the close relationship. At the wrist, injuries to the median nerve (not ulnar nerve) result in paralysis of the thenar eminence muscles. In supracondylar humeral fracture involving the median nerve, pronation is impaired because the median nerve supplies the pronator teres muscle.

34. C The insertion of the pronator teres muscle is proximal to and far from the flexor retinaculum; it is inserted to the middle of the radius at the point of greatest lateral curvature. This makes pronator teres the most efficient pronator of the forearm. By virtue of the ulnar artery and ulnar nerve being together as they traverse Guyon's canal (the space that lies superficial to the flexor retinaculum), the artery and nerve are usually injured by the same injury. Guyon's canal is in the medial aspect of the wrist. The boundaries of this canal are the pisiform bone, the hook of hamate, and the pisohamate ligament (that connects the pisiform bone with the hamate). Trauma to the ulnar artery may result in the formation of a thrombus, aneurysm, damage to the intima of the artery, or in severe cases, transection of the artery. The palmar cutaneous branch of the median nerve is also prone to injury because it is similarly superficial to the flexor retinaculum.

35. B The ulnar artery is palpable lateral to the flexor carpi ulnaris tendon. The radial artery is palpable in the "anatomical snuffbox." The median nerve provides the innervation of all the muscles of the thenar eminence. The radial artery is palpable lateral to the flexor carpi radialis tendon.

36. A Anatomically, the scapular "head" is the thickened portion at the lateral angle; this lateral angle bears the glenoid cavity where the scapula articulates with the humerus, forming the glenohumeral joint; the glenoid fossa at its head lies in between the acromion and coracoid processes. The two processes of the scapula are the coracoid and acromion processes. The acromion process has a direct relationship with the lateral end of the clavicle (acromioclavicular joint). The acromion process is at the lateral end of the scapular spine, which is on the dorsal surface of the scapula; the acromion process also forms the tip of the shoulder. There is a shallow anterior concavity in the body (blade) of the scapula; this is the subscapular fossa (also called the costal surface) of the scapula.

37. C The medial end of a clavicle is attached to the manubrium sterni, while the lateral end is the acromial end. Clavicles have a somewhat S-shape. Clavicles are most prone to fracture at the middle third of their length; this is because this part of the clavicle is not only the thinnest portion but also lacks ligamentous support, unlike the medial and lateral thirds of the bone.

38. A It is the lesser tubercle that is located on the anterior portion of the upper part of the humerus; the greater tubercle is located laterally. It is the tendon of the biceps brachii that passes in the groove between the greater and lesser tubercles. The anatomical neck of the humerus is the depression or groove that surrounds the position of attachment of the shoulder joint capsule; it separates the humeral head from the tubercles. The surgical neck is further distal, the boundary between the humeral head and humeral shaft, and in proximity to the axillary nerve, and is the site where fractures frequently occur, exposing not only the axillary nerve but also the posterior circumflex humeral artery to damage [48].

39. D The coronoid fossa is located on the anterior surface of the humerus. The deltoid tuberosity is on the lateral side of approximately the mid-shaft of the humerus. The olecranon fossa receives a process of the ulna, i.e., the olecranon process. The epicondyles provide attachment to muscles and ligaments.

40. D Both flexion and extension movements at the elbow involve the trochlear and capitulum. The ulna is shorter than the radius. The radial tuberosity is the attachment of the distal end of the biceps brachii tendon. The pivoting motion of the head of the radius during

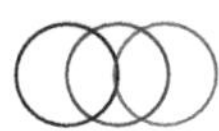

pronation causes the radial shaft to cross over the ulna. The olecranon process is a part of the ulna and to it is attached the tendon of the triceps brachii.

41. B The eight bones are carpals, not metacarpals. The fourteen phalanges are two for the thumb and three for each of the other fingers. Normally, there are five metacarpals and five fingers for each palm. The carpus has an anterior concavity that permits nerves and tendons to pass through.

42. B The deltoid and supraspinatus are abductors. Only the pectoralis major is a flexor, not the pectoralis minor. The pectoralis major can also adduct a raised arm. Pectoralis minor is involved in protraction and stabilization of the shoulder; it also plays a role as an accessory muscle of respiration as it elevates the ribs during inspiration.

43. A The coracobrachialis, from its name, is related to the coracoid process and the brachium (arm); its proximal attachment (origin) is the coracoid process of the scapula, and its distal attachment (insertion) is the medial aspect of the middle third of the humerus. The primary actions of the coracobrachialis are flexion and adduction of the arm at the glenohumeral joint; the secondary actions that this muscle performs are stabilization of the proximal end of the humerus in the glenoid fossa when the arm is abducted and resistance against a downward pulling force applied to the arm. The musculocutaneous nerve, with roots C5–C7, (which carries motor fibers to muscles and sensory fibers to skin) innervates the coracobrachialis. The arterial blood supply to this muscle is from two sources—the brachial artery and the anterior circumflex humeral artery. The anterior circumflex humeral artery arises from the third part of the axillary artery. The actions of teres major are extension and adduction. The thoracodorsal nerve provides nerve supply to latissimus dorsi. The suprascapular nerve supplies the supraspinatus and infraspinatus.

44. B The pectoralis major and teres major rotate the arm medially. The latissimus dorsi and pectoralis major have the same insertion—the intertubercular groove (sulcus) of the humerus; however, while the pectoralis major tendon is attached to the lateral lip/crest of the sulcus, the teres major tendon is attached to the medial lip/crest of the sulcus, and the latissimus dorsi tendon lies on the floor of the groove. The three muscles (pectoralis major, teres major, and latissimus dorsi) work in tandem to adduct and medially rotate the humerus—and thus, the arm [49]; the intertubercular groove (or sulcus) is synonymous with the bicipital groove. The coracobrachialis and pectoralis major cause flexion. The deltoid and teres minor have the same nerve supply—axillary nerve. The teres minor and infraspinatus rotate the arm laterally.

45. D The supinator rotates the forearm laterally. The musculocutaneous nerve supplies the biceps brachii and the coracobrachialis muscles. The brachialis is the strongest flexor of the elbow [50]. The brachioradialis is one of the muscles employed during flexion at the elbow.

46. C The nerve supply of the brachialis consists of the musculocutaneous nerve and the radial nerve; of these two nerves, the musculocutaneous nerve provides the main motor innervation. The brachialis is a deep-seated arm muscle and pure arm flexor at the elbow joint [50]. The radial nerve supplies the brachioradialis and supinator, which are extensor muscles; the radial nerve also supplies the triceps brachii. The pronator quadratus lies not between the proximal ends of the radius and ulna but between their distal ends. The triceps brachii has the olecranon process of the ulna as its insertion.

47. C While the surgical neck, greater tubercle, intertubercular sulcus, anatomical neck, and the head of the humerus are in the proximal portion of the humerus, the deltoid tuberosity is in the shaft of the humerus.

48. D The median antebrachial vein, median cubital vein, and accessory cephalic vein are superficial veins of the forearm; others include the basilic and cephalic veins at the level of the forearm—the basilic and cephalic veins extend superiorly and so are found in the arm [51]. Among the veins in the upper limb, the cephalic vein is the longest—it commences laterally, just after the venous network on the dorsum of the hand, and usually terminates by emptying into the axillary vein. There may be an abnormal communication between the cephalic vein and the external jugular vein [52].

Brachial veins are paired deep veins in the arm; brachial veins are venae comitantes of the brachial artery since they accompany the brachial artery. The merger of the radial vein and ulnar vein at the cubital fossa creates the brachial veins [53]. The radial vein, ulnar vein, and the brachial veins that they form are deep veins. The basilic vein (like the cephalic vein) is a superficial vein. The basilic vein commences in the forearm medially, just after the dorsal venous network of the hand; the basilic vein continues as a superficial vein proximally in the arm up to the middle 1/3 of the arm; at this point, it becomes a deep vein by penetrating the deep fascia of the arm. The basilic vein and paired brachial veins join at the inferior border of the teres major, where they form the axillary vein.

When the axillary vein crosses the lateral border of the first rib, its name changes to subclavian vein. In the upper chest, at the level of the sternoclavicular joint, the subclavian vein and the internal jugular vein join to form the brachiocephalic vein on the right and on the left [54]. "Brachiocephalic" is derived from "brachium" (arm) and "cephalus" (head)—this vein drains the upper limb, the head, and the neck. The right and left brachiocephalic veins unite to form the superior vena cava posterior to the manubrium sterni at the level of the costal cartilage of the right first rib. The superior vena cava empties venous blood into the right atrium [55].

49. C The brachial artery is in the anterior compartment of the arm, which consists of the biceps brachii, brachialis, and coracobrachialis. This artery is the major artery that provides blood supply to the arm. There are two muscles that constitute the posterior compartment of the arm: the triceps brachii and anconeus. The two muscles are arm extensors and receive their innervation from the radial nerve; the triceps brachii from the C6, C7, and C8 roots and the anconeus via the C7, C8, and T1 roots [56].

50. A Regarding having a good grip with the fingers, the action of the wrist extensors is required. With the wrist flexors, the wrist extensors create a stable base to enable the intrinsic and extrinsic flexor muscles of the digits (fingers) to perform maximally. From the report following their study titled "Factors Affecting Grip Force: Anatomy, Mechanics, and Referent Configurations," Ambike et al. showed the presence of multiple muscle groups that exert different actions on the wrist-grip system, which potentially permits various muscle activation patterns compatible with just about any task [57]. The actions of gripping and other actions at the wrist joint have multiple muscles in common. Wrist flexion and production of grip force are achieved by contributions from flexors of the distal phalanges of the digits: flexor digitorum profundus (distal interphalangeal joints of second to fifth digits) and flexor pollicis longus (interphalangeal joint of the thumb) [58, 59]. Contribution toward wrist extension and grip relaxation is by extensor digitorum communis [57].

 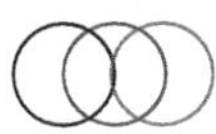

The hand is served by extrinsic muscles and intrinsic muscles. The intrinsic muscles of the hand are the muscles that originate from and insert in the hand; they, therefore, have their proximal attachments and distal attachments within the hands—these attachments are to bones, fasciae, and ligaments. The muscles of the hand are grouped into at least four compartments: the thenar compartment, hypothenar compartment, adductor compartment, and central palmar compartment. The muscles in the thenar compartment are the opponens pollicis, abductor pollicis brevis, and flexor pollicis brevis [58]. "Brevis" refers to their being "short, brief" and the word is appended to the name of a muscle when there is a long (longus) equivalent.

Hypothenar muscles are in the hypothenar compartment and form the hypothenar eminence. The four muscles are the opponens digiti minimi, abductor digiti minimi, flexor digiti minimi brevis, and palmaris brevis. The muscles in the hypothenar compartment serve the smallest of the digits (digiti minimi, fifth digit) [58]. The adductor compartment contains the adductor pollicis. The other intrinsic muscles are the lumbricals and interossei. The interossei are between the metacarpal bones. There are three palmar interossei (between the second and fifth metatarsals), and they cause adduction of the fingers; the dorsal interossei cause abduction of the fingers [58].

Thumb opposition is primarily the action of abductor pollicis brevis; other muscles that assist in performing this action are opponens pollicis, flexor pollicis brevis, and adductor pollicis. The thumb exerts a counterforce that stabilizes the gripped object on the anterior surfaces of the palm and fingers. During grip, both intrinsic and extrinsic hand muscles are put to use [60].

Figueroa-Jacinto et al. carried out a study in which the participants were asked to push with a single arm on a flat surface at elbow height. The practicality of the work has a bearing on object location, available space for placing hands, and the amount of physical space right from the design stages of workplaces and household spaces. The findings of their study indicated that when an individual is required to press or support their body on a flat surface, spaces should allow enough space to fit the palm, particularly if exertion of maximum force is needed. If an individual had the option of utilizing the entire hand to apply pressure on a surface, that option would be the preferred one [61]. Therefore, the results of their work may help in appreciating and predicting hand postures and finger loads based on object orientation and the required force [61].

CHAPTER 14

ANSWERS AND NOTES FOR MCQs ON LOWER LIMB

1. C The stratum lucidum has cells that are clear; this layer is an extra layer of epidermis in thick skin like the palms and soles. The stratum lucidum makes the epidermis have five layers in the palms and soles, unlike where there is thin skin; in the palms and soles, the layers of the epidermis (from the outermost to innermost) are as follows: stratum corneum, stratum lucidum, stratum granulosum, stratum spinosum, and stratum basale [1]. The stratum corneum consists of many layers of non-nucleated cells; these keratinized cells are both non-nucleated and flattened. Stratum spinosum has many layers of cells and is located beneath the stratum granulosum. There is only one layer of stem cells in the stratum basale; these essentially cuboidal cells produce keratinocytes. The stratum basale is also known as stratum germinativum [2].

The functions of skin are as follows: Protection of the body from a hostile external environment, which includes a myriad of chemicals in water, air, and soil; mechanical forces; all types of pathogens (disease-causing microorganisms); and ultraviolet radiation from the sun. Other functions of the skin include enabling us to appreciate and respond to various sensations like touch, temperature (heat and cold), pain, deep pressure, and vibration [1]. These sensations are from stimulation of a variety of nerve endings in the skin. The skin carries out endocrine functions, particularly the synthesis of vitamin D (calciferol). Vitamin D_3 (cholecalciferol) is synthesized in human skin from 7-dehydrocholesterol [3]. Vitamin D is essential for the gastrointestinal absorption of calcium. The skin is also an important player in immunity as it elaborates bioactive substances like cytokines; the skin also produces pheromones, sweat, and sebum [3]. Clinically, the skin is a diagnostic indicator of certain disease conditions; this is because the state of hydration (like dehydration with loss of skin turgor), degree of smoothness (e.g., cracked heels), characteristics of skin pigmentation (e.g., vitiligo, congenital melanocytic nevi), loss of or alteration in hair (e.g., tinea capitis, trichotillomania), and degree of elasticity are pointers to various diseases which may be minor conditions or severe ones like squamous cell carcinoma, basal cell carcinoma, and melanomas [4].

2. B Regarding temperature regulation, the set point for body temperature is controlled by the hypothalamus. Vasodilatation takes place in blood vessels of the skin to release heat from the body. Constriction of the deeper blood vessels diverts blood to the skin, which helps to eventually release the heat via the skin in a hot environment. An increased heartbeat encourages heat loss from the skin. When a person is subjected to heat stress, there is an increase in inotropy; this increase ensures that stroke volume is maintained or increased with an increase in cardiac output and blood flow. An increase in heart rate results from direct action of heat locally in the sinoatrial node area; there is a combination of removal of parasympathetic neural activity and an enhancement of cardiac sympathetic neural activity. The overall effect is an increase in cardiac output from the increase in both stroke volume and heart rate during exposure to heat stress [5]. In the skin, there is loss of heat. The structure of skin as the organ with the largest surface area and in direct contact with the exterior enhances heat loss in high external temperatures and makes a considerable contribution to the control of body temperature.

DOI: 10.1201/9781003783961-16

 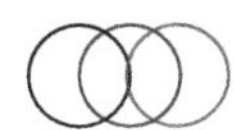

Sweat evaporation from the skin surface is vital for human thermoregulation, especially during periods of strenuous physical work or when people engage in any activity for prolonged periods in hot environments indoors or outdoors [6]. When people need to use personal protective equipment that covers the entire body, the body's core temperature is subjected to a sharp rise; a similar situation occurs when there is heat stress from vigorous exercise, which may result in heat exhaustion or heat stroke.

The ability to satisfactorily increase heat loss through cutaneous vasodilation and sweating is a determinant of temperature regulation in human beings when they are subjected to heat stress. Intrinsic factors like biological sex and age, and supervening conditions like significant injuries and diseases, have the capacity to cause changes in the natural physiological control at various levels. The changes may take place at thermal afferent signaling, central integration of thermal afferents, efferent signaling, or function of thermoregulation at the end-organ. There are also morphological features that, in combination with these intrinsic changes via passive effects on heat loss from the amount of surface area and heat storage from the composition of the mass or tissue, determine the response to heat exposure [7].

3. A Sebaceous glands are holocrine glands; in holocrine glands, glandular secretion is the result of disintegration of the entire cell for release of the formed secretion. Sebaceous glands produce fatty material. They are important in keeping hair waterproof and pliable. Sebaceous glands are usually connected to hair follicles, but sometimes they open directly to the skin surface, e.g., the lips and corners of the mouth [8]. One to four sebaceous glands are associated with one hair. In parts of the body where sebaceous glands are not associated with hair, their ducts open directly onto the skin surface; this also occurs in tarsal (Meibomian) glands of the eyelids. Sebaceous glands are not present on the palms and soles. With aging, sebaceous glands tend to assume an enlarged appearance in sebaceous hyperplasia—a benign condition. Sebaceous hyperplasia is cosmetically displeasing and may resemble basal cell carcinoma; this similarity may cause the physician to initiate investigations and treatment that are not only unnecessary, but cause the patient alarm and anxiety. Sebaceous adenomas may also arise from sebaceous glands [8].

4. A Sweat glands are synonymous with sudoriferous glands [9]. They arise from the deeper part of the dermis. Sudoriferous glands (sweat glands) may be eccrine, apocrine, or apoeccrine. All three types of sweat glands stay in the dermis. The gland comprises cells that secrete and a central lumen—it is into this lumen that their secretion (in this case, sweat) enters. While eccrine glands access the skin surface directly, apocrine glands open indirectly via hair follicles with which they are associated. This explains why eccrine glands can be found almost anywhere on the human skin, whether non-glabrous (hair-bearing) skin or glabrous (hairless, non-hair-bearing) skin. They are especially numerous on the palms and soles. Apocrine glands are in limited areas like the axilla, external ear canal, areola, and anogenital region. A coiled, secretory unit is at the deep end of a tubular duct in both eccrine glands and apocrine glands. In the secretory unit of eccrine glands, the epithelium is lined by cuboidal cells, while in apocrine glands, they are lined with either cuboidal cells or columnar cells [9]. Their activity tends to decrease with advancing age [10]. Apoeccrine glands develop from eccrine glands. They are similar to apocrine glands in that they are limited in distribution. These glands are found in the axillary region. Apoeccrine glands are more similar to eccrine glands in that the distal (upper) part of the duct connects to and empties sweat directly onto the skin surface. Apoeccrine glands produce large amounts of salt water secretions that are like eccrine sweat [11].

5. A The right lymphatic duct drains lymph from the right upper quadrant of the body. Lymphatic drainage of the rest of the body is carried out by the thoracic duct. The right lymphatic duct and the thoracic duct empty into the right and left subclavian veins, respectively. A typical lymph node consists of densely packed B and T cells, plasma cells, and macrophages. Lymph is essentially water; a small percentage is made up of protein, glucose, fat (in chyle), lymphocytes. Lymph enters lymph nodes via vessels that are narrower than the ones by which they exit nodes.

6. A The popliteal artery gives rise to genicular arteries. The saphenous veins are superficial veins and are useful in some emergency interventions. The vertical superficial lymph nodes drain lymph from only a part of the lower limb. The position of the great saphenous vein is constant/consistent at 2.5 cm (one fingerbreadth) anterior to (in front of) the most prominent part of the medial malleolus.

7. A The great saphenous vein (also called the greater saphenous vein, or long saphenous vein) is a preferred vein for performing venous cutdown. The position of this vein is relatively predictable, just as it is superficial. Cutdown on the great saphenous vein is an aseptic procedure. Venous cut-down to achieve resuscitation of patients in shock is mostly done using the great saphenous vein. When percutaneous venous access is unsuccessful, it is imperative to perform a venous cutdown; this is usually in patients who are in hemorrhagic or other forms of hypovolemic shock—the patient may be elderly, a younger adult, a child, or an infant. Other indications for venous cutdown include cardiac arrest without a palpable femoral pulse, patients with unavailability of access to the central line, extensive burns, individuals who require urgent treatment but have been abusing drugs by the intravenous route and all significant peripheral veins have become thrombosed, vascular operations requiring a vein patch, and vascular lower extremity bypass operations that require a vein conduit, like for femoral-popliteal bypass [12].

Contraindications to performing a cutdown are as follows: trauma to the cutdown site, massive pelvic injury with potential iliac vein avulsion, an active infection over the site that should be used for the procedure, evidence or history of coagulopathies, and availability of less-invasive methods of venous access. When none of the great saphenous veins are available for use because of involvement in injury, the basilic vein in the upper extremity may be a useful alternative for access since it is a superficial vein, although it is not as large as the great saphenous vein, which has a diameter of 4 mm at the standard site for cutdown in an adult patient [12].

8. A Peripheral arterial disease of the femoral artery is responsible for intermittent claudication of the lower limb (thigh and calf). The femoral artery is a continuation of the external iliac artery; the femoral artery continues as the popliteal artery. In the thigh, the femoral artery traverses the femoral triangle. The femoral artery is a common site of cannulation for various procedures; the same applies to its accompanying vein. The femoral artery supplies the anterior compartment of the thigh. The femoral artery is the main provider of arterial blood to the lower limb. The femoral artery, in conjunction with the deep femoral artery, its largest branch, supplies the muscles of the anterior, medial, and posterior compartments of the thigh. The alternative name for the deep femoral artery is the profunda femoris [13]. The femoral artery enters the thigh by passing inferior to the inguinal ligament at the mid-inguinal point; this point is an anatomical and clinical reference point—it is the halfway point between the anterior superior iliac spine and the pubic symphysis. The femoral artery gives off additional

 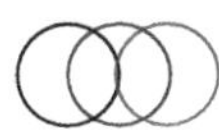

branches—the medial and lateral circumflex femoral arteries. The femoral artery courses around the femoral head and supplies surrounding muscles [13].

Femoral artery cannulation may be performed for diagnostic purposes or for interventional and therapeutic procedures. Diagnostic and monitoring procedures that are commonly performed using femoral artery cannulation include the following: Repeated blood sampling, continuous arterial pressure monitoring, cardiac catheterization, and angiography [14]. Regarding interventional and therapeutic procedures, the following are examples: Hemodialysis (although usually via the femoral vein), repair of congenital heart defects, placement of stents in narrowed coronary or peripheral arteries, angioplasty in patients with myocardial infarction for whom opening of blocked or stenosed coronary arteries is the objective, transcatheter aortic valve replacement in patients with aortic valve disease, initiation of cardiopulmonary bypass for minimally invasive cardiac surgery, and mechanical circulatory support insertion of devices like intra-aortic balloon pumps, Impella (temporary heart pumps), or venoarterial extracorporeal membrane oxygenation (V-A ECMO). The choice of the femoral artery approach for procedures requiring large-bore access is because the artery has a satisfactorily large diameter, which allows more ready access than arteries in other locations [14].

Contraindications pertaining to the access site for the use of novel femoral vascular closure devices include bacterial infection around the access site, multiple attempts to access the site in any part of the artery, obtaining access above the inguinal ligament or via deep femoral arteries, and obtaining access via the lateral surface of the artery wall [15].

9. C Apart from the descending genicular artery, branches of the femoral artery include the profunda femoris artery, superficial epigastric artery, superficial circumflex iliac artery, superficial external pudendal artery, and deep external pudendal artery. The popliteal artery is a continuation of the femoral artery; the sural artery and anterior tibial artery are branches of the popliteal artery—not of the femoral artery. The anterior tibial artery supplies the anterior crural compartment; at the ankle anteriorly, this artery becomes the dorsalis pedis artery [16].

10. A The blood supply to structures of the knee joint is by the popliteal artery [17]. The gastrocnemius and other muscles of the leg receive their blood supply from the popliteal artery via its anterior and posterior tibial branches. The musculocutaneous system of the upper lateral thorax and the scapula obtain their arterial supply from the axillary artery. The external carotid artery supplies the scalp via the superficial temporal artery that supplies the temporal and frontal regions, the posterior auricular artery that supplies the scalp superior and posterior to the auricle, the occipital artery that supplies the posterior part of the scalp [18]. In addition, the internal carotid artery supplies the scalp via its ophthalmic artery, which gives off the supraorbital and supratrochlear branches.

11. D There are six genicular arteries, the most proximal being the descending genicular artery that arises from the distal femoral artery. Genicular arteries supply the knee joint by forming an anastomosis of arteries [19]. The descending genicular artery supplies the patellar network. The anterior tibial artery, posterior tibial artery, and fibular artery, by their malleolar branches, provide the arterial supply to the ankle joint. Genicular artery embolization (GAE) is a new treatment modality for symptomatic osteoarthritis of the knee [19]. Chronic inflammation of the cartilage in osteoarthritis stimulates neoangiogenesis (formation of new blood vessels) and growth of sensory nerve fibers, which help in the development of knee pain. Genicular artery embolization selectively reduces areas of hypervascularity with a resultant decrease in pain [20, 21].

12. D The cuneiform is a short bone, while the frontal bone is a flat bone. The patella is a sesamoid bone; sesamoid bones reduce friction where tendons pass over bony prominences.

The patella is the largest sesamoid bone in the human body. It is anterior to the knee joint and is embedded in the tendon of the quadriceps femoris muscle. By virtue of its distinctive position in the lower extremities, the patella allows its joint (the patellofemoral joint) to have a greater mechanical advantage and enables the quadriceps to bear additional loads yet with less friction [22]. In the knee, the patellofemoral joint (patellofemoral connection is a bone-to-bone articulation); this bony articulation is between the posterior surface of the patella and the patellar surface or trochlear groove of the femur (which is the V-shaped surface of the distal end of the femur). This articulation on a smooth-surfaced cartilaginous surface allows the patella to glide in the superior direction during knee extension; it also allows the patella to glide inferiorly during knee flexion—the patella performs the function of a fulcrum and increases both the efficiency and leverage of the quadriceps femoris muscle. From extension to 90° of flexion, the patella holds the quadriceps femoris tendon away from the femur; when there is further flexion, there is formation of an extensive "tendo-femoral" contact area [22].

The patella provides a unique link between the tendon of the quadriceps femoris and the patellar ligament; the sesamoid bone enables flexion to the extension of the lower extremities. Its presence and the added advantage the patella provides allow the quadriceps tendon to carry forces that greatly exceed the average body weight. When knee movement progresses from flexion to extension, the patella shifts load-bearing to the patellofemoral and tendo-femoral connections [22].

When the knee is in full extension, the patella is the only extensor that achieves contact with the femur and functions as a pulley [23, 24].

The tendo-femoral connections of the knee joint consist of the joint/combined tendon of the quadriceps femoris, the patella, and the tibia. Proximally (superiorly), the quadriceps femoris tendon links the quadriceps femoris muscle to the patellar base (which is the superior pole of the patella). Distally (inferiorly), the continuation of the tendon links the apex of the patella (which is the inferior pole of the patella) to the tibial tubercle (the anterior surface of the proximal [upper] part of the tibia). This lower extension of the patellar tendon, which is between two bones (the lower end of the patella and the upper end of the tibia), is anatomically a ligament (patellar ligament; ligaments link bones); however, since it is the continuation of the quadriceps femoris tendon, it is still referred to as a tendon in clinical settings—patellar tendon reflex when eliciting the "knee jerk" in a hospital setting [25]. Tears of this tendon/ligament do occur but are uncommon. When it occurs, the injury is usually in men in their third or fourth decades of life (twenties and thirties) and individuals who have systemic conditions that present a negative impact to the integrity of tendons. In patients who have complete patellar tendon ruptures, primary repair is the standard of treatment [26].

The most frequently injured quadriceps muscle is rectus femoris muscle; this is by virtue of its superficial location compared with the other three members of the group. Contusion and rupture of this muscle occur frequently in sports [27]. Rectus femoris tears from trauma and rigorous exercise may occur at the proximal or distal attachments of the muscle. When it is partial, conservative treatment usually suffices, especially with restrictions in position and modification of activities. Rehabilitation of torn muscles may be achieved by physical therapy. Myositis ossificans and acute rectus femoris strain are other conditions that affect this thigh muscle.

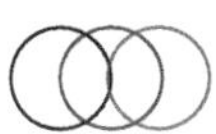

13. B The landmark for identification of the sciatic nerve is midway between the ischial tuberosity and the greater trochanter of the femur [28]. The femoral nerve lies lateral to the femoral pulse. The greater trochanter of the femur is palpable on the lateral surface of the thigh. Inferiorly, the rectus femoris inserts conjointly with the other quadriceps muscles on the base of the patella. The quadriceps femoris conjoined tendon is formed by the tendons of the rectus femoris, rectus lateralis, rectus intermedius, and rectus medialis [29]. Sportspeople who are prone to rectus femoris injury are those who engage in sports that require repetitive kicking and sprinting, especially in football globally [27]. The greater trochanter is a bony landmark; it provides a reference point for the measurement of joint motion. When the greater trochanter changes from its original location, conditions with abnormal movement like femoral anterior glide syndrome may be identified [30]. In patients with femoral anterior glide syndrome, there is a movement impairment with anterior hip pain that is worsened by flexion and extension of the hip. There is an alteration in gliding of the femoral head in the acetabulum from persistent overloading and irritation of the structures in the hip joint [31].

14. B The distal part of the femur is pulled upward when there is a fracture of the neck of the femur. The tibia is subcutaneous medially; open fractures of the shaft of the tibia are expected because of the subcutaneous disposition of the bone. Open fractures of the tibial diaphysis are severe injuries; they are frequently associated with severe soft-tissue injury. There is a high risk of infection, wound complications, and nonunion of the fractured ends of the fractures when there is concomitant contamination of the fracture site and devitalization of the soft tissue at the fracture site [32]. Of the mechanisms/causes of open fractures, the most frequent is trauma from road traffic accidents with automobile collisions. Other examples are gunshots, sports, direct blows/assaults, and falls. High-velocity impact is highly likely to cause open fractures.

15. B The Achilles tendon is superior to the calcaneus. The medial malleolus is at the distal end of the tibia, while the lateral malleolus is the distal end of the fibula. The posterior tibial artery is palpable midway between the medial malleolus and the Archilles tendon. The dorsalis pedis artery is a continuation of the anterior tibial artery. The artery runs in the subcutaneous tissue of the dorsal midfoot; it lies between the tendon of the extensor hallucis longus and the extensor digitorum longus muscles. The dorsalis pedis artery is not present in about 10% of individuals. It is important to note that blood pressure monitoring using this artery may show higher readings than in other peripheral sites [33]. The major branches of the dorsalis pedis artery are as follows: two or three medial tarsal arteries, lateral tarsal artery, arcuate artery, first dorsal metatarsal artery, and deep plantar artery—a terminal branch. The deep plantar artery enters the sole and, by uniting with the lateral plantar artery, completes the deep plantar arch.

The dorsalis pedis artery is a major landmark for palpating the pedal pulse when performing a physical examination on patients. This artery is also a veritable distal target for peripheral bypass surgery, as it is used for saving a lower limb in patients with complications from ischemic foot [34]. Reports from research show that the dorsalis pedis artery may arise from the peroneal (fibular) artery rather than be the continuation of the anterior tibial artery [35, 36]. The dorsalis pedis artery is important clinically because it enables clinicians to assess patients with peripheral artery disease by physical examination using palpation or by determining the ankle-brachial index [37, 38].

16. A The tibia is the shinbone. The tibia is also medial to the fibula. The patella is synonymous with the knee cap. The femur is the longest bone in the body. The findings from the study conducted by Noussios et al. in Northern Greece showed that the vertical diameter of femoral head has an acceptable percentage of error of 14.39% and can be used as a safe criterion for sex identification of human skeletal remains. The values in adult males are higher in the male sex than in the female sex [39].

17. B The hip joint capsule extends from the neck of the femur, making the head intra-articular. The blood supply to the head of the femur is through the ligamentum capitis, which attaches to the fovea capitis of the femoral head. The hip joint permits less freedom of movement than the shoulder joint. There are some disorders and diseases associated with the hip joint capsule; an example is femoroacetabular impingement (FAI) syndrome, which is a painful disorder of the hip. This condition features pathologic contact between the femur and acetabulum during hip movements like repetitive flexion [40].

18. B Of the listed muscles—flexor digitorum superficialis, soleus, gastrocnemius, and iliopsoas—the iliopsoas is the muscle involved in flexing the hip during marching. Flexor digitorum superficialis is a prime mover in flexion at the wrist. The soleus plantar flexes the foot. The gastrocnemius flexes the knee as well as plantar flexes the foot. The gastrocnemius flexes both the knee and foot because it is a bi-articular muscle—it crosses two joints (knee joint and ankle joint). Proximally, the origin of the gastrocnemius is superior to the knee joint; distally, the insertion is inferior to the ankle joint; the two heads at the proximal end of gastrocnemius are attached to the medial and lateral condyles of the femur—this design makes the muscle able to flex the knee joint. Distally, the gastrocnemius and the soleus converge to form the tendo-Achilles (Achilles tendon); this robust tendon is attached to the posterior surface of the calcaneus. Therefore, the proximal attachment allows contraction of the gastrocnemius to flex the hip, while the distal attachment permits contraction of gastrocnemius to cause plantarflexion of the foot at the ankle joint [41]. The design of the gastrocnemius muscle makes it a complex muscle that enables humans to maintain orthostatism, walk, run, and assume various postures. Gastrocnemius affects not only the entire lower limb but also movements of the hip and the lumbar region [42].

19. B The superior gluteal nerve is the nerve that provides innervation of the gluteus medius; the same nerve provides the nerve supply to gluteus minimus and tensor fasciae latae. The gluteus medius originates from the outer aspect of the ilium; the specific proximal attachment is the iliac crest. This is its superior boundary; the inferior boundary is the middle gluteal nerve, while the gluteal line is the posterior border. The insertion of the gluteus medius is the lateral surface of the greater trochanter of the femur; the site of the linea aspera is further inferior on the femur. The gluteus medius works in cooperation with the gluteus minimus and tensor fasciae latae to achieve efficient abduction of the thigh at the hip joint [43].

20. D Gluteus maximus paralysis still allows the individual to walk on a perfectly flat surface. Contraction of the gluteus maximus happens in the stance phase, which is between the heel touching the ground and the foot being flat on the ground or any other flat surface. The gluteus maximus counters further flexion of the hip and initiation of extension. The utility of this large muscle is in climbing up the steps of a staircase or getting up from a seated position [44]. The origin of the gluteus maximus is the posterior surface of the ilium, posterior to the posterior gluteal line and the lateral mass of the sacrum; additional points of origin are the lumbar fascia and sacrotuberous ligament [45].

 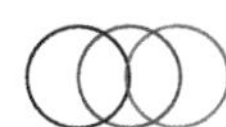

The gluteus maximus has two points where it inserts. The distal attachment of the superficial fibers of the gluteus maximus is the iliotibial tract; the insertion of the deep fibers is the gluteal tuberosity of the femur between the adductor magus and vastus lateralis muscles [46]. The arterial supply for gluteus maximus is by the superior gluteal artery and the inferior gluteal artery. Both arteries access the muscle at its center. The inferior gluteal artery descends along the greater trochanter, accompanied by the sciatic nerve. Rupturing the inferior gluteal artery results in gluteal compartment syndrome and sciatic nerve palsy [47]. Accidental injury to the inferior gluteal artery during the administration of an intramuscular injection makes the artery prone to formation of a pseudoaneurysm. The artery supplies the superficial skin and anastomoses with the perforating arteries of the lower limb. Ultrasound imaging highlighted gluteal activity differences of medial knee displacement in limbs during gait; the displacement may contribute to inadequacy in hip stabilization during daily repetitive task. These findings from the study by DeJong et al. potentiate the use of ultrasound imaging as a visual tool for either screening or intervention [44].

21. C The adductor magnus is a thigh muscle. The hip muscles listed on this MCQ are gemellus inferior, piriformis, and gluteus minimus. The gemellus superior is also a hip muscle. Structures in the gluteal region are muscles (gluteus maximus, gluteus medius, gluteus minimus, and piriformis), arteries (superior gluteal artery, inferior gluteal artery, and pudendal artery), nerves (superior gluteal nerve, inferior gluteal nerve, and sciatic nerve), and bones and ligaments (greater trochanter, ischial tuberosity, and sacrotuberous ligament) [48]. The muscles of the gluteal region are essential for humans to maintain stability in the upright position and for efficient movements from one place to another, including running [49, 50].

22. D The patella articulates with the femur, with the anterior surface of the distal femur. Muscles and ligaments are attached to the medial and lateral epicondyles.

23. A With regard to the muscles that move the thigh, psoas major and iliacus belong to the anterior group. The gluteal muscles are in the posterior group. The pectineus is an adductor; others are adductor longus, adductor magnus, and gracilis. The gracilis is a muscle of knee flexion. The tensor fasciae latae abducts, flexes, and rotates the thigh medially. The tensor fasciae latae is in the proximal anterolateral thigh; it lies between the superficial and deep fibers of the iliotibial band. The belly of the tensor fasciae latae usually terminates prior to the greater trochanter of the femur. The proximal attachment of the tensor fasciae latae consists of the anterior superior iliac spine and the anterior aspect of the iliac crest. The muscle descends on the anterolateral aspect over the thigh, maintaining a superficial course toward the greater trochanter of the femur. The distal attachment of the muscle is the iliotibial track/band; the band consists of the fascial aponeurosis of the gluteus maximus and the tensor fascia latae. The iliotibial band courses along the lateral aspect of the thigh. The attachment of the muscle via the iliotibial band is the Gerdy tubercle of the lateral condyle of the tibia. The tensor fasciae latae works in combination with other muscles (gluteus maximus, gluteus medius, and gluteus minimus) to achieve movements of the hip like flexion, abduction, and internal rotation. Via the attachment of the iliotibial band to the tibia, this muscle is also involved in flexion and lateral rotation of the knee. Of clinical relevance is the fact that the tensor fasciae latae assists in maintaining stability of the pelvis during standing and walking. The tensor fasciae latae is useful in reconstructive surgery, as portions of it serve as flaps. The tensor fasciae latae muscle flap is a reliable flap when used to cover ulcers in the ischial and trochanteric region after radical debridement. The tensor fasciae latae flap can be transferred with its sensitive nerve supply; this approach reduces the chances of ulcer recurrence [51].

24. D The sartorius is the longest muscle in humans. Like the gastrocnemius, the sartorius is a bi-articular muscle; in the case of the sartorius, the joints it crosses are the hip joint and the knee joint. The proximal attachment of the sartorius is the anterior superior iliac spine, where this origin is shared with the tensor fascia latae. The distal attachment of the sartorius is the superomedial aspect of the shaft of the tibia close to the tubercle (tuberosity) of the tibia. The two additional tendons at this insertion of the sartorius are the tendons of gracilis and semitendinosus; the conjoined tendons are pes anserinus. Functionally, the sartorius is peculiar in being a hip flexor and knee flexor [52]. At the hip, the sartorius not only causes flexion but also achieves external rotation. At the knee, the sartorius causes flexion and internal rotation. The name, sartorius, is derived from "sartor," which is derived from the Latin word "sarcire" and refers to the seated position of a tailor who is on duty; the position is figure-of-four with the hips and knees flexed. Collaborating constructively with other muscles, the sartorius allows the leg to be moved into the figure-of four position [52]. Therefore, by flexing both the leg and thigh, the sartorius causes flexion at the knee joint and at the hip joint. The biceps femoris belongs to the posterior compartment of the thigh; it is a hamstring muscle. The semitendinosus flexes and rotates the leg medially. The semitendinosus becomes tendinous in the mid-position of the thigh. The semimembranosus is a hamstring muscle.

25. D The linea aspera is in the shaft of the femur. The linea aspera (rough line) is a longitudinal crest or bony ridge along the posterior shaft of the middle third of the femur. This irregular crest has two lips [53]. The medial condyle and lateral epicondyle are at the distal end of the femur. The greater trochanter is at the proximal end of the bone.

26. C The vastus lateralis is part of the quadriceps femoris, which forms the anterior (i.e., extensor) compartment of the thigh. The vastus lateralis extends the knee just like the rest of the quadriceps muscle group (vastus medialis, vastus intermedius, and the rectus femoris) [52]. The rectus femoris additionally flexes the hip. Since the vastus lateralis performs extension and not flexion, it is unlikely to have been injured during the trauma. The sartorius, semimembranosus, semitendinosus, and popliteus flex the knee, and any of them could have been involved in the injury.

27. D The sartorius is the muscle utilized in crossing the legs. It flexes both the hip and the knee as it crosses both joints; it also laterally rotates the tibia and medially rotates the femur. The biceps femoris flexes the knee but extends the hip. The vastus intermedius extends the knee. Other muscles that flex the knee are the hamstrings; the hamstrings have long and short heads of the biceps femoris, semitendinosus, and semimembranosus. The popliteus also engages in knee flexion action, but it is principally an internal rotator of the tibia [54].

28. D Like other sesamoid bones, the presence of the patella within the tendon helps to reduce stress on that tendon and increase efficiency of the associated muscle during movements.

There are many sesamoid bones in the human body. Sesamoid bones frequently provide extra strength to related muscles; this advantage allows weight-bearing actions and support to the stability of the tendons in which sesamoid bones are embedded or to which they are closely related. In conjunction with the tendon(s) that a sesamoid bone

 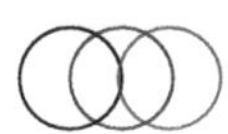

is associated with, a synovial joint is formed. At the knee, the patella amplifies joint leverage and the extensor properties. An injured patella seriously hampers the leverage and extensor capabilities at the joint, and this is particularly limiting to sportspeople and other active people [55, 56].

There are two broad categories of sesamoid bones, type A and B.

Type A sesamoid bones are adjacent to a joint and are a constituent of the synovial joint capsule. Type A sesamoid bones include the sesamoid bones associated with the hallucis muscle tendons, pollicis muscle tendons, and the patella. *Type B sesamoid bones* lie over bony prominences; they are separated from the bony prominence by a bursa situated beneath. The sesamoid bone of the peroneus (fibularis) longus tendon is an example of Type B sesamoid bone [57].

Sesamoid bones in other parts of the lower limb are the fabella (usually in proximity with the lateral head of the gastrocnemius), the hallux sesamoid pair (one each on the medial side and the lateral side of the first metatarsal bone), cyamella (buried in the tendon of the popliteus muscle), and os peroneum (located inside the peroneus longus tendon) [55].

Another type of sesamoid bone is the fibrocartilaginous sesamoid; this type of sesamoid provides marked flexibility and elasticity—flexibility from the fibrous component and elasticity from the cartilage tissue [58].

There are also sesamoid bones in the upper extremities, especially in the hand and wrist. There are usually five sesamoid bones per hand. Two sesamoid bones are present in the tendons of the flexor pollicis brevis and adductor pollicis. A third sesamoid bone is in the interphalangeal joint. The fourth and fifth sesamoid bones are located in the distal portion of the second metacarpal bone and the distal portion of the fifth metacarpal joint [59].

29. C The knee joint has two menisci. The two condyloid joints are between the tibia and femur. The gliding joint is between the femur and patella. The knee joint is associated with the patellar and oblique popliteal ligaments; others are the tibial collateral ligament, fibular collateral ligament, and arcuate popliteal ligament.

30. A The bursa associated with the knee joint is anatomically close to the largest sesamoid bone (the patella) and is called the suprapatellar bursa; the others are the prepatellar bursa and the infrapatellar bursae (superficial and deep). The bursae that are in the lower limb but are not anatomically close to the largest sesamoid bone are the tibial collateral ligament bursa, fibular collateral ligament bursa, the gastrocnemius-semimembranosus bursa, pes anserine bursa, and iliotibial bursa. The bursae that are present around the knee are in two groupings: the bursae around the patella and the ones beyond the patella [60, 61].

31. C Regarding bursae, the most important weight-bearing locations are the knees. A bursa contains fluid and is found either between skin and tendon or tendon and bone; in these locations, they reduce friction between the adjacent moving structures. The characteristic sites are the vicinity of large joints like the shoulder, elbow, hip, and knee. Bursae are also found in other sites that are not large joints. Examples of sites that are not large joints include the hand and wrists (radial bursa and ulnar bursa) and the foot and heel (subcutaneous medial malleolus bursa, retrocalcaneal bursa, subcutaneous calcaneal bursa, bursae near the big toe, intermetatarsal bursae). Trauma, infection, overuse, and hemorrhage are causes of inflammation of a bursa [60]. Other etiological factors regarding bursitis are inflammatory arthropathy and systemic diseases, of which collagen vascular disease is a good example. Bursitis may also be idiopathic [62]. Occupational characteristics may lead to the development of bursitis; examples of such occupation-related bursitis are prepatellar bursitis (housemaid's knee) and superficial infrapatellar bursitis (clergyman's knee).

32. D Some knee joint ligaments are intra-articular; the two cruciate ligaments cross each other as they go from tibia to femur. Rotation is possible when the knee is flexed. The tibial collateral ligament is synonymous with the medial collateral ligament.

33. B The knee joint normally contains not more than 0.5 mL of synovial fluid. Ball-and-socket joints allow movements in all planes. Synovial fluid has the consistency of uncooked egg albumin. Menisci are within synovial joints, e.g., the knee joint.

34. A The common peroneal nerve is part of the popliteal fossa. The popliteal artery is a deep structure. The gastrocnemius forms the lower boundaries.

35. C The medial border of the sartorius forms the lateral boundary of the femoral triangle. The femoral triangle is bounded superiorly (proximal border) by the inguinal ligament, not the inguinal canal. The medial boundary is formed by the lateral border of the adductor longus muscle. The intersection between the medial border of the sartorius and lateral border of the adductor longus muscle forms the apex of the femoral triangle inferiorly.

The floor of the femoral triangle is formed by pectineus, iliopsoas, adductor longus, and adductor brevis. In the clinical setting, the femoral triangle provides access to the femoral vein for central venous catheterization. From the medial aspect of the femoral triangle to the lateral border, the structures are readily remembered when the acronym "VAN" is used, with V representing the femoral vein, A stands for the femoral artery, and N refers to the femoral nerve [63]. The femoral triangle is a triangular depression that is a subfascial space in the superomedial aspect of the upper one-third of the anterior surface of the thigh [63].

36. A The adductor canal (Hunter's canal, subsartorial canal) is a tunnel that is distal to the anteromedial thigh and serves as a passageway for neurovascular structures. Depending on the sex of an adult, the average length of the adductor canal ranges between 8.5 and 11.5 cm [64].

The borders of the adductor canal are as follows: (a) The anterolateral border (margin) is formed by vastus medialis. (b) The adductor longus and magnus muscles constitute the posterolateral border. (c) The medial border (roof) is formed by the vasto-adductor membrane; superficial to the vasto-adductor membrane is the sartorius. (d) The proximal border is the apex (inferior border) of the femoral triangle at the intersection of the medial border of the sartorius and medial border of the adductor longus. (e) Regarding the distal border of the adductor canal, this termination is regarded as the adductor hiatus; among the five fibrous openings in the adductor magnus muscle, the adductor hiatus is the largest. The popliteal artery is the continuation of the superficial femoral artery (i.e., femoral artery) as it crosses the adductor hiatus distally [64]. The adductor hiatus allows femoral vessels to pass from the adductor canal superiorly into the popliteal fossa inferiorly [65].

37. D The plantaris courses deep to the gastrocnemius and constitutes the inferolateral border of the popliteal fossa; the plantaris and the lateral head of the gastrocnemius therefore form the inferolateral border of the popliteal fossa. The deepest component of the roof of the popliteal fossa is the deep fascia, also referred to as the popliteal fascia. Before

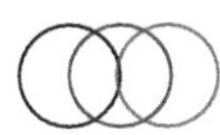

this deep fascia are skin, followed by superficial fascia. The semimembranosus and semitendinosus form the superomedial boundary. The superolateral boundary is made up of the biceps femoris muscle (short and long heads).

The popliteal fossa has more boundaries than the ones addressed in this MCQ. The lower border has inferomedial and inferolateral parts; the inferomedial part of the lower border is formed by the medial head of the gastrocnemius and inferolateral portion of the lower border is formed by the lateral head of the gastrocnemius. The floor of the fossa includes the popliteal surface of the femur, the capsule of the knee joint, popliteal ligament, and the fascia, which encases the popliteus muscle [66].

The shallow depression that lies posterior to the knee joint is referred to as the popliteal fossa. The popliteal fossa contains essential structures for lower extremity functionality. The constituents, which include vascular, nervous, lymphatic, and adipose structures, are prone to developing swellings, masses, and other abnormalities. Apart from patients complaining of pain in the posterior aspect of the knee from a variety of pathological conditions, they may present with bursae, Baker cyst (popliteal cyst), lymphadenopathy, thrombophlebitis, popliteal artery aneurysm, and neoplasia [66].

38. C The tibia is essentially a vertical, erect bone; the fibula is a smaller (thinner) bone than the tibia. Unlike the case of the tibia, the proximal (upper) part of the fibula is not involved in the formation of the knee joint [67]. There are two malleoli—the medial malleolus and lateral malleolus. The medial malleolus is the inferior end of the tibia, and the lateral malleolus is the distal (inferior, lower) end of the fibula. The lateral malleolus is readily palpable through skin, just like the medial malleolus. The proximal end of the fibula is the fibular head. The articulation between the tibia and fibula proximally is just inferior to the lateral condyle of the tibia. The medial and lateral condyles of the tibia have concave surfaces. The palpable prominence of the lower end of the tibia provides attachment for ligaments that are part of the deltoid ligament complex; this large, triangular ligament links the medial aspect of the lower end of the tibia with the bones at the medial aspect of the ankle—these bones are the talus, calcaneus, and navicular. The deltoid ligament (medial ankle ligament) complex consists of four ligaments in two layers (superficial and deep); the three ligaments in the superficial layer are the tibio-navicular ligament and tibio-calcaneal ligament. The ligaments that form the deep layer are the anterior tibiotalar ligament and posterior tibiotalar ligament—they link the lower end of the tibia directly with the talus bone [68]. The muscles that have tendons that pass behind the medial malleolus are the tibialis posterior, flexor digitorum longus, and flexor hallucis longus—these are efficiently held by the flexor retinaculum. They pass posterior to the medial malleolus to the foot.

39. D Osgood–Schlatter disease is painful swelling of a bony projection of the tibia inferior to the knee. Alternative names for Osgood–Schlatter disease are osteochondrosis, tibial tubercle apophysitis, and traction apophysitis of the tibial tubercle. Apophysis is a bony projection to which muscle attaches by its tendon; in the tibia, it is the tibial tubercle; in the femur, it is the greater trochanter. Tibial tubercle apophysitis causes anterior knee pain in athletes whose skeleton is not mature. In children and adolescents, apophysis serves as a secondary ossification center in the non-weight-bearing part of the bone [69]. Anterior knee pain in Osgood–Schlatter disease is characteristically atraumatic (no evidence of trauma) and of insidious (a gradual) onset. Physical examination of the patient demonstrates tenderness over the distal attachment of the patellar tendon (the tibial tuberosity). Osgood–Schlatter disease is a self-limiting condition. The etiology is repetitive extensor mechanism stress from activities like sprinting and jumping [70].

The proximal portions of the tibia are the medial and lateral condyles. The tibia is articulated at its upper end with the medial and lateral condyles of the femur. The tuberosity is on the anterior surface of the tibia.

40. A The upper surfaces of the tibia are concave and have an intercondylar eminence. The tibia provides an attachment anteriorly for the patellar ligament. The talus has a direct articulation with the tibia. This direct articulation between the tibia and the dome of the talus, along with the articulation between the fibula and the talus, form the talocrural joint, which is the main ankle joint (or true ankle joint); it is a syndesmotic uniaxial hinge joint. Movements that this joint allow are dorsiflexion and plantarflexion; however, in plantarflexion, it permits other movements including inversion and eversion [71]. Avascular necrosis of the talus may result from fracture of the talus. Fractures of the talus usually occur in the talar neck because that is the weakest part of the bone. Tarsal tunnel syndrome is another clinical condition associated with the talus. Arterial blood supply to the talus is from three main arteries—the peroneal artery, posterior tibial artery, and anterior tibial artery. Innervation of the medial side of the talus is from the posterior tibial nerve and saphenous nerve. The deep peroneal nerve innervates the dorsal portion of this bone. Its dorsolateral aspect receives innervation from the medial dorsal cutaneous nerve—a branch of the superficial peroneal nerve. The nerve supply to the lateral side of the talus is from the intermediate dorsal cutaneous nerve, which is a branch of the superficial peroneal nerve [72].

41. C The fibula is at the lateral side of the leg. The upper part of the fibula is the head and articulates with the tibia just inferior to the lateral condyle. At its inferior end, the fibula is a part of the ankle joint. This thin bone provides minimal weight-bearing function when compared with the tibia [73]. However, by the anterior tibiofibular ligament and posterior tibiofibular ligament, it contributes to stability of the ankle joint. The ligaments restrict excessive eversion and inversion movements while enhancing the hinge motion—the major motion of the ankle joint. The fibular shaft provides sites for attachment of muscles and ligaments. The muscles include the fibularis longus and fibularis brevis. The ligaments are the calcaneofibular ligament, anterior talofibular ligament, and posterior talofibular ligament.

42. A The fibula is the calf bone; it articulates with the ankle at the lateral malleolus. The tibia is medial to the fibula and does not enter the knee joint. An ankle fracture is a fracture of the distal tibia or fibula that forms the ankle joint, usually associated with ligament and soft tissue injury. Older persons are usually involved in injuries that result in lower limb fractures, specifically the ones that affect the tibia and fibula. Ankle fractures have associated injuries to ligaments and soft tissues. Selection of internal fixation methods for the management of fractures of the distal portion of the fibula should depend on the type of ankle fracture and the patient's peculiarities—like presence or absence of osteoporosis, quality of skin, and the state of surrounding soft tissues [74].

43. B Most of the toes have three phalanges—except the great toe. The great toe has two phalanges; the great toe has no middle phalanx. As a variant, the little toe may be bi-phalangeal, lacking the middle phalanx. Phalanges articulate proximally with metatarsals. Regarding the lateral toes (II–V) in humans, there is extreme reduction in the length of toes when compared with the great toe (hallux). The length reduces fairly regularly from the second to the fifth toes. This is one of the specific morphological features of the human foot in comparison with other primates, particularly other hominoids [75].

 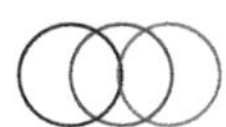

44. C The calcaneus is useful for body weight support. The posterior surface of the calcaneus has a circular convex structure with three distinct facets. Other than the two bony protrusions on the lateral surface of the calcaneus, this surface is a wide, flat surface; the protrusions are the peroneal tubercle (fibular trochlea) anteriorly and a bony elevation posteriorly for the attachment of the calcaneofibular ligament. On the medial surface of the calcaneus is the sustentaculum tali [76]. The blood supply to the calcaneus is from calcaneal anastomosis formed by branches of the posterior tibial and fibular arteries. Lymphatic drainage is principally to the popliteal and inguinal lymph nodes; it eventually enters the thoracic duct [76]. The nerve supply to the calcaneus is provided by the tibial nerve and sural nerve. The tibial nerve provides the medial calcaneal branches; the sural nerve gives off the lateral calcaneal branches [76]. The instep is the location of the metatarsals. The heads of the metatarsals are at their distal ends. The longitudinal arch spans between the heel and the toe. The talus is freely movable, articulating with the lower end of the tibia.

45. B The human foot is a complex and essential part of our anatomy and function; the design of the foot makes it possible for us to stand and move, turn, run, and perform various activities while in the erect position. The foot consists of bony, muscular, tendinous, ligamentous, vascular, and nervous tissues. Each of these may be involved in damage or pathological conditions. The foot is anatomically divided into three parts—the hindfoot, midfoot, and forefoot. There are 30 joints and at least 26 bones in the foot [77, 78]. The bones of the foot are grouped into tarsus (tarsal bones), metatarsus (metatarsal bones), and toes (phalanges) [79].

Seven bones form the tarsus; of these seven, two comprise the hindfoot. The two bones that make up the hindfoot are the talus and the calcaneum; the talus "sits atop" the calcaneus. The calcaneus is the largest of the bones of the tarsus [78]. By the distal ends of the two leg bones (tibia and fibula), the ankle joint is formed with the body of the talus (talar dome). There are three borders for the ankle joint (lateral, medial, and superior) formed, respectively, by the lateral malleolus, medial malleolus, and talar dome, which together comprise the C-shaped space referred to as the ankle mortise [80, 81].

46. B The talus is small only when compared with the calcaneus; it is, therefore, the second largest tarsal bone. The posterior part of the talus is the posterior process, which comprises the lateral tubercle, medial tubercle, and a groove for the tendon of flexor hallucis longus. The portion of the talus that is anterior to the posterior process consists of the trochlea, neck, and head; the head of the talus is, consequently, the most distal part of the talus, and it creates articulation with the navicular at the medial aspect of the transverse tarsal joint. Being at a level higher than the other tarsal bones, the talus slopes infero-medially to end at the head, which is covered with cartilage to articulate with the navicular as described [78, 82]. The calcaneus helps to support the weight of the body.

47. B The calcaneus forms the base of the heel. The metatarsus consists of five bones. The metatarsus articulates with the tarsal bones proximally. The head of a metatarsal bone is the distal part of the bone. Injuries attributable to stress to the metatarsal bones are common among military recruits, runners, and ballet dancers. Since magnetic resonance imaging and nuclear bone scans are more sensitive in picking up stress fractures in these bones, they are the preferred modality of assessment of patients with suspected fractures from exposure to repetitive stress. The usual sites of stress fractures in the foot and ankle are the head of the talus (subchondral), the tuberosity of the calcaneus, the navicular, the base of the first and fifth metatarsal bones, and the diaphysis to the neck of the second to fourth metatarsal bones [83]. While fatigue fractures result from healthy bone being subjected to repetitive stress, repeated stress to abnormally weakened bones causes insufficiency fractures. Stress fractures of metatarsal bones may, therefore, be of the fatigue fracture or insufficiency fracture variety [84].

The navicular articulates with the talus posteriorly. The navicular is wedge-shaped in the midfoot. This bone articulates with five tarsal bones, of which there are three cuneiforms, the talus, and the cuboid. The joints are syndesmoses. The navicular occasionally undergoes stress fracture. The navicular has four sides and two ends; the four sides are anterior, posterior, dorsal, and plantar aspects, while the ends are the medial and lateral ends [85].

48. D The transverse arch extends across the foot. Each of the metatarsals aligns with its corresponding phalanx. The talus is the only ankle bone that is freely movable. Movement of most of the tarsal bones is limited.

The arches of the foot make the sole of the human foot concave; the arches are present at birth. The three arches of the foot are (a) the transverse arch or anterior arch, (b) the medial arch or internal longitudinal arch, and (c) the lateral arch or external longitudinal arch. Arching of the foot makes humans unique and contributes to the ability of humans to be in the upright position. It contributes to weight bearing and weight distribution. An arched foot does not allow a complete footprint, unlike the case with a palm print. The medial part of the calcaneum, the talus, the navicular, the three cuneiform bones (lateral cuneiform, intermediate cuneiform, and medial cuneiform), and the metatarsals (save the lateral two, i.e., the first metatarsal, second metatarsal, and third metatarsal) constitute the medial longitudinal arch. This arch provides both stability and a supportive base when the foot performs weight-bearing action [86].

The bones that make up the lateral longitudinal arch are the calcaneus, cuboid, fourth metatarsal, and fifth metatarsal. The lateral longitudinal arch is lower than the medial longitudinal arch. The calcaneus and talus are involved in the formation of the two longitudinal arches. The lateral longitudinal arch forms "the small arc of a big circle" [86]. Two approaches for evaluating the human footprint are manual and instrumental. The manual method is tedious, while the instrumental method is expensive. Examples of the instrumental method used for assessing footprint and footprint abnormalities are digital photography, radiography, ink imprints, optical podoscopes, baropodometry, pedography, and platinum scanners [87]. From their research work, Gutiérrez-Vilahú et al. concluded that the Photoshop CS5 software method is reliable and valid for the study of footprints in young people with Down syndrome [88].

49. D The soleus causes plantar flexion; the gastrocnemius does the same. The tibialis posterior causes inversion; the peroneus longus causes eversion. Dorsal flexion results from the action of the tibialis anterior and extensor digitorum longus.

50. A The calcaneus is the most likely bone involved in the scenario of pain on stepping on the floor after waking up in the morning. Plantar heel pain may be from various causes; these etiologies may be local (from within the heel), referred (from outside the heel), or systemic (from diseases that affect other parts of the body but target the heel). Local causes include calcaneal stress fractures, plantar fasciitis, local tumors, atrophy of the plantar heel fat pad, plantar warts, and osteomyelitis. Other local causes may be neurological, such as posterior tarsal tunnel syndrome arising from entrapment of the tibial nerve, entrapment of the medial calcaneal nerve (branch of the tibial

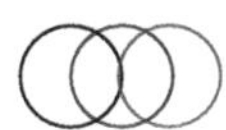

nerve proximal to the ankle flexor retinaculum)—the entrapment of this nerve may be from tight fascia, scarring from previous surgical intervention in the area, or from varicosities. The Baxter nerve (inferior calcaneal nerve) may also be compressed with resultant plantar heel pain.

Systemic diseases like seronegative spondyloarthropathies and rheumatoid arthritis can cause plantar heel pain. Metastases from cancers like gastric cancer, bronchogenic cancer, and bladder cancer can cause plantar heel pain. Referred pain from sacroiliac radiculopathy may also result in plantar heel pain.

In this 42-year-old obese patient with plantar heel pain, the cause may be a calcaneal spur, which is evidence of osteoarthritis involving the calcaneus. Obesity and his occupation may have contributed to it. Other risk factors for plantar heel pain include inappropriate footwear and protracted standing [89].

Chapter 15

ANSWERS AND NOTES FOR MCQs ON HEAD AND NECK

1. B The ossicles are small bones in the middle ear. Bones that are not rich in red marrow contain yellow marrow; yellow marrow is essentially fat, which has replaced red marrow as the individual grows into adulthood. Examples of bones that contain both red marrow and yellow marrow, but principally yellow marrow, in adults are the long bones of the upper extremity and long bones of the lower extremity. These are the humerus, radius, and ulna in the upper extremity and the femur, tibia, and fibula in the lower limb. In these long bones there is still red marrow, but its presence is limited to their proximal ends, principally the proximal ends of the humeri and femori. The diaphysis (middle portion of long bones) contains yellow marrow in adults [1]. Bone marrow has a high blood supply and has been found to have lymphatic drainage, although it was previously thought to lack lymphatic drainage. Part of the vascularization of the marrow of long bones is provided by the nutrient artery, which accesses the bone via the nutrient canal at the middle portion of the shaft. An anastomosis of arteries that arises from the periosteal arteries enters the marrow and penetrates cortical bone to provide the remainder of the arterial supply to long bones.

Hematopoiesis (synthesis of blood cells—erythrocytes, leukocytes, and platelets) is derived from two Greek words, *haima* for "blood" and *poiein* for "to make." The synonym is hemopoiesis. Blood islands of the yolk sac are the initial sites for hematopoiesis. During gestation, the liver and spleen take over blood cell synthesis. After birth, the primary site for hematopoiesis is the bone marrow. Other sites where hematopoiesis occurs are sites for extramedullary hematopoiesis; the most common site for extramedullary hematopoiesis is the spleen [1].

Bones that remain rich in red marrow include the sternum, ribs, vertebrae, and pelvis. This is why the sites for bone marrow biopsy are usually the sternum and the iliac crest; specifically, the posterosuperior aspect of the iliac crest is preferred for both bone marrow aspiration and biopsy because of its easier accessibility for the clinician and comfort and safety for the patient. The sternum is a last resort for bone marrow aspiration and is infrequently used for bone marrow biopsy [2].

Bone marrow fat is actively involved in storage of energy, metabolism of bone, endocrine function, and metastasis of tumors to bone. It is, therefore, far from being inert but is a metabolically active organ. Bone marrow fat is a significant depot of fat; only subcutaneous fat and visceral fat exceed it in amount of fat in the human body. Via direct cell contact and the secretion of adipocyte-derived factors, bone marrow adipocytes exert an influence on hematopoiesis. They also affect the progression of diseases like leukemia, multiple myeloma, and aplastic anemia [3].

2. B A synarthrosis is an immovable joint. Joints are synonymous with articulations. Joints make bone growth possible. They may be classified by the degree of movements possible. Joints are made up of bones and connective tissue; embryogenically, they are derived from mesenchyme. Development of bones may be direct or indirect. Direct development is via intramembranous ossification; indirect development is by

DOI: 10.1201/9781003783961-17

endochondral ossification. During intramembranous ossification, osteogenic cells result from direct differentiation of mesenchymal cells. Regarding endochondral ossification, hyaline cartilage is first formed by differentiation of mesenchymal cell, which is followed by the hyaline cartilage becoming replaced by bony tissue. The mesenchymal cells between the developing bones give rise to the connective tissue of the joint. In embryonic development of synovial joints, paraxial blastema forms hyaline cartilage; later, the articular capsule is formed. The cavity of a synovial joint is created by cell death within each interzone. The synovial joint cavity contains synovial fluid, which is also synthesized by mesenchymal cells [4]. The articular cartilage is a remnant of the hyaline cartilage that metamorphoses into long bones; this occurs between gestational weeks 6 and 8 by the process of endochondral ossification. Articular cartilage is formed at the end of epiphyses in the synovial joint cavity and decisively assists in the smooth movement that normal functioning synovial joints are known for [5, 6].

3. A Fibrous joints typically lie between bones that make close contact; syndesmosis is the type with an interosseous ligament (like the interosseous ligament between the tibia and fibula). Suture is the type found only between flat bones of the skull, and gomphosis is the type found between the root of a tooth and the jawbone.

A region where two bones make contact is a joint. Joints may be classified by two schemes—histological or functional. Histological classifications of a joint include the fibrous joint, cartilaginous joint, or synovial joint; this classification is based on the principal connective tissue that constitutes the joint. Functional classification of joints produces three types of joints: immovable synarthroses (immovable joints), amphiarthroses (slightly movable joints), and diarthroses (freely movable joints). In the singular form, the names of these joints end with "is" rather than the "es" for plural. The two classification schemes for joints therefore produce synarthroses, which are fibrous joints, amphiarthroses, which are cartilaginous joints, and diarthroses, which are synonymous with synovial joints [7, 8].

4. D Rotational movement is not possible at condyloid joints, e.g., at the metacarpophalangeal joint. All synovial joints are diarthroses. There are, however, a variety of synovial joints based on the function that the joint is designed to allow—i.e., the type of movement that the joint should permit. The arrangement of the ligaments that connect the bones in the articulation determines the range of movement. Synovial joints may be classified according to the movement types that are possible in the joint. The movement type makes a joint a hinge joint, saddle joint, planar joint, pivot joint, condyloid joint, or ball-and-socket joint [4].

Regarding condyloid joints, also referred to as ellipsoid joints, the articulation is between the shallow depression that is present in one of the bones and the rounded structure of another bone or other bones. The design of a condyloid joint makes it a biaxial joint—allowing movement in two axes. Condyloid joints allow four movements—flexion, extension, abduction, and adduction, e.g., at the metacarpophalangeal joint of the fingers, except the thumb [4]. The thumb is different because, apart from having a metacarpophalangeal joint that allows a wide range of movement, its carpometacarpal joint (which is proximal) allows a further and greater range of movement since it is a saddle joint—the combination of the movements at the metacarpophalangeal joint and the carpometacarpal joint is what gives the thumb the unique opposition movement. Opposition is the movement that allows the thumb to reach and contact the tips of the four medial fingers (second to fifth) of the ipsilateral (its) hand.

The pivot joint is exemplified by the anterior arch of the atlas and dens (odontoid process) of the axis. A pivot joint occurs where one bone must articulate with another bone that possesses a cylindrical end; this joint is covered in a ring formed by ligaments. This type of joint is uniaxial and permits rotational movement around just one axis, with the movable bone contribution to the joint moving inside the ring. In the chosen example of the joint formed by the atlas and axis, the first cervical vertebra (C1) forms a fixed base for the second cervical vertebra (C2) to use its vertical superior projection (odontoid process, dens) to rotate in just one axis (transverse axis); this movement of the axis within the atlas turns the head sideways to the left and right and is supported by ligaments, principally the transverse ligament of the atlas. This movement occurs in the atlantoaxial joint. The proximal radioulnar joint—discussed in an earlier chapter on the upper extremity—is another example; in this second example, the rotational movement in the joint allows pronation and supination of the forearm [4].

A ball-and-socket joint is a spheroidal joint. In a ball-and-socket joint, there is articulation between the rounded head of one bone and the concave receptacle of another bone; the former is the ball and the latter is the socket. This type of synovial joint is multiaxial (with multiple axes for movement); apart from rotation, the range of movement includes flexion, extension, abduction, and adduction. This type of synovial joint occurs only in two locations: the hip and shoulder. The ball-and-socket joint of the lower extremity (the acetabulofemoral joint, hip joint) has a deep socket formed by the acetabulum; in conjunction with the arrangement of the surrounding ligaments, there is a limitation to the movement of the femur in this joint. This is different from the shoulder joint, where the shallowness of the socket provided by the glenoid cavity allows a wide range of motion of the arm/humerus [4].

In a hinge joint, articulation is between the convex end of one bone and the concave edge of another. Hinge joints are uniaxial joints. Flexion and extension are characteristically the movements that occur at hinge joints like the knee joint, ankle joint, elbow joint, and interphalangeal joints.

Two saddle-shaped bones articulate to create a saddle joint; one of the bones is concave in one direction and convex in another. A saddle joint is biaxial; a saddle joint is exemplified in the upper limb by the joint formed between the trapezium (a carpal bone) and the first metacarpal bone. This saddle joint permits the thumb to flex and extend (movements that are parallel to the palm); it also allows the thumb to abduct and adduct (movements that are perpendicular to the palm). This joint makes it possible for opposition of the thumb to be achieved [4].

A planar joint is synonymous with a gliding joint. It is formed between two similarly sized bones that make contact at their flat surfaces; the movements in a planar (gliding) joint mirror the movements on a slide. Surrounding ligaments limit movements at these joints, although they are multiaxial joints. Examples of planar joints are the acromioclavicular joint, intertarsal joints, and intercarpal joints. The joint formed between the calcaneus and the cuboid on the lateral aspect of the foot (i.e., the calcaneocuboid joint) is different from the joints formed between other tarsal bones, as it is a saddle joint [4].

5. D Supraclavicular fossa is a part of the posterior triangle. The level of the cricoid cartilage is the sixth cervical vertebra. The isthmus of the thyroid gland overlies the third to fifth tracheal rings. The suprasternal notch corresponds to the level of the intervertebral disk between the second and third thoracic vertebrae (T2/T3) [9]. The suprasternal notch (jugular notch) is also the surface landmark for initial assessment of the tip of a

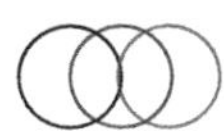

well-placed endotracheal tube in newborns [10]. This initial assessment of the position of the tip of an endotracheal tube by palpation may be further and better assessed by ultrasonography. The suprasternal notch may also serve as a valuable reference for chest compression depth in adults during cardiopulmonary resuscitation (CPR). The depth of chest compression during this life-saving procedure can be assessed by measuring the external anteroposterior diameters of the chest at the suprasternal notch and at the lower half of the sternum [9].

6. A The trachea is not palpable behind the lower part of the manubrium sterni because the palpating finger does not reach there; rather, it is at or above the suprasternal notch. The sternocleidomastoid muscle divides the neck into the anterior triangle and posterior triangle. The subclavian artery is palpable on the first rib. Thoracic outlet syndrome is a mechanical space clinical condition in which the brachial plexus, with or without the subclavian vessels, becomes compressed. When subclavian artery compression occurs, there is a structural anomaly with the first rib in almost all cases of this uncommon presentation—nerve compression is the more common reason for thoracic outlet syndrome [11].

Clinical diagnosis of thoracic outlet syndrome is often challenging, making the use of an imaging technique an essential addition to clinical assessment to achieve a reduction in the differential diagnoses and arrive at the definitive diagnosis; this happens when the structure that is compressed and the precise site of compression are identified. Identification of the structure that causes the compression is also important. Cervical plain radiography is the first imaging modality; it is used for assessing for bone abnormalities and to reduce the differential diagnoses. Thereafter, computed tomographic angiography or magnetic resonance imaging is carried out while doing postural maneuvers; these help in finding out what really occurs during which physical or postural activity by the patient [12].

7. D Cavernous sinus thrombosis may result from picking the boil, leading to spread of infection via facial veins to the cavernous sinus; other risk factors for this severe condition are acute sinusitis, periorbital infections, thrombophilia, and immunosuppression. Cavernous sinus thrombosis is a life-threatening condition, and there must be a high index of suspicion with identification of the following clinical features: fever, periorbital swelling, and ophthalmoplegia. Ophthalmoplegia occurs in cavernous sinus thrombosis because of the inflammatory responses to blocked veins that result in pressure effects on the nerves (CIII, CIV, and CVI) that supply the extraocular muscles; the pressure disrupts nerve function and, therefore, the function of the muscles that they innervate. These nerves traverse the cavernous sinus in their course to the eye muscles they serve. A high index of suspicion is critical for making the diagnosis of cavernous sinus thrombosis early and initiating robust management promptly [13]. The posterior triangle of the neck is where the external jugular vein is located. Occipital lymph nodes are in the apex of the posterior triangle. The superficial cervical nodes are found along the external jugular vein. The anterior and lateral part of the neck is the location of the internal jugular vein; this important vein lies within the carotid sheath. Blood from the scalp and deeper parts of the face drains into the external jugular vein; the external jugular vein eventually empties into the subclavian vein [14].

8. B The posterior cervical chain of lymph nodes becomes enlarged in trypanosomiasis; this particular lymphadenopathy (Winterbottom's sign) is present in this parasitic infection caused by *Trypanosoma brucei gambiense* [15]. Paralysis of the eleventh cranial nerve, not the eighth, would prevent the patient from shrugging. The anterior border of the masseter is where to palpate the facial artery. The thyroglossal duct is in the anterior triangle of the neck. Another important relationship is the bifurcation of the common carotid artery and the upper border of the thyroid cartilage. The thyroid cartilage covers and protects the anterior and lateral parts of the larynx. The thyroid cartilage extends vertically between the hyoid bone superiorly and the cricoid cartilage inferiorly. The thyroid cartilage is the largest of the main six cartilages (although the total number of cartilages of the larynx is nine). The thyroid cartilage is like a book that is opened halfway, with the back facing anteriorly. The meeting point of the two halves in the middle is the laryngeal prominence, better known as the Adam's apple.

9. B The internal jugular vein and the inferior belly of the omohyoid are not neck midline structures. The body of the hyoid bone, the thyroid cartilage, and the isthmus of the thyroid gland are midline structures in the neck. The isthmus of the thyroid gland is at the level of the second and third tracheal rings. The thyroid gland is in the anterior triangle. There are right and left lobes, which are the large lobes linked by an isthmus. There is also a smaller lobe referred to as the pyramidal lobe ("tubercle of Zuckerkandl"); the pyramidal lobe may be absent. On the posterior surfaces of each of the right and left lobes of the thyroid gland lie the superior parathyroid gland and inferior parathyroid gland (a total of four parathyroid glands). The vascular supply of the thyroid gland is hereby described for the right lobe and left lobe.

The right lobe of the thyroid gland receives arterial blood supply from the right inferior thyroid artery and the right superior thyroid artery. The right inferior thyroid artery arises from the thyrocervical trunk, which originates from the right subclavian artery [16]. The thyrocervical trunk gives off the supraclavicular artery, superficial cervical artery, and the right inferior thyroid artery. The right superior thyroid artery arises from the right external carotid artery and courses downward toward the upper part of the right lobe of the thyroid gland; on its way to the thyroid gland, it gives off the right superior laryngeal artery. Since the right inferior thyroid artery ultimately originates from the subclavian artery and the superior thyroid artery ultimately takes its origin from the common carotid artery, it means that the major arterial supply to the thyroid gland is dual—from the subclavian and carotid arterial systems. Regarding the venous drainage of the right lobe of the thyroid gland, the right superior thyroid vein and right middle thyroid vein empty into the right internal jugular vein, which drains into the right brachiocephalic vein. The right inferior thyroid vein drains directly into the right brachiocephalic vein.

Pertaining to the left lobe of the thyroid gland, the typical arterial supply is via the left inferior thyroid artery and left superior thyroid artery. The left inferior thyroid artery arises from the thyrocervical trunk, which arises from the left subclavian artery. The left superior thyroid artery arises from the left external carotid artery. The left superior thyroid vein empties into the internal jugular vein, just as the left middle thyroid vein does. The left inferior thyroid vein drains directly into the left brachiocephalic vein.

The thyroid ima artery is a third artery that is present in just about 10% of the population; while this artery usually arises from the brachiocephalic trunk, it may arise from many other arteries (large or small) like the arch of the aorta, brachiocephalic trunk up to the pericardiacophrenic artery, and internal thoracic artery; this variable artery provides arterial blood supply to the isthmus of the thyroid and the anterior surface of the gland [17].

The primary innervation of the thyroid gland is provided by the autonomic nervous system. Branches of the vagus nerve provide the parasympathetic input to the thyroid gland. Sympathetic fibers to the thyroid gland are from the superior, middle, and inferior cervical ganglia of the sympathetic trunk [18]. The autonomic nervous system achieves thyroidal vascular tone modulation.

10. D Supraclavicular lymph nodes and occipital lymph nodes are in the posterior triangle of the neck. The thyroid gland, superior thyroid artery, and sternohyoid muscle are structures in the anterior triangle of the neck. The posterior triangle of the neck consists of anterior, posterior, and inferior borders plus the roof, floor, and apex. The posterior border of the sternocleidomastoid muscle forms the anterior border of the posterior triangle of the neck. The anterior border of the posteriorly located trapezius forms the posterior border of the posterior triangle. The middle 1/3 of the clavicle forms the inferior border of the posterior triangle of the neck. The roof of this triangle is composed of both a superficial and a deeper part. The structures in the superficial part of the roof consist of skin, subcutaneous tissue, platysma muscle, and superficial nerves and blood vessels. The structure that makes the deeper part of the roof of this triangle consists of the investing layer of the deep cervical fascia that lies between the trapezius posteriorly and the sternocleidomastoid anteriorly. The floor of the posterior triangle has muscular and fascial components. The muscular part consists of splenius capitis, levator scapulae, scalenus medius, and scalenus posterior; the fascial part consists of the prevertebral layer of deep cervical fascia. Where the sternocleidomastoid and trapezius muscles meet at their attachment to the superior nuchal line of the occipital bone forms the apex of the posterior triangle [19].

11. C The mylohyoid (or diaphragma oris) is a muscle of the floor of the mouth; it does not play a part in facial expression. The buccinator, platysma, and levator labii superioris alaeque nasi play roles in making various expressions of the face. The mylohyoid is a flat, triangular, paired muscle with its proximal attachment at the mandible, close to the molar teeth. Its distal attachment is the hyoid bone. The mylohyoid elevates the hyoid bone and the oral cavity but depresses the mandible. The mylohyoid nerve arises from the inferior alveolar nerve, which is a branch of the mandibular division (the lowest of the three divisions) of the trigeminal nerve. The mylohyoid nerve provides motor nerve supply to the mylohyoid muscle. The mylohyoid artery, a branch of the inferior alveolar artery that itself arises from the internal maxillary artery, provides arterial supply to the mylohyoid muscle [20]. The mylohyoid muscle may be considered a muscular hammock that provides support to the floor of the mouth. This muscle also proves to be essential to achieving normal speech and swallowing.

12. B The superficial temporal artery is useful in carrying out pulse monitoring manually during anesthesia. In 2015, Bhaskar et al. reported two cases where superficial temporal artery pressure monitoring proved especially useful during cardiac surgery; they considered their work on selective use of superficial temporal artery pressure monitoring as unprecedented or the first to be reported [21].

The synonym of Bell's palsy is idiopathic facial nerve paralysis. Bell's palsy is a neuropathy and targets the facial nerve (the seventh cranial nerve, CN VII). When classical, the patient with Bell's palsy presents with unilateral facial weakness, reduced wrinkling of the forehead, nasolabial fold flattening, drooping of the corner of the mouth, in addition to drooling—all affecting one side of the face. With or without treatment, most patients fully recover within 6 months [22]. Bell's palsy is a lower motor neuron palsy of acute onset, idiopathic origin, and benign character [23]. The trigeminal nerve subserves facial skin sensation. Sagging of the right angle of the mouth is a result of right facial nerve palsy. Facial nerve branches have a relationship with the parotid gland.

Regarding the parotid gland, it is the largest of the major salivary glands; the major salivary glands are three paired salivary glands—parotid glands, submandibular glands, and submental glands. The location of the parotid gland is the retromandibular fossa; it is the main occupant of this space. Structures that border the parotid gland are the zygomatic arch (superiorly), the masseter muscle (anteriorly), and the sternocleidomastoid muscle (posteriorly). Its superficial lobe extends anteriorly and covers the ramus of the mandible and the posterior part of the masseter [24]. The parotid gland, like all salivary glands, has three major cell types: acinar cells, ductal cells, and myoepithelial cells. Their fundamental structure consists of ducts and secretory portions. The ducts are branched and open into the oral cavity while the gland's secretory endpieces (acini) synthesize saliva [25]. Salivary glands are exocrine glands.

13. A The muscles of mastication are the temporalis, masseter, lateral pterygoid, and medial pterygoid. Orbicularis oculi is one of the muscles of facial expression. The orbicularis oculi is a sphincteric muscle of the eyelids. The major function of the orbicularis oculi is closure of the eyelids, but it also supports drainage of lacrimal fluid (tears) [26]. Kitagawa et al. report a case of muscle fiber blending of orbicularis oculi with those of orbicularis oris. Both are sphincter muscles and both affect facial expression. The fibers that allowed the blending of these two orbicularis muscles that are anatomically distant although still on the face (i.e., eyes and mouth) were the fibers of the distal insertion of the levator labii superioris and levator anguli oris [27]. This is a rarity. The result of this variation could affect the usual expressions that follow the contraction of the sphincter muscles [27].

14. D The trapezius causes shrugging movement by its upper fibers; its lower fibers depress, i.e., move the scapula and shoulder downward. The rhomboid major links the medial part of the scapula with the upper thoracic vertebrae and therefore adducts the scapula. The serratus anterior helps in making a thrusting motion since it pulls the scapula antero-inferiorly. The pectoralis minor assists in achieving forceful inhalation by raising the upper ribs. The levator scapulae connects the cervical vertebrae (above) to the upper scapula (below) and, when it contracts, elevates the scapula. The proximal attachment of the levator scapulae is to the transverse processes of the first to fourth cervical vertebrae (C1–C4), while the distal attachment is at two sites—the superior angle and the medial border of the scapula [28].

15. D The dorsal scapular nerve innervates the rhomboid major. The eleventh cranial nerve is the accessory nerve—it innervates the trapezius. The dorsal scapular nerve also provides innervation for the levator scapulae; the nerve supply of the serratus anterior is the long thoracic nerve.

16. B The sternocleidomastoid is in the lateral part of the neck. Its fibers run inferosuperiorly inserting at the base of the skull posterior to the ear (at the mastoid). Contraction of the muscle turns the face to the contralateral (opposite) side. Working together, the pair of sternocleidomastoids can elevate the sternum or flex the head toward the chest [29].

17. D The trachea lies anterior to the esophagus. It is cylindrical but flexible. It is about 12.5 cm in an adult. There are 20 tracheal rings, but their open ends face posteriorly. The cartilaginous rings protect the trachea from collapsing. The major reason the C-shaped hyaline cartilage rings of the trachea are incomplete is to make an allowance for the trachea to narrow or get wider. Particularly when swallowing in the process of having a meal, esophagus expansion is feasible despite the presence of the trachea anteriorly [30].

18. C Tracheostomy prevents asphyxiation and allows adequate ventilation of the patient. The trachea spans between the end of the larynx and the bifurcation of the trachea into the right and left main (primary) bronchi. The tracheal rings are C-shaped and may be up to twenty; the rings are of hyaline cartilage.

19. B By contracting and relaxing, the trachealis allows modulation of airflow through the trachea. The trachealis spans the posterior space created by the open ends of the tracheal rings. In adults, the diameter of the trachea is about 2.5 cm. The inner surface of the trachea is lined by ciliated pseudostratified columnar epithelium. The bifurcation of the trachea into the right main bronchus is at a slightly higher level than the left; the right main bronchus is also wider than the left, and the angle it makes with the trachea is smaller than the angle the left primary bronchus makes with the trachea (about 20° versus 40°–60°); consequently, aspiration of tracheal contents tends to enter the right lung via the right bronchus rather than the left lung via the more angulated left main bronchus. The small angle that the right main bronchus makes with the trachea makes this bronchus essentially a "continuation" of the trachea [31].

20. A The trapezius enables a person to carry out multiple actions at the shoulder joint: elevation, lateral rotation, depression, and retraction. The trapezius has upper, middle, and lower fibers. Each of these parts contributes to the multiple movements that the muscle allows. The upper fibers allow the trapezius to elevate the scapula to produce the shrugging movement at the shoulder; these fibers also enable the trapezius to rotate the scapula superiorly, like when abducting the arm from the 90° position further superiorly to the 180° position. The middle fibers of the trapezius retract the scapula; the result is moving the scapula posteriorly and toward the spine, which is in the midline; these fibers also keep the scapula stable with support from the serratus anterior, which, in combination, enables the scapula to abut (stay against, adjoin) the rib cage posterolaterally. The action of the lower fibers of the trapezius is to depress the scapula (pull it inferiorly, downward); the lower fibers of the trapezius also assist the upper fibers and the serratus anterior in carrying out their primary functions. Overall, these motions of the trapezius lead to scapular rotation against the levator scapulae and the rhomboid muscles. This rotation, in combination with the action of the deltoid muscle, is paramount for the propulsion of objects.

The cervical plexus is formed by the ventral rami of the first four cervical spinal nerves (C1 to C4); it contributes to the sympathetic trunk and provides communications/linkages with the seventh cranial nerve (CN VII, facial nerve), tenth cranial nerve (CN X, vagus nerve), and eleventh cranial nerve (CN XI, spinal accessory nerve). The cervical plexus also gives off the following main cutaneous spinal nerve branches: the lesser occipital nerve, greater auricular nerve, transverse cervical nerve, and supraclavicular nerve—these are sensory nerves. It is the supraclavicular nerve that supplies the skin over the upper chest, neck, and shoulder (and, therefore, provides sensory innervation to the skin over the trapezius muscle). The spinal accessory nerve (CN X1, eleventh cranial nerve, by the cervical spinal nerve roots C1–C5 or C1–C6) provides the motor supply to the trapezius [32]. The brachial plexus is formed from the ventral rami of spinal nerves from the cervical and upper thoracic levels (C5–C8, and T1). Cervical is from "cervix" = neck; brachial is from "brachium" = arm.

21. B The cavernous sinus is a vascular sinus. The frontal sinus, sphenoidal sinus, maxillary sinus (antrum), and ethmoidal sinus are air sinuses.

22. C The temporalis is inserted into the coronoid process and anterior ramus of the mandible. The masseter elevates the mandible. The trigeminal nerve provides innervation to all muscles of mastication.

23. D By virtue of its location, the occipitalis does not participate in movements that lead to facial expression. Muscles that are associated with facial expression are orbicularis oculi, platysma, and epicranius.

24. A The orbicularis oris closes and protrudes the lips, e.g., in kissing. When expressing surprise, the epicranius is in use; the zygomaticus is involved in smiling. Paralysis of the buccinator prevents blowing.

25. D The lateral pterygoid, one of the muscles of mastication, pulls the jaw from side to side. The frontalis and occipitalis are scalp muscles, while the digastric is a muscle of the floor of the mouth. The mylohyoid is in use when the floor of the mouth is elevated; this muscle also elevates the hyoid bone. Among other actions, the platysma causes tension of the skin of the neck and lower face when it contracts. Levator palpebrae superioris alaeque nasi dilates the nostril and elevates the upper lip.

26. B Mastoid air cells (also called air cells of Lenoir) are in the mastoid process of the temporal bone. They are enclosed pockets/cavities of air. They are not part of the paranasal sinuses, which are found in the frontal, ethmoidal, maxillary, and sphenoid bones.

27. D The sphenoid bone has a sinus that opens into the nasal cavity through the spheno-ethmoidal recess. The characteristics of the mucous membranes of paranasal sinuses are like those of the nasal cavity mucous membrane. The structure of paranasal sinuses helps to reduce the weight of the skull by virtue of containing air. All paranasal sinuses drain into the nasal cavity via the ostia of the superior meatus, middle meatus, and sphenoethmoidal recess. The access of the frontal sinus, anterior ethmoidal sinus, and maxillary sinus into the nasal cavity is the middle meatus. The sphenoidal sinus drains through the sphenoethmoidal recess (which is superior to the superior meatus) into the nasal cavity. The posterior ethmoidal sinus opens via the superior meatus into the nasal cavity. The sphenoethmoidal recess is above the superior turbinate; the superior meatus is located between the superior turbinate and the middle turbinate; the middle meatus is between the middle turbinate and inferior turbinate. The inferior meatus, which is inferior to the inferior turbinate, does not drain the paranasal sinuses but the lacrimal apparatus via the nasolacrimal duct.

28. D The anterior fontanel is diamond-shaped. It is formed between two frontal bones and two parietal bones. The space is occupied by a membrane. The anterior fontanel represents the junction between the coronal suture and sagittal suture. The anterior fontanel allows growth and development of the skull and its contents. It normally closes at about 18 months after the birth of the child.

29. C Regarding the front seat passenger who did not wear a seat belt and hit their head on the windscreen (windshield) during a road traffic accident that involved vehicular impact with a stationary object, the frontal bone is likely to be fractured. Frontal

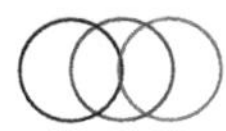

bone fractures with an accompanying frontal sinus fracture occur from motor vehicle accidents (MVAs), assaults, falling objects, falls, and trauma with penetrating injuries, e.g., gunshot wounds. The frontal cranial bone is thicker than bones in the lateral part of the face and resists trauma more than those bones. However, when the force from trauma is adequate to cause injuries to the frontal bone and accompanying frontal sinus injuries occur, a multidisciplinary team approach may be the standard way to achieve efficient management [33]. It is, therefore, necessary to call in specialists from other teams or refer the patient to a center where the specialists are available; this is to prevent complications and achieve no (or minimal) reduction in the quality of life of the patient from distortion of normal facial architecture.

30. C The vestibule is the space between the lips and cheeks in front and the teeth behind. The buccinator is in each cheek; the muscle in the lips is the orbicularis oris. The vermilion is the reddish or lighter part of the lips; it is highly vascular, richly innervated, and devoid of sweat glands or hair. Each of the lips has a frenulum linking the lip to the gum; the upper lip has the superior labial frenulum, and the lower lip has the inferior labial frenulum.

31. D The tongue has both serous lingual glands and mucous lingual glands that produce saliva. The tongue is essentially a muscular organ. The tongue is covered with nonkeratinized stratified squamous epithelium. The body of the tongue is the anterior 2/3, while the root is the posterior 1/3; while the body is in the oral cavity, the root is in the oropharynx. The tongue has taste buds, which are in three of the four types of papillae. Fungiform papillae occupy the tips and sides of the tongue; foliate papillae are at the sides of the tongue; vallate papillae form a V with the apex of this arrangement posteriorly disposed. Filiform papillae, though the most numerous, do not play a part in gustation [34].

32. C Molars and premolars crush and grind food using their broad surfaces. Canines are pointed, and this enables them to puncture and shred food. Incisors have cutting edges and are adapted for biting off food. The occlusal surfaces of teeth are the surfaces that meet to occlude the oral cavity when the teeth meet (occlusion). The teeth that have occlusal surfaces are the premolars and molars. The occlusal surfaces make it possible for the cusps, fissures, and grooves in the upper and lower premolars and molars to interlock and provide satisfactory grip and alignment for chewing and grinding food. Functional occlusal surfaces, therefore, enhance mastication and the eventual process of food digestion by significantly reducing the size of food and at the same time increasing the overall surface area of crushed food when compared with the initial form of the food.

The mandible is the largest bone in the skull of humans; it constitutes the lower jawline and shapes the contour of the inferior third of the human face. By virtue of its degree of mobility, the mandible is required in mastication and occlusion [35]. The muscles of mastication are the temporalis, masseter, medial pterygoid, and lateral pterygoid; these muscles allow a wide range of movements that are primarily of six types. The six types of mandibular movement are opening, closing, protrusion, retrusion, rightward jaw translation, and leftward jaw translation.

33. A Paralysis of the lateral rectus muscle results in medial squint. Correct associations include the following: the lacrimal gland and the superolateral wall of the orbit, ptosis and paralysis of the levator palpebrae superioris, and fracture of the floor of the orbit and "dislocation" of the eyeball into the maxillary sinus.

34. D The inferior oblique rotates the eye upward and away from the midline. Ciliary muscles are smooth muscles. The levator palpebrae superioris opens the eye. The lateral rectus rotates the eye away from the midline.

35. D The radial muscle fibers of the iris receive sympathetic nerve fiber supply; this aspect of the autonomic nervous supply to the iris causes pupillary dilatation (mydriasis). The trochlear nerve is the fourth cranial nerve (CN IV); it supplies the superior oblique. The abducens nerve—the sixth cranial nerve (CN VI)—supplies the lateral rectus. The third cranial nerve (CN III), the oculomotor nerve, subserves the inferior oblique; it also innervates the superior, inferior, and medial recti. The seventh cranial nerve (CN VII) is the facial nerve.

36. A The third cranial (oculomotor) nerve supplies both the levator palpebrae superioris and inferior oblique. It is the superior oblique that rotates the eye both downward and laterally. Therefore, the superior and inferior oblique muscles abduct the eye, i.e., rotate the eye outward. However, the superior oblique depresses the eye, and the inferior oblique elevates the eye; this apparently counterintuitive action is explained by the unique pulley (trochlea) location and actions on the tendons of these two oblique extrinsic muscles of the eye. Ciliary muscles relax the suspensory ligaments. Circular muscles of the iris constrict the pupil. The oculomotor nerve supplies most of the extrinsic eye muscles of the eye (except the superior oblique and lateral rectus).

37. A The lens is normally transparent. The choroid is the vascular middle layer of the wall of the eye and lies between the outer sclera and the inner retina; unlike a normal lens, which is transparent, a normal choroid is pigmented and has rich vascularization. The cornea is a part of the sclera; it is the transparent anterior part of the sclera that refracts light. The pupil is an opening in the iris.

38. B Colorless vision in dim light is provided by rods only. The retina contains more rods than cones; while there are 3 million cones, there are about 100 million rods. There are three sets of cones. The cones are concentrated in the fovea centralis, the area of sharpest vision; there are no rods in this part of the macula lutea. The fovea centralis is in the center of the macula lutea. The macula lutea is a small, flat spot sited precisely in the center of the posterior portion of the retina. As the fovea is responsible for high-acuity vision, there is a high concentration of cone photoreceptors in the fovea centralis because this is where perception of high-resolution images occurs; the fovea is endowed with approximately 50 cone cells per 100 micrometers squared in area and is elliptical horizontally. While the diameter of the macula is about 5.5 mm, the diameter of the fovea is just 0.35 mm [36].

39. C Horizontal movement of the two eyes to look at an object at the left involves concomitant contraction of the left lateral and the right medial recti. Superolateral movement of the eye is from contraction of the inferior oblique muscle. Tenderness when applying pressure to the tragus is an indicator of inflammation of the external ear. The lobule is the soft inferior end of the pinna; the helix is the upper rim of the earlobe.

40. B Central retinal artery and vein emerge from the optic disk. Tears gain access to the nose via the inferior meatus. Accommodation leads to constriction of the pupils. It is the pulling of the auricle superoposteriorly (upward and backward) at auroscopy (otoscopy) that straightens the external auditory meatus and enhances examination of

 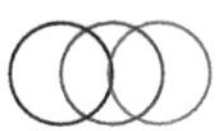

the tympanic membrane [37]. Upward and forward displacement tends to obliterate the meatus. Instrumental examination using plain otoscopy, pneumatic otoscopy, digital otoscopy, smartphone-enabled otoscopy, or micro-otoscopy (using a microscope) helps to assess a patient with relevant suspected ear conditions. The conditions that may be identified by otoscopy include otitis externa, impacted cerumen (earwax), aural foreign bodies, perforation of the tympanic membrane, acute and chronic otitis media, trauma, cholesteatoma, sclerosis of the tympanic membrane (tympanosclerosis, myringosclerosis), or external auditory canal exostoses [38].

41. D The mastoid bone should also be examined as in cases of otitis media as a differential diagnosis; this is because mastoiditis is a complication of otitis media. At otoscopy, a hyperemic, bulging tympanic membrane is an indicator of acute otitis media; this is because of fluid accumulating in the middle ear from increased secretion in this inflammatory/infective condition. The handle of the malleus normally runs posteroinferiorly. The finding of a cone of light below the tip of the handle of the malleus is normal.

42. A The opening of the middle ethmoidal sinus is into the middle meatus. The largest of the turbinates is the inferior turbinate. The laryngeal orifice is anterior to the esophagus.

43. C The clinical scenario of the MCQ is, "The parents of a pupil receive a telephone call that their 9-year-old son fell just after playing with classmates. They had held hands, creating a circle, and had run in a circular direction. The affected child was unwilling to join the group for this physical exercise." The most likely site of dysfunction in the child is the semicircular ducts since they are responsible for maintaining equilibrium during angular acceleration or deceleration. The utricle and saccule are responsible for static equilibrium and linear acceleration. The utricle and saccule are therefore responsible for enabling an individual to appreciate the specific orientation of the head when the body is stationary; they also maintain linear equilibrium when the person is moving essentially in a straight line, e.g., in a train or bus journey.

44. C Regarding a member of a church choir who develops weakness, a dry cough, and hoarseness of the voice, all in the past 3 days, the most likely site of infection is the vocal cords of the larynx. This patient's pathological condition is laryngitis. Recurrent laryngeal nerves arise from the vagus nerve (tenth cranial nerve, CN X) on the right side and left side. The level of the origin of the left recurrent laryngeal nerve is inferior to the aortic arch (at the T4/T5 vertebral level), which is lower than the T1/T2 level for the inferior surface of the right subclavian artery, where the right recurrent laryngeal artery loops over just after its origin from the right vagus nerve [39]. The two vagus nerves arise at the same vertebral level, but the left vagus nerve gives off the left recurrent laryngeal nerve at a level that is lower than the level at which right vagus nerve gives off the right equivalent.

Innervation of the majority of the intrinsic muscles of the larynx is by the recurrent laryngeal nerve or by its terminal portion—the inferior laryngeal nerve. The exception, the cricothyroid muscle, obtains its innervation from the external laryngeal nerve. Recurrent laryngeal nerves are branches of the vagus nerve; the vagus nerve carries motor, sensory, and parasympathetic fibers to the larynx. After they loop over the respective major arteries, these nerves ascend on the tracheoesophageal groove; they course on the posteromedial aspect of the thyroid gland and innervate the trachea, esophagus, and most of the intrinsic laryngeal muscles [40].

The internal laryngeal nerve and the superior laryngeal artery descend to the thyrohyoid membrane, where the internal laryngeal nerve fans out across the epiglottis and innervates the mucous membrane of the larynx below the vocal cords. The left recurrent laryngeal nerves course upward to the trachea and esophagus, then enter the larynx; the point of entry is posterior to the cricothyroid joint. The right recurrent laryngeal nerves branch off the vagus in the base of the neck, course lateral to the trachea, and enter the larynx between the cricoid cartilage and thyroid cartilage. It is normal for the internal and inferior laryngeal nerves to link at Galen anastomosis [40].

The larynx comprises a cartilaginous skeleton, ligaments, muscles, and a mucous membrane lining. The skeleton of the larynx consists of nine cartilages; the cartilages are one thyroid cartilage, one cricoid cartilage, one epiglottis, two arytenoid cartilages, two corniculate cartilages, and two cuneiform cartilages [40]. Possession of multiple joints between the cartilages makes the cartilage movable. The joint between the cricoid cartilage and thyroid cartilage (cricothyroid joint) links the thyroid cartilage to the cricoid arch. The cricoarytenoid joint provides the link between each arytenoid cartilage and the cricoid cartilage. The arycorniculate joint is the connection between the arytenoid cartilage and the Santorini cartilages. The corniculate cartilages are synonymous with cartilages of Santorini; these small, elastic, cone-shaped cartilages articulate with the apices of the arytenoid cartilages [40].

45. B Each palatine tonsil is embedded between the palatopharyngeal arch posteriorly and the palatoglossal arch anteriorly. The soft palate is muscular and glandular, boneless, and lies posterior to the hard palate. The palate (hard and soft palate) separates the oral cavity inferiorly from the nasal cavity superiorly. The uvula is a conical, midline projection of the soft palate; it is visible posteriorly when examining the oral cavity.

46. D Pharyngeal constrictors force food downward during deglutition. They are circular and there are three: the superior, middle, and inferior constrictors, and form the superficial layer of pharyngeal muscles. Both superficial and deep layers are skeletal muscles [41]. In the pharynx, the longitudinal muscles form the deep muscle layer, while the superficial muscle layer consists of circular muscles—it is important to note that this is the opposite of the arrangement of the muscle layers (of smooth muscles) in the intestines [42]. In the stomach, there is a third layer of muscles that churns food—this is the oblique layer, which is also of smooth muscle. In the pharynx, the outer circular layer and inner longitudinal layer constitute the muscular wall, which is entirely of skeletal muscles. The circular muscles in the outer layer are called the superior pharyngeal constrictor, middle pharyngeal constrictor, and inferior pharyngeal constrictor. The longitudinally disposed muscles of the inner layer are called palatopharyngeus, salpingopharyngeus, and stylopharyngeus [43].

Palatopharyngeus comprises two divisions: longitudinal and transverse. The proximal attachment of the palatopharyngeus is the hard palate; the distal attachment of this muscle is the pharyngeal wall. The palatopharyngeus spans the whole length of the pharynx. Its wide distribution shows that it causes elevation of the pharynx or depression of the soft palate; it additionally functions as a nasopharyngeal sphincter when the pharyngeal isthmus is closed [44].

Regarding the salpingopharyngeus, the proximal attachment is the cartilaginous part of the pharyngotympanic tube (Eustachian tube, auditory tube), and the distal attachment (insertion) is the palatopharyngeus muscle in the lateral pharyngeal wall. The function of the salpingopharyngeus is elevation of the pharynx and a contribution to opening of the Eustachian tube during deglutition (swallowing). The nerve supply to the salpingopharyngeus is the vagus nerve (CN X). In the conclusion of the article of their research work, Perta et al. stated as follows: "Though both the superior origin and inferior course of SP are highly variable, the size of the SP muscle is dependent on characteristics known to affect muscle fibers, such as the relationship between age and body weight. Given the consistent and quantifiable presence of the SP muscle, its potential role in velopharyngeal function for speech and swallowing is reconsidered" [45].

Stylopharyngeus is the third of the listed inner longitudinal muscles of the pharyngeal wall (with the circular constrictor muscles external to them). This thin and long muscle is attached proximally to the styloid process of the temporal bone; distally, by joining with fibers of the palatopharyngeal muscle, it attaches to the posterior border of the thyroid cartilage [46].

47. C The subclavius causes fixation and depression of the clavicle at the sternoclavicular joint. Platysma causes tension of skin of the lower face and anterior neck. The platysma also depresses the mandible and angle of the mouth. The sternocleidomastoid causes elevation of the clavicle and manubrium sterni at the sternoclavicular joint. Sternocleidomastoid also causes contralateral rotation of the neck and ipsilateral flexion at the cervical spine. Contraction of the sternocleidomastoid also achieves head and neck extension at the atlanto-occipital joint and superior cervical spine, and neck flexion at the inferior cervical vertebrae [47].

48. C Regarding the arterial blood supply to the head and neck, the artery that is not derived from the common carotid artery is the thyrocervical trunk. The thyrocervical trunk arises from the aortic arch. Direct branches of the common carotid artery are the internal carotid artery and external carotid artery. After the bifurcation of the common carotid artery, the external carotid artery gives off the following branches: ascending pharyngeal artery, superior thyroid artery, lingual artery, facial artery, occipital artery, posterior auricular artery, maxillary artery, transverse facial artery, and superficial temporal artery.

Most of the blood supply to the head and neck region is through the carotid arteries and vertebral arteries. There are two common carotid arteries and two vertebral arteries. While the right common carotid artery arises from the brachiocephalic artery (which is a branch from the aortic arch), the left common carotid artery arises directly from the aortic arch. The origin of the left common carotid artery is, therefore, in the thorax, while the origin of the right common carotid artery is in the neck [48]. It is also in the neck that the right common carotid artery and the left carotid artery bifurcate into the internal carotid artery and external carotid artery—this occurs at the level of the carotid sinus. At the bifurcation of each common carotid artery, there is a dilated/bulbous structure just inferior to the angle of the mandible and medial to the sternocleidomastoid muscle; it is rich in baroreceptors [49]. Baroreceptors are sensitive to blood pressure, and they are involved in blood pressure control. The internal carotid artery continues to the interior of the brain, where it provides arterial supply to the brain. The external carotid artery, by its branches, supplies the face and neck [48].

49. D With respect to the grouping of muscles in the neck, the scalene muscles are in the lateral aspect of the neck and are situated deep to the sternocleidomastoids. Strap muscles are the infrahyoid muscles—located below the hyoid bone. Innervation of the trapezius is by the spinal accessory nerve (CN XI, eleventh cranial nerve). The prevertebral muscles are deep-seated muscles.

The scalene muscles are three (scalenus anterior, scalenus medius, and scalenus posterior). The proximal attachment of the anterior scalene is the anterior tubercles of the transverse processes of the third to sixth cervical vertebrae; the distal attachment is the scalene tubercle of the superior surface of the first rib. With regard to the middle scalene muscle, its proximal attachment consists of the transverse processes of the last six cervical vertebrae, between the anterior and posterior tubercles; the distal attachment (insertion) is the superior surface of the first rib, posterior to the sulcus of the subclavian artery. The origin of the scalenus posterior is the posterior tubercles of the transverse processes of the last three or last four cervical vertebrae; the distal attachment is the anterior surface of the second rib [50].

The anterior and middle scalene muscles are the usual reference points for defining the posterior interscalene gap (fissura scalenorum); it is through this space that the brachial plexus traverses [51]. The study findings, documented by Harry et al., showed this to occur in just 60% of cases. Scalenus minimus (a fourth and small, inconstant scalene muscle found just posterior to the anterior scalene) was present in 46% of instances, with bilaterality in 14 cadavers. The most common variation was the situation where the C5 and/or C6 ventral rami penetrated the anterior scalene [52].

50. B The visceral compartment/space is a central, tubular anatomical part of the neck that has the middle layer of the deep cervical fascia/pre-tracheal fascia, which encloses vital organs and structures. Regarding the visceral compartment of the neck, the carotid artery is not a part; the carotid artery is an important constituent of the carotid sheath. The thyroid gland, esophagus, and larynx belong to the visceral compartment of the neck. Other structures in the visceral compartment of the neck are paratracheal lymph nodes and recurrent laryngeal nerves. In this compartment, there is a further differentiation into three layers. The endocrine layer comprises the thyroid gland and the parathyroid glands. The alimentary layer has the cervical esophagus. The respiratory layer contains the hypopharynx, larynx, and trachea.

This anatomic space/compartment in the neck has relationships; the relationships are with structures above it (superiorly), below it (inferiorly), in front of it (anteriorly), behind it (posteriorly), and on both sides (laterally). The structures are as follows: the hyoid bone or the skull base—superior, the superior mediastinum up to the level of arch of the aorta—inferior, the infrahyoid strap muscles—anterior, the buccopharyngeal fascia and retropharyngeal space—posterior, and the major neurovascular structures in carotid sheaths bilaterally [53].

Chapter 16

ANSWERS AND NOTES FOR MCQs ON NEUROANATOMY

1. B Oligodendrocytes produce nerve growth factor; they also form the myelin sheath. Oligodendrocytes are the final product of the process of oligodendrocyte precursor cells synthesizing glial cells. Oligodendrocytes are in the white matter. Oligodendrocytes perform multiple functions in the central nervous system, one of which is production of the myelin sheath. The myelin sheath is comprised essentially of lipids, which make up 70% of the myelin sheath; the remainder, i.e., 30%, is protein material such as myelin basic protein and proteolipid protein [1]. Oligodendrocytes project their cell membranes to surround axons in the white matter; they can concomitantly wrap around up to 50 axons; the myelin sheath provides insulation for axons [2].

Astrocytes are involved in phagocytosis [3]. Of the ependyma (neuroglia, neuronal support cells), the cuboidal and columnar epithelial cells line the brain ventricles and spinal cord central canal. Multipolar neurons are common in both the brain and spinal cord. In the spinal cord, the motor neurons are multipolar neurons (interneurons, association neurons) [4]. The sensory neurons in the peripheral nervous system are not multipolar neurons but pseudounipolar neurons. The cell body of a neuron is synonymous with soma; soma has a nucleus and organelles. Dendrites receive afferent signals, while axons carry efferent signals; dendrites may also be involved in independent signaling and protein synthesis. Axons end at the axon terminal. It is at an axon terminal that neurotransmitters, neurohormones, and neuromodulators are released. Kinesin and dynein are proteins involved in axonal transport. A multipolar neuron consists of one axon, one or more collateral branches, and a minimum of two dendrites; other types of neurons are anaxonic neurons, bipolar neurons, and pseudounipolar neurons [5]. Pseudounipolar neurons have one axon from the soma; the axon has two branches, one of which receives input while the other sends the signal to the central nervous system for processing [6].

2. A The cell body is also known as the perikaryon or soma. The nucleus is spherical. The nucleolus is a conspicuous nuclear structure; depending on the type and function of the cell, the nucleolus may occupy up to about one-third of the nucleus. Each actively growing mammalian cell contains 5 to 10 million ribosomes in its nucleus; these large numbers are required for efficient protein synthesis. The nucleolus is the subcellular structure of the nucleus where ribosomal RNA (rRNA) transcription, processing, and assembly of ribosome subunits occurs [7]. One axon may be associated with numerous dendrites. The axon hillock, a conical projection of the soma, is believed to be the origin of the axon.

3. B Axon terminals are part of the axon of a neuron—but not part of the cell body (soma). At axon terminals, synaptic connections are made with other neurons. The soma (perikaryon) differs from the axon by possessing rough endoplasmic reticulum, which all axons lack. A part of the perikaryon projects into the axon; since axons lack rough endoplasmic reticulum, they do not have ribosomes; and because they do not have ribosomes, axons cannot synthesize proteins. All proteins in axons arise from the soma of the neuron [8].

DOI: 10.1201/9781003783961-18

Axons and dendrites are the two types of protrusions from the protoplasm of the soma of neurons. Some features that differentiate axons from dendrites are as follows: Structurally, axons lack rough endoplasmic reticulum, while dendrites contain them. In terms of length, axons are longer than dendrites. Functionally, axons usually transmit signals while dendrites receive signals [8]. Axons may have collaterals, which are bifurcations; however, every neuron has just one axon. An axonal branch that exceeds 10 micrometers qualifies to be called a collateral [9]. In axons that have collaterals, both the axon and collateral have tapered ends—these tapered ends are referred to as telodendrons. It is the telodendron that eventually forms a synapse with another neuron at the body (soma), dendrite, or axon—or muscle fiber in muscle tissue. Synonyms of synapse are synaptic knob or button.

4. A The two parts of the human nervous system are the peripheral and central nervous systems. Nerve fibers transmit electrochemical changes—nerve impulses. Synapses are the interneuronal spaces essential in information exchange.

5. B The dura mater lines the internal periosteum of skull bones. The dural reflection, tentorium cerebelli, divides the brain into a supratentorial part with the cerebrum and an infratentorial part with the cerebellum; it thus has the occipital lobe of the cerebrum superiorly and the cerebellum inferiorly. The arachnoid mater is the thin, web-like, avascular membrane between the dura mater and pia mater. "Arachnoid" means "akin to or pertaining to the spider, an arachnid"—and cobwebs are products of the spider. The spinal cord anterior fissure is deep; the posterior sulcus is shallow.

The spinal cord is a long cylindrical continuation of the central nervous system; it is inside the central cavity in the vertebral column. The approximate length of the spinal cord in males and females, respectively, are 42.3 cm and 38.9 cm [10]. In its cervical and lumbar regions, the spinal cord has two fusiform enlargements called the cervical enlargement and lumbosacral enlargement, respectively. The brachial plexus formation and exit from the spinal cord account for this prominence in cervical spinal level; in the lumbar region, the lumbosacral enlargement (at L2 to S3 levels) is due to the lumbosacral plexus of nerves bound for the lower limb [10]. The greatest transverse diameter of the spinal cord is at the level of the C5 segment [11].

6. D The funiculi are synonymous with the columns of white matter (anterior, lateral, and posterior). The spinal cord extends between the foramen magnum and the L1/L2 intervertebral disk levels. Cervical and lumbar enlargements are where nerves to the upper and lower limbs, respectively, arise. The filum terminale is a thin cord of fibrous connective tissue between the conus medullaris and the superior aspect of the coccyx. The epiconus is the part of the terminal end of the spinal cord that directly continues with the conus medullaris; while the epiconus consists of the portion of the spinal cord that contains L4, L5, and S1 segments, the filum terminale immediately commences with the next sacral segment (S2) and covers S2, S3, S4, S5, and all segments of the coccyx [12]. The filum terminale is approximately 20 cm in adults; it is a delicate strand of fibrous tissue that stabilizes the spinal cord via the connection between the conus medullaris and the coccyx. The cauda equina is the continuation of the lumbosacral nerve roots [13].

Cerebrospinal fluid (CSF) fills the subarachnoid space, which surrounds the external surface of the spinal cord between the arachnoid mater and pia mater. CSF is also in the central canal within the spinal cord; this small central canal is in continuity with the ventricles in the brain. Vertebral foramina in the entire length of the vertebral column form the central canal. The spinal cord and associated structures are within the vertebral (spinal) canal of the vertebral column; all these structures are bathed by circulating CSF.

7. C Corticospinal tracts control the voluntary movements carried out by skeletal muscles. Corticospinal tracts are synonymous with pyramidal tracts. (The fasciculus cuneatus is related to decussation at medulla oblongata. The fasciculus gracilis relates to the posterior column. Spinocerebellar tracts are ascending tracts; others are the spinothalamic tracts, the fasciculus gracilis, and fasciculus cuneatus. The reticulospinal tract and rubrospinal tract are extrapyramidal tracts [14].)

8. B The primary motor areas (in the precentral gyrus) are just anterior to the central sulcus, which separates the frontal lobe from the parietal lobe; it is also referred to as the sulcus of Rolando. The visual area is in the posterior part of the occipital lobe. The auditory area is in the posterior, dorsal part of the temporal lobes. The association areas include the frontal lobes and lateral portions of the temporal, occipital, and parietal lobes [15]. Broca's area is related to the frontal lobe, above the lateral sulcus. Broca's area is involved in the planning, coordination, and programming of speech by allowing the primary motor cortex and the appropriate peripheral nerves to control mouth, tongue, and laryngeal muscle movements [16]. Broca's area, therefore, coordinates the transformation of information that is processed in various parts of the cerebral cortex prior to articulating them in speech by the actions of the primary motor cortex and required peripheral nerves [17].

9. D The aqueduct of Sylvius is just a communication for the flow of cerebrospinal fluid (CSF) between the third and fourth ventricles [18]. The largest ventricles are the two lateral ventricles. The diencephalon consists of structures between the cerebral hemispheres and above the brainstem: thalamus, hypothalamus, optic tracts and chiasma, infundibulum, posterior pituitary gland, mamillary bodies, and the pineal gland [19]. The cerebellum is not a part of the brainstem; the medulla oblongata is. The limbic system enables a person to associate feelings with experiences, good or bad [20, 21].

10. D The frontal and temporal lobes occupy the anterior and middle cranial fossae, respectively. The cerebellum is in the posterior cranial fossa. The spinal cord is not in any of the cranial fossae.

11. A The peripheral nervous system is also involved in sensory, integrative, and motor functions. Oligodendrocytes and microglia are found in the central nervous system; other glial cells are the star-shaped astrocytes and ependymal cells [22]. Although microglia and astrocytes are basically different in origin and function, they frequently contribute to the development of neurons, axons, glia, blood vessels, and synapses. Challenges that lead to dysfunction of microglia or astrocytes during brain development are expected to play a role in the disorders that pertain to the development of the nervous system even later in life [23].

12. A The abducens nerve terminates in the lateral rectus muscle. It arises from the inferior pons and traverses the superior orbital fissure. When paralyzed, the affected eye cannot be rotated laterally; at rest, the muscles opposing the lateral rectus rotate the eye medially.

13. C The nuclei of the last four cranial nerves are in the medulla oblongata; therefore, these nerves arise from or terminate in the medulla oblongata. They are the glossopharyngeal nerve (IX), vagus nerve (X), accessory nerve (XI), and hypoglossal nerve (XII).

14. D A neuron is not a glial cell. A neuron consists of the body, dendrites, and axon. Glial cells include the following: astrocytes, Schwann cells, oligodendrocytes, ependymal cells, and microglia [22].

15. B Astrocytes have the shape of a star. They have many processes. The origin of microglia is a monocyte; microglia are immune effector cells. They have a sparse distribution in the nervous system. Each Schwann cell myelinates just one axon. Schwann cells are present in the peripheral nervous system. They are like oligodendrocytes, which are in the central nervous system, in the sense that both cell types are able to do myelination of axons [24]. Ependymal cells are epithelial cells that line the surfaces of all ventricles; they play a role in maintaining the integrity of the blood–brain barrier [25].

16. B Astrocytes provide the substrates that neurons require for the production of adenosine triphosphate (ATP). Regarding the function of glial cells, while it is correct that oligodendrocytes myelinate the axons in the central nervous system, it is incorrect for Schwann cells; Schwann cells are in the peripheral nervous system, and that is where they do myelination. The resident macrophages in the central nervous system are microglia. Ependymal cells are the glial cells that function as a source of neural stem cells (progenitor cells).

17. B When there is enlargement of the ventricles or there is an inflammatory process, the ependymal cells and subependymal astrocytes collaboratively create ependymal granulations. In the mature brain, ependymal cells have structural and enzymatic characteristics required in scavenging and detoxifying a wide range of substances in the cerebrospinal fluid; this makes ependymal cells create a metabolic barrier at the interface between brain tissue and cerebrospinal fluid [26]. The most abundant cells in the central nervous system are astrocytes; of the glial cells, microglia are the fewest [22]. The cells that provide the layer of cells that creates a semi-permeable layer in the central nervous system are ependymal cells; ependymal cells are the glial cells that line the ventricles and fluid-filled compartments in the central nervous system [22]. Both Schwann cells and oligodendrocytes produce myelin basic protein; this protein is a requirement for the synthesis, structure, and stability of the myelin sheath, which these glial cells form in the peripheral nervous system and central nervous system, respectively.

18. B Microglia are the glial cells that possess elongated nuclei with little cytoplasm [22]. Astrocytes have numerous foot processes; these foot processes are important in forming the blood–brain barrier [22]. Ependymal cells are the epithelial cells that line the ventricular system [22]. Schwann cells and oligodendrocytes are equivalent glial cells, but they are not synonymous. Their equivalence is in the fact that they perform a similar function—myelination of axons; however, the site of this action is different [22]. The fact that oligodendrocytes are linked to one another and to astrocytes via gap junctions is an indication that glial cells may provide a functional "syncytium" in white matter tracts [27, 28].

19. D The preganglionic neurons of the sympathetic nervous system arise from the first thoracic (T1) to the second lumbar (L2) segments. The cell bodies of preganglionic neurons are distributed in four regions of the gray matter in the spinal cord; the distribution is bilateral and symmetrical [29]. The four regions of the gray matter in the spinal cord where cell bodies of preganglionic neurons are distributed are the ventral horn, dorsal horn, lateral horn, and intermediolateral nucleus; for the sympathetic nervous system,

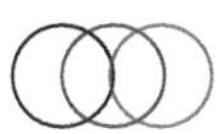

the sites are the lateral horn and intermediolateral nucleus in the indicated segments (which may include L3). Prior to synapsing, the first-order neurons of the sympathetic autonomic nervous system are short; synapsing occurs on the postsynaptic neurons in sympathetic ganglia [30]. The neurotransmitter at the preganglionic synaptic junction is acetylcholine; this is the same in the postganglionic synaptic junction—in the entire sympathetic nervous system it is, therefore, uniformly acetylcholine [31].

20. C Postganglionic neurons get to their effector sites, where they release epinephrine or norepinephrine (neurotransmitters) in most of the sites. The sympathetic nerve supply to sweat glands utilizes acetylcholine as its postganglionic neurotransmitter; the same applies to the arrectores pili muscle of hair follicles [32]. Alpha-2 adrenergic receptors operate by decreasing the cyclic adenosine monophosphate (cAMP) pathway, while it is Alpha-1 adrenergic receptors that work through the inositol triphosphate and calcium ion (IP3/Ca^{2+}) signaling pathway. Beta-2 and Beta-1 adrenergic receptors work by increasing the cyclic adenosine monophosphate pathway [33].

21. A The parasympathetic autonomic nervous system (ANS) causes inhibition of glucose output that glucagon induces. Increased glycogenolysis and gluconeogenesis in the liver (a function at the alpha-1 and beta-2 receptors) are among the actions of the sympathetic ANS. In the kidneys, an increase in renin secretion, (β-1) receptor activity, increases renin secretion with a resultant increase in intravascular volume. In the gastrointestinal tract, the reduced motility in the stomach and the intestines results in a slowing down of digestion while energy is redirected to other parts of the body; in the gallbladder, there is a combination of reduced contraction of the wall and an increase in the tone of the sphincter of Oddi from sympathetic ANS activity. Stimulation of beta-1 and beta-2 receptors results in an increased cardiac output from an increased heart rate and force of contraction.

22. C The sympathetic trunk contains the ***para***vertebral ganglia. The sympathetic trunk is a chain (sympathetic chain) of sympathetic ganglia that spans between the base of the skull and the coccyx; the chain lies to the right and to the left of the vertebral column; "para" refers to their being beside/around the vertebral column. The ***pre***vertebral ganglia are in front of the vertebrae in the abdomen and the abdominal aorta; they consist of celiac ganglia, superior mesenteric ganglia, and inferior mesenteric ganglia that are associated, respectively, with the celiac trunk, superior mesenteric artery, and inferior mesenteric artery, which are the main branches of the abdominal aorta. The sympathetic ganglion cells are, therefore, distributed in the sympathetic chain (paravertebral ganglia) and prevertebral ganglia (collateral ganglia). The sympathetic preganglionic neurons that control the ganglia in the sympathetic division of the autonomic nervous system in charge of motor activity of the viscera are located in the lateral gray horn of the thoracic segment of the spinal cord up to the upper part of the lumbar segment of the spinal cord (T1 to L2 or L3).

23. D Activity of the sympathetic autonomic nervous system on some viscera results in the following: in the urinary system, relaxation of the detrusor muscle, contraction of the urethral sphincters, and an attendant decrease in urine output; in the genital system, ejaculation during sexual stimulation; in the immune system, immune suppression; and in the bronchial tree, bronchodilation. Other examples of activation of the sympathetic system include relaxation of the ciliary muscle causing a flattening of the lens and contraction of the radial smooth muscle fibers of the iris leading to mydriasis—a more flattened lens and a wider pupil allow distant vision when response to stress is required; arteriolar dilatation and exercise-induced metabolic activity leading to an increase in skeletal muscle blood flow during exercise; dilatation of coronary arteries, vasoconstriction of large arteries, and venoconstriction of large veins; and increased metabolism and increased lipolysis. Changes that occur in response to stress are responses produced by stimulation of the sympathetic autonomic nervous system [30, 34]. The changes that take place during the activation of this "fight or flight" system lead to an increase in the use of energy and an inhibition of digestion.

24. A Regarding the parasympathetic division of the autonomic nervous system, the preganglionic neurons are in the brainstem and sacral segment of the spinal cord. In the parasympathetic division, ganglia of motor neurons are located in or close to the organs they control; the motor neurons are more widely distributed in ganglia than is the case with the sympathetic autonomic nervous system. The receptors in the parasympathetic division respond to one autonomic neurotransmitter—acetylcholine. Regulation of the visceral motor system is by sensory feedback from visceral afferent fibers. The hypothalamus and brainstem tegmentum are the main centers that control the visceral motor system and modulate homeostasis [33]. The hypothalamus controls sleep, hunger, and thirst.

25. C Dysfunction in or damage to the lateral nucleus of the hypothalamus results in a decrease in appetite. Challenges in other parts of the hypothalamus produce the following results: in the paraventricular nucleus, a decrease in the secretion of oxytocin; in the posterior nucleus, excessive heat dissipation; in the suprachiasmatic nucleus, circadian rhythm dysfunction; in the anterior nucleus, poor heat dissipation; in the ventromedial nucleus, an increase in appetite; in the arcuate nucleus, dysfunction of the tuberoinfundibular pathway; and in the supraoptic nucleus, central diabetes insipidus due to loss of ability to produce antidiuretic hormone [35].

26. B The twelfth cranial nerve (CN XII) is not a part of the craniosacral outflow of the parasympathetic autonomic nervous system; the main anatomical areas are the craniosacral outflow, which consists of cranial nerves III, VII, IX, X, and S2–S4 spinal segments; it also covers the sites of ganglia, which are either close to or in the target visceral organs. The parasympathetic system plays a major role during conditions reminiscent of "rest and digest" [36, 37].

27. A Multifunctional enteric neurons do not work alone; rather, they work in cooperation with other cells like enteric glial cells, enteroendocrine cells, macrophages, and interstitial cells [38]. Enteric glial cells may be identified, visualized, and isolated using techniques like immunofluorescence, enzymatic digestion, and confocal microscopy (an advanced imaging technique). Enteric glia are important factors in health and disease; moreover, there is a sophisticated communication between the gut and the brain. Improvement in knowledge of the relationships between the gut and the brain could lead to breakthroughs in treatments of complex gastrointestinal and neurodegenerative diseases [39]. Enteroendocrine cells exert systemic hormonal effects, especially to achieve modulation of blood glucose levels and appetite. Enteroendocrine cells suppress appetite by producing peptide YY (PYY), cholecystokinin (CCK), and glucagon-like peptide-1 (GLP-1) after a meal to signal satiety via the vagus nerve to the brain. On the other hand, enteroendocrine cells stimulate appetite during hunger by releasing ghrelin in the stomach [40]. They are also involved in intestinal stem cell function and proliferation, absorption of nutrients, and creation of the mucosal barrier [40].

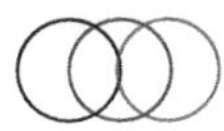

28. C Oculomotor nerve (CN III): Testing for pupillary light reflex, some extraocular muscle movements, eyelid movements, and accommodation is correct. The parasympathetic nerve fibers to the ciliary muscle of the ipsilateral (same side of the) eye are through CN III. Pointing light from a pen torch results in constriction—this is a normal reflex reaction to light. The person performing the test on extraocular eye muscles must remember that testing eye movements in the six cardinal directions actually examines two nerves apart from CN III. The oculomotor nerve supplies only the following muscles: superior rectus, inferior rectus, medial rectus, and inferior oblique. Therefore, the test should specifically cover the movements of the first three listed muscles (which are direct and easy to assess) in addition to the movement of the eye that the inferior oblique causes—upward and outward for that eye (superolateral movement), which, when broken down, is elevation and extortion of the examined eye. CN III also innervates the muscle of the upper eyelid; this muscle (levator palpebrae superioris) causes elevation of the upper eyelid in its full extent when there is no muscle weakness; when there is weakness, there is ptosis with drooping of the eyelid. The other action that CN III performs is accommodation; accommodation and pupillary constriction involve the intrinsic muscles of the eye. The eye "accommodates" changes in the distance of objects and allows the lens to adjust its shape to successfully focus on either distant or near objects—and those in between. The ciliary muscle is involved. When the circular fibers of the ciliary muscle relax, there is a tightening of the suspensory ligament of the lens. It should be noted that the zonular fibers of the suspensory ligament of the lens run along the equator of the eye; this means that when these fibers tighten (and become taut) to make the lens focus on a distant object, they "pull" the lens away from its center to the periphery (toward the eyeball)—the result is relaxation of the lens with a tendency to flattening. Since the natural lens is biconvex, becoming flattened reduces the refractive power of the eye lens and allows rays from afar to focus on the retina rather than behind it. The opposite happens when accommodation is for seeing near objects clearly.

CN I (Olfactory nerve): The correct way of testing is asking the patient to identify the smell of a familiar object by bringing the object close to one nostril at a time with the person's eyes closed in each instance—while the other nostril is occluded; the result indicates normal sense of smell, altered sense of smell, or loss of smell (anosmia) in one side of the nose or both sides.

CN II (Optic nerve): Testing vision entails a more detailed screening, which should cover the following: pupillary light reflex, visual acuity using a Snellen chart (for distant vision) and Ishihara chart (for near vision), accommodation, crude visual field assessment by confrontation, extraocular eye muscle movements by following a nearby moving object, and fundoscopy by using an ophthalmoscope.

CN IV: Assessing for CN IV means assessing for the movement that the superior oblique muscle causes; the movement is downward and inward; the breakdown of this movement is depression and intorsion (inward rotation of the examined eye) [41].

29. C Ophthalmic nerve (CN V1): The first division of the trigeminal nerve is the ophthalmic nerve (V1)—note that it is written V1, not VI. CN V1 is the first division of the fifth cranial nerve; CN VI is the sixth cranial nerve; cranial nerves are written in Roman numerals (I, V, VI, IX, X, etc.). The ophthalmic division of the trigeminal nerve is an entirely sensory nerve and serves corneal reflex and appreciation of sensations—there is no motor function. The parts of the face that this trigeminal nerve division serves are the ipsilateral eye, forehead, upper eyelid, and side of the nose. Examination of sensation is for light touch and pain, for which a small amount of cotton wool and the tip of a pin (for a slight pinprick) are the tools, respectively. The "pretest" is performed on another exposed part of the skin to enable the person who is being tested to know the feeling that is being tested and respond when they appreciate it during the test proper. The test is performed on the areas that the ophthalmic nerve supplies, and the patient's eyes are closed; it is performed on both sides of the face to know whether it is the right or left nerve that is involved, where there is involvement. The pinprick should be performed after light touch; a patient may respond to light touch but not appreciate pain. In a patient who complains of not feeling pain, it is good to ask the patient who appreciates a pinprick if what they feel is dull pain or sharp pain. During the tests for sensation, the patient should state with a "Yes" when they appreciate the touch or pain. If the patient does not indicate, the clinical examiner may confirm by asking the patient if they feel the sensation when and without applying touch or pain—all with the patient's eyes closed. Normal is when the tested feeling is present on both sides and to the same expected degree. Abnormal is when there is an absence or reduction in sensation on either or both sides. For assessing corneal reflex, the patient looks up and away from the wisp of cotton wool that is used to touch the side (margin) of the cornea, just beyond the corneo-scleral junction. The clinical examiner watches both eyes when the test is performed because corneal reflex is a consensual reflex. In a cornea with normal sensation (afferents carried by the ophthalmic nerve), both eyes blink rapidly when the cornea experiences light touch; the blink is a reaction by the action of the efferent fibers carried by the facial nerve, which innervates the orbicularis oculi. Damage to just one side results in the absence of corneal reflex on that side [42].

Maxillary division (CN V2): Sensory innervation of the skin over the ipsilateral upper lip, cheek, and upper jaw is by this second division of the trigeminal nerve. The same procedure described above is applied to the appropriate areas of facial skin that CN V2 innervates.

Mandibular division (CN V3): This is the third, most inferior, and largest division of the trigeminal nerve. CN V3 is a mixed (sensory and motor) nerve, unlike CN V1 and CN V2. The mandibular division of the trigeminal nerve carries sensory fibers that supply general sensation to the inferior 1/3 of the face, the lower jaw, the mucous membrane of the oral cavity (the inner lining of the cheeks, gingiva (gums) of the lower jaw, the lower teeth, the anterior 2/3 of the tongue, and the floor of the mouth). CN V3 also provides motor innervation to all muscles of mastication by its various branches [43]. The motor component of CN V3, therefore, supplies the masseter muscle, temporalis muscle, lateral pterygoid muscle, medial pterygoid muscle, mylohyoid muscle, and the anterior belly of the digastric muscle.

During the jaw clench test, the main muscles that are "put to the test" when the patient clenches their teeth are the masseter muscle (supplied by the masseteric nerve) and temporalis muscle (motor supply by deep temporal nerves); the symmetry, strength, and bulk of these two muscles are tested by palpating them on both sides. Weakness on one side indicates a lesion on that side. With regard to the jaw opening test, the patient opens their mouth fully, and the clinical examiner applies pressure against the open jaw; the degree of resistance by the jaw reflects the integrity of innervation and power of the muscles that open the mouth. Among the muscles that open the mouth, the lateral pterygoid is the most important; the lateral pterygoid obtains its motor nerve supply from the lateral pterygoid nerve—one of the branches of CN V3. The others that assist the lateral pterygoid muscles are the mylohyoid (supplied by the mylohyoid nerve), the anterior belly of the digastric (motor supply also by the mylohyoid nerve), and the geniohyoid (motor supply by hypoglossal nerve, CN XII). The third test of the motor function of CN VI is jaw reflex; in this test, the mouth is partially opened and a percussion hammer is used to strike the jaw lightly. When the test is normal, the jaw jerks by reflex.

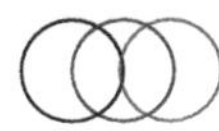

30. A The facial nerve's sensory fibers are able to pick up the six available types of taste, including umami and oleogustus. Sweet, sour, salty, bitter, umami, and oleogustus are the six modalities of gustation. To test for taste, the following are examples of what may be applied to the tongue: sweet (sugar, glucose, mineral drink), sour (liquid from an unripe citrus fruit), salty (common salt), bitter (coffee grains and liquid from cabbage, broccoli, kale, bitter leaf, bitter melon, dandelion green, etc.), umami (savory, glutamate-containing items like meats, seafoods, eggs), and oleogustus (the unpleasant, rancid, unpalatable taste) in certain foods is from free fatty acids that they contain. Examples are rancid foods and aged cheese; oleic acid and linoleic acid are useful in experimental conditions. For assessing a person's ability to appreciate taste, three swabs of sweet, salty, and sour usually suffice; these are applied to each side of the surface of the anterior 2/3 of the protruded tongue. The patient is asked to identify the taste, and the results from the two sides are matched with the constituents of the applied swab [44].

The motor portion of the facial nerve supplies all the muscles of the face. The major muscles for facial expression are the frontalis, orbicularis oculi, buccinator, orbicularis oris, platysma, the posterior belly of the digastric, and the stapedius muscle. The stapedius is one of the muscles that are innervated by the facial nerve. The stapedius is located in the middle ear; this muscle helps reduce vibrations from loud noises by contracting reflexively in response to a person hearing high-intensity sounds at about or exceeding 85 dBa. The stapedius may be tested in the clinical setting by using an acoustic reflex test; this test measures the involuntary contraction of the stapedius muscle in response to loud sounds. This test need not be done because, on clinical grounds, the diagnosis of hyperacusis may be made if the patient answers the question regarding how they respond to loud sounds; if the response shows that such sounds are abnormally loud to them (or the person accompanying the patient provides the information that the patient usually complains of sounds being excessively loud even if every other person assesses the sounds as just being loud). To confirm the diagnosis, an audiologist may perform the acoustic reflex test using the specialized equipment, electroacoustic immittance audiometer. Acoustic reflex is absent in patients with damage to the facial nerve on the ipsilateral side; if, however, the reflex is present although the patient has clinical evidence of one-sided facial nerve paralysis, it means that the facial nerve lesion is distal to (after) the point of the facial nerve giving off the branch to the stapedius muscle. This test is, therefore, useful in localizing damage to the facial nerve. The test is useful in ruling out the presence of a tumor in the parotid gland [45]. In all patients who have intratemporal facial paralysis that arises proximal to (before) the stapedius muscle, the stapedius reflex is expected to be absent; when the reflex returns, it is an early indicator of recovery, and this usually precedes recovery of movement of the face [45]. Testing a person's ability to blow a balloon assesses CN VII integrity; this simple test targets the orbicularis oris and buccinator (both muscles are innervated by lower deep branches of the buccal nerve, a branch of CN VII). Balloon-blowing involves controlled exhalation, and it has proved to enhance lung ventilation, airway clearance, and respiratory muscle strength in patients with respiratory challenges [46].

In patients who have peripheral lesions (nuclear lesions, infranuclear lesions), there is a partial to total paralysis of the face; such patients present with smoothing of the brow (from paralysis of the frontalis muscle), open eye (from paralysis of the orbicularis oculi), flat nasolabial fold (from paralysis of levator labii superioris alaeque nasi), and drooping of the mouth ipsilateral to the lesion (from paralysis of many muscles: orbicularis oris, buccinator, zygomaticus major, and zygomaticus minor, and risorius, levator anguli oris, and depressor anguli oris).

In patients who have supranuclear lesions (also commonly referred to as central lesions), there is a sparing of the brow and eyelid musculature; there is flattening of the nasolabial fold and drooping of the mouth contralateral to the lesion.

31. B **CN VI (Abducens nerve):** Regarding testing for CN VI, the evaluation must include movements that the lateral rectus muscle causes; this is because this extraocular eye muscle is innervated by the abducens nerve; the lateral rectus moves the ipsilateral eye laterally while the medial rectus moves the contralateral eye medially concomitantly. The clinician assessing this cranial nerve must observe the two eyes to determine if the normal abduction by the lateral rectus occurs at the same time as the adduction of the opposite eye takes place (caused by the medial rectus).

CN VIII (Vestibulocochlear nerve): In the Rinne test, the mastoid process is tested before the external auditory meatus. The base of a struck and activated tuning fork is placed on the skin over the mastoid process and the patient is asked to indicate when they stop hearing the vibrations; immediately thereafter, the prongs of the tuning fork are placed close to the external auditory canal. The patient is asked if they can hear the sound that they heard earlier when the base of the tuning fork was placed on the mastoid process. If the answer is in the affirmative, it is normal since sound conduction through air (the untouched ear) is, in people with normal hearing, better than through bone (although the mastoid bone is in proximity with the hearing apparatus). In sensorineural hearing loss, air conduction of sound waves is still greater than bone conduction of sound waves, but the overall conduction is less than in normal hearing. On the other hand, the Rinne test shows that bone conduction of sound waves is greater than (or equal to) air conduction of sound waves, i.e., conduction of sound waves through bone is better than (or the same as) it is through air in patients who have conduction hearing loss.

Summary: When there is anything that obstructs conduction of sound waves by the normal and more efficient direct means through the tympanic membrane, the alternative indirect route through bone becomes better for airwaves to gain access to the hearing mechanism in the cochlea [47].

In normal hearing, the Weber test shows equal hearing with both ears. This test entails applying the base of a tuning fork to the patient's forehead or top of the head to make the closest contact with skull bone. Sensorineural hearing loss demonstrates better hearing with the normal ear. If the patient has conductive hearing loss, the affected ear hears better because the airwaves pass through skull bone (frontal or parietal) to the cochlea in that ear more readily than the normal ear that still prefers to have conduction of the generated sound waves through air via the unaffected external auditory canal and the normal tympanic membrane.

CN IX (Glossopharyngeal nerve): Evaluation of this cranial nerve entails assessing the gag reflex, swallowing, and movement of the palate. Patients who have lesions of the glossopharyngeal nerve experience difficulty in swallowing; CN IX provides motor innervation to only one pharyngeal muscle—the stylopharyngeus—which assists in elevating the larynx and pharynx during deglutition (swallowing). The patients also have impaired appreciation of taste over the posterior one-third of the tongue and the palate. There is also sensory impairment over the same areas that they have a deficit in taste but with the inclusion of sensory impairment in the tonsils and oropharynx. They lose gag reflex and also have dysfunction of the parotid gland since there is parasympathetic denervation of the parotid gland; the result is a reduction in saliva secretion with dryness of the mouth (xerostomia) as evidence.

Prior to any obvious physical examination, the clinician should listen to the patient as the patient speaks during the consultation. What to look out for includes hoarseness,

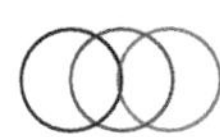

whispering speech, and nasal speech. The patient may mention that they have a challenge with "choking" or aspirating/regurgitating liquids through the nostrils.

With the mouth open, inspection of the palatal arch on each side should be done for symmetry or asymmetry. If required, the base of the tongue should be gently depressed using a tongue spatula/blade; if this is not done well, the patient may not want to continue with the test. The clinician should request that the patient say a long "ahhh" while inspecting the palatal arches as they contract to constrict and elevate when normal. An observation of the soft palate is similarly made; when normal, the soft palate swings postero-superiorly to close off the nasopharynx from the oropharynx. When there is CN IX paralysis, there is no palatal arch elevation or constriction on the affected side. Prior to testing for the gag reflex, the clinician should notify the patient and briefly explain the procedure. The clinician should use a tongue blade to touch the palatal arches, one after the other, and observe for gagging in each instance.

32. D **CN X (Vagus nerve):** The uvula stays in the midline as it is elevated when there is no paralysis of CN X. Paralysis of the vagus nerve causes uvula deviation to the normal side; this is because the intrinsic muscle (musculus uvulae) in the unaffected side contracts, moving the uvula toward its side. The musculus uvulae is the only intrinsic muscle in the uvula; it is a pair of muscle bundles. The function of this muscle is to shorten, widen, and tense the uvula; this action assists with normal speech; it also prevents food from accessing the nasal cavity during deglutition.

The five muscles that make up the soft palate are the musculus uvulae, levator veli palatini, tensor veli palatini, palatoglossus, and palatopharyngeus. The primary innervation to the muscles of the soft palate is CN X, with the exception of the tensor veli palatini, which receives motor supply from the mandibular division of the trigeminal nerve (CN V3) [48].

CN XI (Spinal accessory nerve): Assessing just the trapezius is not adequate for evaluating CN XI; this is because the accessory nerve also supplies innervation to another significant muscle, the sternocleidomastoid. It is palpation of the sternocleidomastoid muscle and trapezius muscle that are relevant for assessing CN XI function; what the examiner looks for are muscle bulk, tone, and power.

CN XII (Hypoglossal nerve): Inspecting a protruded tongue does not provide the essential information about CN XII integrity. Other tests are inspection of the tongue when it is at rest; palpation of the external surface of the cheek to provide resistance against the tongue pressed against the inner wall of each side of the cheek—this assesses tongue power; and assessment of articulation—the patient with hypoglossal nerve paresis or paralysis would have difficulty in moving the tongue to articulate words like "no, no, no" without slurring. Damage to the nucleus of CN XII or nerve fibers of CN XII results in tongue deviation toward the lesioned side; the ipsilateral genioglossus muscle may be weak or flaccid, impairing the muscle's ability to protrude its half of the tongue; the contralateral (opposite) side works normally and keeps its side protruded, leaving the damaged side ineffective [49]. This is the deviation-on-protrusion sign.

33. C Appreciation of the exact source or location of pain is by the cerebral cortex. The somatosensory cortex (S1 and S2) enables us to appreciate not only the source of pain but also to pinpoint the location, quality, and intensity/degree of the pain. S1 of the somatosensory cortex resides in the postcentral gyrus; it deals with the sensory-discriminative aspect of pain, which enables the individual to know if the pain is sharp or burning, but pain has other characteristics. In the anterior cingulate cortex and insular cortex dwells the ability to appreciate the affective (emotional) aspect and emotional response to pain [50]. The prefrontal cortex enables an individual to modulate and fine-tune the sensory input and the emotional aspect of pain with a resultant most intelligent or reasonable response to it. Pain processing by the prefrontal cortex relies on its connections to other areas of the cerebral neocortex, hippocampus, thalamus, amygdala, basal nuclei (ganglia), and periaqueductal gray (PAG). When a person is in acute or chronic pain, there are alterations in neurotransmitters, gene expression, glial cells, and neuroinflammation in the prefrontal cortex; these lead to changes in the structure, connectivity, and activity in this part of the brain [51]. Pain impulses ascend in the spinothalamic tract after processing at the dorsal horn of the spinal cord. Mechanical force and temperature changes can stimulate pain receptors. The hippocampus is pivotal for long-term memory.

34. C Impulses arising from taste receptors also travel in glossopharyngeal and vagus nerves. The gustatory cortex is in the parietal lobes. There are four primary kinds of taste cells for the following taste sensations: sweetness, bitterness, sourness, and saltiness, which are all primary taste sensations. With the recognition of two more types of taste over the years, there are now six primary forms of taste. Savory is synonymous with umami and the other is oleogustus, which is the taste of lipids or fats via free fatty acids. Fatty acid translocase (CD36) is a transmembrane glycoprotein; it has a high affinity for long-chain fatty acids that are in the nanometer (nM) range. This molecule is expressed in taste buds in humans and some mammals [52].

It has long been held that receptors for sweetness predominate at the tip of the tongue, while receptors for bitterness are at the back of the tongue. Taste thresholds have been demonstrated to differ at different locations within the mouth where gustatory receptors are found [53]. It is now recognized that it is the density of various taste receptors that differs in various parts of the tongue. The receptors for all taste sensations are distributed all over the tongue. The receptor for sweet taste consists of two proteins (T1R2 and T1R3); the receptor for bitter taste is the proteins TAS2Rs. Perception of bitter-tasting substances in food and drinks is initiated by TAS2Rs; this is a family of G protein-coupled receptors that are expressed on the surface of taste buds. TAS2Rs respond to bitter compounds by triggering neural pathways with resultant appreciation of the gustatory sensation [54]. The question exists whether there is a relationship between gut health and the spatial aspects of taste perception [55].

35. C Olfaction is the chemical sensation of gaseous odorants. Memory of, and emotional reaction to, smell from olfactory impulses are domiciled in the limbic system. However, the piriform cortex is the primary olfactory cortex where initial conscious perception and integration of odor occur. Olfactory receptors are chemoreceptors, and they are in the nasal cavity [56]. Adaptation by olfactory receptors to smell is fast. In conjunction with taste receptors, olfactory receptors enable us to appreciate food; this is because taste and olfaction are modalities of sensation that work in synergy to cause valuable interactions with the environment for our survival. From afar, olfaction enables us to recognize what could endanger us (including what should not be ingested). Taste enables us, at close range, to determine what is nutrient-rich food and what is not [57].

Olfactory receptors (ORs), like gustatory receptors, are G protein-coupled receptors. When an odorant molecule binds to an OR in the nasal epithelium, this binding leads to activation of an olfactory-type G protein and triggers a cascade of signals. Cyclic adenosine monophosphate and ion channels are involved. A neural signal is relayed to the brain [58].

36. B With respect to innervation of the alimentary canal, the muscular layer of the canal is adequately supplied by fibers of sympathetic and parasympathetic nerves. Impulses from the parasympathetic nerves increase activities of the digestive system. The sacral region of the spinal cord contributes to the parasympathetic supply of the distal half of the large intestine. In humans, parasympathetic neurons that innervate the descending/distal colon are in the sacral segment of the spinal cord; the sensory neurons are present in the dorsal root ganglia; the vagus nerve supplies the gastrointestinal tract up to the transverse colon [58, 59]. Contraction of sphincter muscles is a sympathetic nerve action.

37. C Parasympathetic stimulation of salivary glands results in a large amount of watery saliva. The submandibular, sublingual, and parotid glands are major salivary glands. The major salivary glands are in pairs. They produce saliva through serous cells and mucous cells. The mucosa of the cheeks and palate contains hundreds of minor salivary glands scattered all over them; these are, respectively, the buccal and palatine salivary glands.

38. B The frontal lobe is responsible for many functions—motor, language, and cognition. The cognitive processes include personality, self-awareness, social and moral reasoning, executive function, attention, affect, mood, and memory [60]. Cognition is a higher-level function of the brain; it covers areas (domains) like attention, memory, intelligence, judgment, and executive functions like the ability or inability to execute plans or to execute solutions to problems. Affect is the way or method in which a person expresses their feelings; this could be by "body language," facial expressions, or the tone of voice when they speak. While affect is objective (external), mood is subjective (internal).

Regarding memory, the prefrontal cortex (a part of the frontal lobe) plays a key role in holding and manipulating memory in the short term and retrieving information required for use from memory storage; it works in conjunction with other parts of the brain that form a network pertaining to memory. Working memory entails actively maintaining information in the short term and manipulating memory [61]. The Broca area is in the left frontal lobe; this part of the frontal lobe is responsible for producing and articulating speech.

39. A Apart from controlling the senses of smell and hearing, the temporal lobe of the cerebrum is responsible for learning, language, emotional behavior, and memory [62]. Declarative memory covers semantic memory and episodic memory; declarative memory is memory regarding everyday functions. Patients with amnesia have a challenge with this form of memory. Declarative memory is believed to primarily depend on the medial aspect of the temporal lobe with structures like the hippocampus [63].

Nondeclarative memory is considered to rely mainly on the corpus striatum, cerebellum, and cortical association areas [64]. Nondeclarative memory has subcomponents; the most significant is procedural memory, which is the formation of memories for carrying out motor activities [63]. Procedural memory also entails associative learning forms and non-associative learning forms. Classical and operant conditioning are examples of associative learning forms. Habituation, priming, and learning of perceptual and cognitive routines are examples of non-associative learning forms [64].

40. C The basal ganglia are synonymous with basal nuclei. The organization of the basal ganglia is as follows: The caudate nucleus and putamen form the striatum, the putamen and globus pallidus form the lentiform nucleus. The striatum and lentiform nucleus form the basal ganglia (nuclei). The basal nuclei are involved in the control of motor activities [65].

41. C The primary somatosensory area is the post-central gyrus—the most anterior gyrus of the parietal lobe just posterior to the central sulcus [66, 67]. The post-central gyrus appreciates and interprets sensations from the contralateral side of the body. Somatosensory sensations include heat, cold, pressure, movement, stretch, pain, and touch [68].

42. A The premotor area is also called the motor association area. It is in the frontal lobe. This is where decision-making, planning, and preparation for motor activity reside [69]. Transmission of the neural intention is sent to the primary motor area (cortex), which is in the precentral gyrus of the frontal lobe, located just anterior to the central sulcus.

43. A In the 65-year-old male who develops tremors when he is at rest and getting up from a chair is slow and clumsy, the most likely part of the brain with a lesion is the basal nuclei; this patient has Parkinson's disease. Tremor management in patients with Parkinson's disease tends to be challenging because response to dopaminergic agents may be poor when compared with the expected results, especially in patients who have tremor-dominant Parkinson's disease; response to these medications is better in patients who have the akinetic/rigid subtype of Parkinson's disease [70].

In a patient with cerebellar disease, the tremors occur when they are about to commence a motor activity and progressively worsen to the extent that there may be past-pointing or overshooting the target of the action/activity; in cerebellar disorders, the tremors are coarse and of a higher amplitude, unlike the fine tremors of low amplitude that characterize Parkinson's disease [71]. In the study by Kovács et al., tremor in patients with acute cerebellar lesions was a feature in postural positions and intentional positions, but never when the patients were at rest. Involvement of the anterior lobe and lobule VI of the cerebellum appears to be related to high tremor intensity. Pathological tremor that acute lesions of the cerebellum induce tends to improve rather than become worse [71].

44. B In hydrocephalus, there may be obstruction, poor absorption, or overproduction of cerebrospinal fluid; in each case, development of hydrocephalus is related to the ventricles. In a child who develops hydrocephalus from bacterial meningitis, the part of the brain to which the pathology is related is the ventricular system. The ventricular system of the brain consists of a series of linked intracerebral cavities filled with cerebrospinal fluid (CSF) that provide a cushioning effect for the brain [72]. Regarding the ventricular system, the following structures are involved in the circulation of CSF: two lateral ventricles, one third ventricle, and one fourth ventricle, for a total of four ventricles [72]. Secretion of cerebrospinal fluid occurs mainly in the choroid plexus of the lateral ventricles [72].

In the ventricular system, the flow of CSF is unidirectional; the direction is rostral-to-caudal. The flow of CSF commences at the lateral ventricles. From the lateral ventricles, cerebrospinal fluid flows through the interventricular foramina (of Monro) into the third ventricle. From the third ventricle, CSF flow goes through the cerebral aqueduct (of Sylvius) into the fourth ventricle. CSF continues its flow through the **m**edian aperture (foramen of **M**agendie) and the paired **l**ateral foramina (of **L**uschka) out of the ventricular system and into the subarachnoid space at the level of the base of the brain [73].

Outside the ventricular system, CSF is contained in the subarachnoid space. The subarachnoid space lies between the arachnoid membrane and pia mater. The arachnoid membrane is adherent to the dura mater and forms the outer layer of the subarachnoid space. The arachnoid membrane consists of fibroblasts; tight junctions link fibroblasts. Claudin 11 is in tight junctions. Tight junctions seal the CSF compartment. Arachnoid trabeculae protrude into the subarachnoid space and fuse with the pia mater, which is

 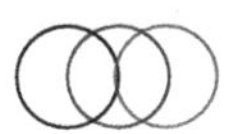

a single-cell layer closely applied to the foot processes of astrocytes and the surfaces of brain parenchyma [73].

Apart from cushioning the brain and the spinal cord, CSF provides buoyancy and contributes to maintenance of chemical homeostasis and elimination of waste products. Arachnoid villi and arachnoid granulations reabsorb CSF into the dural sinuses, principally the superior sagittal sinus; to a lesser degree, the transverse sinuses; and eventually into the venous circulation. Alternative/additional means of CSF reabsorption consist of the dural lymphatic vessels, perineural pathways along cranial nerves, and spinal nerve root sheaths; in some of these, the lymphatic drainage system is involved in CSF reabsorption [73].

45. C Pontine hemorrhage may result in unconsciousness with associated bilateral pinpoint pupils in the patient. A recently well adult but currently unconscious patient found to have pinpoint pupils bilaterally during physical examination by the attending physician in the emergency room most likely has a lesion in the brainstem at the level of the pons. Unopposed parasympathetic action from disruption of the descending sympathetic fibers results in extreme miosis with pupillary aperture that is usually less than 1 mm.

Pontine hemorrhage constitutes about 10% of intracerebral hemorrhages. Although a high mortality rate makes pontine hemorrhage the most harmful form of intracerebral hemorrhage, patients with mild forms of this condition do survive, especially those with small posteriorly located hematomas—they may, however, have some neurological deficits. The overall mortality rate of primary pontine hemorrhage is about 40%–50% [74]. Primary pontine hemorrhages have a predilection for the middle pons and the junction of the basis pontis (large ventral [anterior] part of the pons) and tegmentum [75].

46. A The cerebellum is involved in coordinating movements and maintaining muscle tone, posture, and balance. It coordinates the motions at various joints. The actions of the cerebellum, therefore, ensure smoothness in the contraction of skeletal muscles to achieve accuracy of the intended tasks [76].

47. B The pituitary gland (hypophysis) is in the saddle-shaped sella turcica; the sella turcica is a depression in the sphenoidal bone (sphenoid). Superior and anterior to the pituitary gland is the optic chiasm. Anteriorly, an additional structure that is related to the pituitary gland is the second cranial nerve (CN II, optic nerve), which extends from the eyes in front to the optic chiasma on its way to the visual cortex in the occipital lobe of the brain. Lateral to the hypophysis is the cavernous segment of the internal carotid arteries on both sides. The pituitary gland is surrounded by the cavernous sinus on both sides, with the anterior and posterior intercavernous sinuses lying in a closer relationship with the hypophysis than the main cavernous sinus. In the lateral wall (between the two dural layers) of the cavernous sinus are three cranial nerves (CN III, CN IV, and CN V); regarding CN V, its first and second divisions (V1 and V2) lie in the lateral wall of the cavernous sinus, while the mandibular branch (CN V3) is not in the cavernous sinus but runs inferior to the sinus to exit the skull through the foramen ovale. The abducens nerve (CN VI) is the only cranial nerve that runs inside the cavernous sinus. The basilar venous plexus lies just posterior to the pituitary gland [77].

The sellar region consists of the hypophysis (pituitary gland) and sella turcica. The pituitary fossa is surrounded by the bony walls of the sella turcica; the anterior wall is formed by the tuberculum sellae; the posterior wall is created by the dorsum sellae; the sulcus chiasmaticus is anterosuperior to the tuberculum sellae. The posterior clinoid process is formed by the rounded margins of the dorsum sellae; the anterior equivalent (anterior clinoid process) is formed by the anterolateral margins of the sella turcica [77].

48. C Inflammation of the ipsilateral facial nerve is responsible for Bell's palsy. The facial nerve passes through the stylomastoid foramen. Temporary paralysis of the facial nerve and its branches accounts for the motor features of Bell's palsy.

49. C The mandibular division is the third and largest division of the fifth cranial nerve (the trigeminal nerve). It is a mixed nerve with both sensory and motor fibers. The motor component of this division (CN V3) of the trigeminal nerve (CN V) originates from the pons, while the sensory component terminates at the pons. Damage to the nerve results in impairment in chewing and loss of sensation. The motor component of the mandibular division of the trigeminal nerve terminates in the masseter, temporalis, lateral and medial pterygoids, mylohyoid, anterior belly of the digastric, and the tensor tympani of the middle ear. The mandibular division receives sensory impulses from the lower part of the face, floor of the mouth, and anterior 2/3 of the tongue except for taste buds; it also receives sensory impulses from the lower teeth, lower gums, and dura mater of the middle cranial fossa [78].

50. C The spinal accessory nerve is the eleventh cranial nerve. It exits from the jugular foramen. The nerve is essentially a motor nerve. It is involved in head, neck, and shoulder movements and swallowing. The ipsilateral side of the paralyzed nerve results in the paralyzed trapezius' inability to cause shrugging movement on the affected right side [79].

The seven parts of the central nervous system are the cerebral hemispheres, diencephalon, midbrain, pons, cerebellum, medulla, and spinal cord. The diencephalon is made up of the epithalamus, thalamus, hypothalamus, ventral thalamus, and the third ventricle. The brainstem consists of the midbrain, pons, and medulla. The forebrain comprises the cerebral hemispheres and the diencephalon. The brainstem provides access to many of the central nervous system's major tracts. The ascending tracts relay sensory signals from the spinal cord and brainstem to the midbrain and forebrain. The descending tracts relay motor impulses from the forebrain and midbrain to motor neurons located in the brainstem and spinal cord. Cranial nerves are numbered using Roman numerals just after CN (for cranial nerve). Regarding the cranial nerves, their nuclei are located in the brainstem in the following locations: CN I, nasal epithelium; CN II, retina; CN III, midbrain; CN IV, midbrain; CN V, pons; CN VI, midbrain; CN VII, pons; and CN VIII, CN IX, CN X, CN XI, and CN XII, medulla oblongata. The vestibular nuclei of CN VIII are in the pontomedullary junction [80]. Three of the cranial nerves are entirely sensory; they are the olfactory nerve (CN I), optic nerve (CN II), and auditory/vestibular (vestibulocochlear) nerve (CN VIII). Five cranial nerves are wholly motor; these nerves are the oculomotor nerve (CN III), trochlear nerve (CN IV), abducens nerve (CN VI), spinal accessory nerve (CN XI), and hypoglossal nerve (CN XII). Four nerves are mixed nerves; these are the trigeminal nerve (CN V), facial nerve (CN VII), glossopharyngeal (CN IX), and vagus nerve (CN X) [81].

REFERENCES

CHAPTERS 1 AND 9 ABDOMEN

1. Kim JY, Dao H. Physiology, Integument. [Updated 2023 May 1]. In: StatPearls [Internet]. Treasure Island (FL): StatPearls Publishing; 2025 Jan. Available from: https://www.ncbi.nlm.nih.gov/books/NBK554386/
2. Yousef H, Alhajj M, Fakoya AO, et al. Anatomy, Skin (Integument), Epidermis. [Updated 2024 Jun 8]. In: StatPearls [Internet]. Treasure Island (FL): StatPearls Publishing; 2025 Jan. Available from: https://www.ncbi.nlm.nih.gov/books/NBK470464/
3. Hodge BD, Sanvictores T, Brodell RT. Anatomy, Skin Sweat Glands. [Updated 2022 Oct 10]. In: StatPearls [Internet]. Treasure Island (FL): StatPearls Publishing; 2025 Jan. Available from: https://www.ncbi.nlm.nih.gov/books/NBK482278/
4. Sugumar K, Gupta M. Anatomy, Abdomen and Pelvis: Inguinal Ligament (Crural Ligament. Poupart Ligament). [Updated 2024 Jan 30]. In: StatPearls [Internet]. Treasure Island (FL): StatPearls Publishing; 2025 Jan. Available from: https://www.ncbi.nlm.nih.gov/books/NBK542321/
5. Nassereddin A, Sajjad H. Anatomy, Abdomen and Pelvis: Linea Semilunaris. [Updated 2023 Jul 24]. In: StatPearls [Internet]. Treasure Island (FL): StatPearls Publishing; 2025 Jan. Available from: https://www.ncbi.nlm.nih.gov/books/NBK555983/
6. Abdulla MA, Fahad SMA. Anthropometric determinations of umbilical position in Iraqi adults. Indian J Plast Surg. 2020 Dec;53(3):394–8. doi: 10.1055/s-0040-1721869. Epub 2020 Dec 26. PMID: 33402770; PMCID: PMC7775206.
7. Smith JC, Watkins GE, Taylor FC, et al. Angioplasty or stent placement in the proximal common iliac artery: is protection of the contralateral side necessary? J Vasc Interv Radiol. 2001 Dec;12(12):1395–8. doi: 10.1016/s1051-0443(07)61696-0. PMID: 11742012.
8. Briggs KB, Rentea RM. Patent Urachus. [Updated 2023 Apr 10]. In: StatPearls [Internet]. Treasure Island (FL): StatPearls Publishing; 2025 Jan. Available from: https://www.ncbi.nlm.nih.gov/books/NBK557723/
9. Kaufmann RL, Reiner CS, Dietz UA, et al. Normal width of the linea alba, prevalence, and risk factors for diastasis recti abdominis in adults, a cross-sectional study. Hernia. 2022 Apr;26(2):609–18. doi: 10.1007/s10029-021-02493-7. Epub 2021 Oct 5. PMID: 34609664; PMCID: PMC9012734.
10. Heylen J, Campioni-Norman D. Bilateral inguinoscrotal hernia with gastric contents and subsequent perforation: Lessons in operative management. Int J Surg Case Rep. 2020;77:853–6. doi: 10.1016/j.ijscr.2020.11.155. Epub 2020 Dec 2. PMID: 33395911; PMCID: PMC8253855.
11. Jiang J, Koay J. Anatomy, Abdomen and Pelvis: Conjoint Tendon (Inguinal Aponeurotic Falx). [Updated 2023 Jul 24]. In: StatPearls [Internet]. Treasure Island (FL): StatPearls Publishing; 2025 Jan. Available from: https://www.ncbi.nlm.nih.gov/books/NBK549772/
12. Omole AE, Mandiga P, Kahai P, et al. Anatomy, Abdomen and Pelvis: Large Intestine. [Updated 2025 Apr 6]. In: StatPearls [Internet]. Treasure Island (FL): StatPearls Publishing; 2025 Jan. Available from: https://www.ncbi.nlm.nih.gov/books/NBK470577/
13. Vernon H, Wehrle CJ, Alia VSK, et al. Anatomy, Abdomen and Pelvis: Liver. [Updated 2022 Nov 26]. In: StatPearls [Internet]. Treasure Island (FL): StatPearls Publishing; 2025 Jan. Available from: https://www.ncbi.nlm.nih.gov/books/NBK500014/
14. Van Wettere M, Bruno O, Rautou PE, Vilgrain V, Ronot M. Diagnosis of Budd-Chiari syndrome. Abdom Radiol (NY). 2018 Aug;43(8):1896–1907. doi: 10.1007/s00261-017-1447-2. PMID: 29285598.
15. Schick MA, Kashyap S, Collier SA, et al. Small Bowel Obstruction. [Updated 2025 Jan 19]. In: StatPearls [Internet]. Treasure Island (FL): StatPearls Publishing; 2025 Jan. Available from: https://www.ncbi.nlm.nih.gov/books/NBK448079/
16. Bazira PJ. Anatomy of the caecum, appendix, and colon. Surgery (Oxford). 2023 Jan; 41(1):1–6. doi: 10.1016/j.mpsur.2022.11.003.
17. Wei Z, Yao J, Wang S, Liu J, Summers RM. Automated teniae coli detection and identification on computed tomographic colonography. Med Phys. 2012 Feb;39(2):964–75. doi: 10.1118/1.3679013. PMID: 22320805; PMCID: PMC3281971.
18. Gilani SN, Bass G, Leader F, Walsh TN. Collins' sign: validation of a clinical sign in cholelithiasis. Ir J Med Sci. 2009 Dec;178(4):397–400. doi: 10.1007/s11845-009-0404-7. PMID: 19685000.

19. Kudzinskas A, Cunha B. Anatomy, Anterolateral Abdominal Wall Nerves. [Updated 2023 Jan 1]. In: StatPearls [Internet]. Treasure Island (FL): StatPearls Publishing; 2025 Jan. Available from: https://www.ncbi.nlm.nih.gov/books/NBK556034/
20. Rao JN, Wang JY. Regulation of Gastrointestinal Mucosal Growth. In: Intestinal Architecture and Development. San Rafael (CA): Morgan & Claypool Life Sciences; 2010.Available from: https://www.ncbi.nlm.nih.gov/books/NBK54098/
21. Chaudhry SR, Bordoni B. Anatomy, Thorax, Esophagus. [Updated 2023 Jul 24]. In: StatPearls [Internet]. Treasure Island (FL): StatPearls Publishing; 2025 Jan. Available from: https://www.ncbi.nlm.nih.gov/books/NBK482513/
22. Rosen RD, Winters R. Physiology, Lower Esophageal Sphincter. [Updated 2023 Mar 17]. In: StatPearls [Internet]. Treasure Island (FL): StatPearls Publishing; 2025 Jan. Available from: https://www.ncbi.nlm.nih.gov/books/NBK557452/
23. Gindea C, Birla R, Hoara P, Caragui A, Constantinoiu S. Barrett esophagus: history, definition and etiopathogeny. J Med Life. 2014;7 Spec No. 3(Spec Iss 3):23–30. PMID: 25870690; PMCID: PMC4391409.
24. Heda R, Toro F, Tombazzi CR. Physiology, Pepsin. [Updated 2023 May 1]. In: StatPearls [Internet]. Treasure Island (FL): StatPearls Publishing; 2025 Jan. Available from: https://www.ncbi.nlm.nih.gov/books/NBK537005/
25. Ogobuiro I, Gonzales J, Shumway KR, et al. Physiology, Gastrointestinal. [Updated 2023 Apr 8]. In: StatPearls [Internet]. Treasure Island (FL): StatPearls Publishing; 2025 Jan. Available from: https://www.ncbi.nlm.nih.gov/books/NBK537103/
26. Steer H. The source of carbon dioxide for gastric acid production. Anat Rec (Hoboken). 2009 Jan;292(1):79–86. doi: 10.1002/ar.20762. PMID: 18951509.
27. Mahadevan V. Anatomy of the pancreas and spleen. Surgery (Oxford). 2019; 37(6):297–301. doi: 10.1016/j.mpsur.2019.04.008.
28. Kogure K, Ishizaki M, Nemoto M, et al. Close relation between the inferior vena cava ligament and the caudate lobe in the human liver. J Hepatobiliary Pancreat Surg. 2007;14(3):297–301. doi: 10.1007/s00534-006-1148-7. Epub 2007 May 29. PMID: 17520206.
29 Ramesh Babu CS, Sharma M. Biliary tract anatomy and its relationship with venous drainage. J Clin Exp Hepatol. 2014 Feb;4(Suppl 1):S18–26. doi: 10.1016/j.jceh.2013.05.002. Epub 2013 May 25. PMID: 25755590; PMCID: PMC4244820.
30. Ensari A, Marsh MN. Exploring the villus. Gastroenterol Hepatol Bed Bench. 2018 Summer;11(3):181–90. PMID: 30013740; PMCID: PMC6040026.
31. Goosenberg E, Aloysius MM, Afzal M. Tropical Sprue. [Updated 2025 Sep 14]. In: StatPearls [Internet]. Treasure Island (FL): StatPearls Publishing; 2025 Jan. Available from: https://www.ncbi.nlm.nih.gov/books/NBK567742/
32. Costa C, Bartilotti Matos F, Carvalho Sá D, Neves Maia J. Tropical sprue: a rare cause of malabsorption syndrome. Cureus. 2024 Feb 6;16(2):e53748. doi: 10.7759/cureus.53748. PMID: 38465131; PMCID: PMC10921071.
33. Nakashima J, Zulfiqar H. Embryology, Rectum and Anal Canal. [Updated 2023 May 1]. In: StatPearls [Internet]. Treasure Island (FL): StatPearls Publishing; 2025 Jan. Available from: https://www.ncbi.nlm.nih.gov/books/NBK551682/
34. Brunt EM, Gouw AS, Hubscher SG, et al. Pathology of the liver sinusoids. Histopathology. 2014 Jun;64(7):907–20. doi: 10.1111/his.12364. Epub 2014 Mar 8. PMID: 24393125.
35. Jones MW, Hannoodee S, Young M. Anatomy, Abdomen and Pelvis: Gallbladder. [Updated 2022 Oct 31]. In: StatPearls [Internet]. Treasure Island (FL): StatPearls Publishing; 2025 Jan. Available from: https://www.ncbi.nlm.nih.gov/books/NBK459288/
36. Yamane M, Ishikawa Y, Asano D, et al. Surgical anatomy of the dorsal pancreatic artery: considering embryonic development. Pancreatology. 2023 Sep;23(6):697–703. doi: 10.1016/j.pan.2023.07.009. Epub 2023 Aug 1. PMID: 37574438.
37. Grover CA, Sternbach G. Charles McBurney: McBurney's point. J Emerg Med. 2012 May;42(5):578–81. doi: 10.1016/j.jemermed.2011.06.039. Epub 2011 Oct 5. PMID: 21982626.
38. Lotfollahzadeh S, Lopez RA, Deppen JG. Appendicitis. [Updated 2024 Feb 12]. In: StatPearls [Internet]. Treasure Island (FL): StatPearls Publishing; 2025 Jan. Available from: https://www.ncbi.nlm.nih.gov/books/NBK493193/
39. Wang AW, Prieto JM, Cauvi DM, Bickler SW, De Maio A. The greater omentum: a vibrant and enigmatic immunologic organ involved in injury and infection resolution. Shock. 2020 Apr;53(4):384–90. doi: 10.1097/SHK.0000000000001428. PMID: 31389904; PMCID: PMC7000303.
40. Meza-Perez S, Randall TD. Immunological functions of the omentum. Trends Immunol. 2017 Jul;38(7):526–36. doi: 10.1016/j.it.2017.03.002. Epub 2017 Jun 1. PMID: 28579319; PMCID: PMC5812451.
41. Liu Y, Hu JN, Luo N, et al. The essential involvement of the omentum in the peritoneal defensive mechanisms during intra-abdominal sepsis. Front Immunol. 2021 Mar 18;12:631609. doi: 10.3389/fimmu.2021.631609. PMID: 33815381; PMCID: PMC8012523.

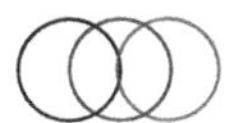

42. Halperin ST, 't Hart BA, Luchicchi A, Schenk GJ. The forgotten brother: the innate-like B1 cell in multiple sclerosis. Biomedicines. 2022 Mar;10(3):606. doi: 10.3390/biomedicines10030606. PMID: 35327408; PMCID: PMC8945227.
43. Mattos MS, Vandendriessche S, Waisman A, Marques PE. The immunology of B-1 cells: from development to aging. Immun Ageing. 2024 Aug;21(1):54. doi: 10.1186/s12979-024-00455-y. PMID: 39095816; PMCID: PMC11295433.
44. Hodge BD, Kashyap S, Khorasani-Zadeh A. Anatomy, Abdomen and Pelvis: Appendix. [Updated 2023 Aug 8]. In: StatPearls [Internet]. Treasure Island (FL): StatPearls Publishing; 2025 Jan. Available from: https://www.ncbi.nlm.nih.gov/books/NBK459205/
45. Alani M, Rentea RM. Midgut Malrotation. [Updated 2023 Jul 31]. In: StatPearls [Internet]. Treasure Island (FL): StatPearls Publishing; 2025 Jan. Available from: https://www.ncbi.nlm.nih.gov/books/NBK560888/
46. Grassi C, Conti L, Palmieri G, et al. Ladd's band in the adult, an unusual case of occlusion: case report and review of the literature. Int J Surg Case Rep. 2020;71:45–9. doi: 10.1016/j.ijscr.2020.04.046. Epub 2020 May 11. PMID: 32438336; PMCID: PMC7240054.
47. Gowda SN, Bordoni B. Anatomy, Abdomen and Pelvis: Levator Ani Muscle. [Updated 2022 Oct 26]. In: StatPearls [Internet]. Treasure Island (FL): StatPearls Publishing; 2025 Jan. Available from: https://www.ncbi.nlm.nih.gov/books/NBK556078/
48. Elmore SA. Enhanced histopathology of the spleen. Toxicol Pathol. 2006;34(5):648–55. doi: 10.1080/01926230600865523. PMID: 17067950; PMCID: PMC1828535.
49. Ochi A, Muro S, Adachi T, Akita K. Zoning inside the renal fascia: the anatomical relationship between the urinary system and perirenal fat. Int J Urol. 2020 Jul;27(7):625–33. doi: 10.1111/iju.14248. Epub 2020 Apr 20. PMID: 32314429; PMCID: PMC7384158.
50. Tang Y, Gao R, Lee HH, et al. Renal cortex, medulla and pelvicaliceal system segmentation on arterial phase CT images with random patch-based networks. Proc SPIE Int Soc Opt Eng. 2021;11596:115961D. doi: 10.1117/12.2581101. Epub 2021 Feb 15. PMID: 34531632; PMCID: PMC8442958.

CHAPTERS 2 AND 10 THORAX

1. Hunter MP, Goldin J, Regunath H. Pleurisy. [Updated 2024 Nov 14]. In: StatPearls [Internet]. Treasure Island (FL): StatPearls Publishing; 2025 Jan. Available from: https://www.ncbi.nlm.nih.gov/books/NBK558958/
2. Johansson ME, Sjövall H, Hansson GC. The gastrointestinal mucus system in health and disease. Nat Rev Gastroenterol Hepatol. 2013 Jun;10(6):352–61. doi: 10.1038/nrgastro.2013.35. Epub 2013 Mar 12. PMID: 23478383; PMCID: PMC3758667.
3. Steenvoorden MM, Tolboom TC, van der Pluijm G, et al. Transition of healthy to diseased synovial tissue in rheumatoid arthritis is associated with gain of mesenchymal/fibrotic characteristics. Arthritis Res Ther. 2006;8(6):R165. doi: 10.1186/ar2073. PMID: 17076892; PMCID: PMC1794508.
4. Tamer TM. Hyaluronan and synovial joint: function, distribution and healing. Interdiscip Toxicol. 2013 Sep;6(3):111–25. doi: 10.2478/intox-2013-0019. PMID: 24678248; PMCID: PMC3967437.
5. Sippl N, Faustini F, Rönnelid J, et al. Arthritis in systemic lupus erythematosus is characterized by local IL-17A and IL-6 expression in synovial fluid. Clin Exp Immunol. 2021 Jul;205(1):44–52. doi: 10.1111/cei.13585. Epub 2021 Mar 16. PMID: 33576004; PMCID: PMC8209560.
6. Logar HB, Medvescek NR, Rakovec P. Standardization of the apex beat in the full left lateral position and its diagnostic value in detecting left ventricular dilatation. Acta Cardiol. 2011 Aug;66(4):459–64. doi: 10.2143/AC.66.4.2126594. PMID: 21894802.
7. Shahoud JS, Burns B. Anatomy, Thorax, Internal Mammary (Internal Thoracic) Arteries. [Updated 2023 Jul 24]. In: StatPearls [Internet]. Treasure Island (FL): StatPearls Publishing; 2025 Jan. Available from: https://www.ncbi.nlm.nih.gov/books/NBK537337/
8. Psallidas I, Helm EJ, Maskell NA, et al. Iatrogenic injury to the intercostal artery: aetiology, diagnosis and therapeutic intervention.Thorax. 2015 Apr;70(8). doi:10.1136/thoraxjnl-2014-206658.
9. McAllister M, Lim K, Torrey R, Chenoweth J, Barker B, Baldwin DD. Intercostal vessels and nerves are at risk for injury during supracostal percutaneous nephrostolithotomy. J Urol. 2011 Jan;185(1):329–34. doi: 10.1016/j.juro.2010.09.007. PMID: 21075386.
10. Haroutounian S, Jensen TS. Neuropathic Pain Following Surgery. In: Nerves and Nerve Injuries. Vol 2: Pain, Treatment, Injury, Disease and Future Directions; 2015. 113–27. doi: 10.1016/B978-0-12-802653-3.00057-9
11. Davoodabadi A, Mosavibioki N, Mashayekhil M, et al. Correlation of rib fracture patterns with abdominal solid organ injury: a retrospective observational cohort study. Chinese J Traumatol. 2022 Jan;25(1):45–8. doi: 10.1016/j.cjtee.2021.07.007.

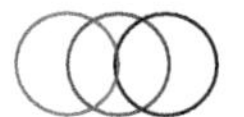

12. Lalloo UG, Ambaram A. Symptoms of Respiratory Disease | Chest Pain. Encyclopedia of Respiratory Medicine. Academic Press; 2006. 189–95. doi: 10.1016/B0-12-370879-6/00520-2.
13. Baxter CS, Singh A, Ajib FA, et al. Intercostal Nerve Block. [Updated 2023 Jul 31]. In: StatPearls [Internet]. Treasure Island (FL): StatPearls Publishing; 2025 Jan. Available from: https://www.ncbi.nlm.nih.gov/books/NBK482273/
14. Saby A, Swaminathan K, Pangarkar S, Tribuzio B. Alleviating thoracotomy pain with intercostal liposomal bupivacaine: a case report. PM R. 2016 Nov;8(11):1119–22. doi: 10.1016/j.pmrj.2016.06.003. Epub 2016 Jun 9. PMID: 27292436.
15. Altalib AA, Miao KH, Menezes RG. Anatomy, Thorax, Sternum. [Updated 2023 Jul 24]. In: StatPearls [Internet]. Treasure Island (FL): StatPearls Publishing; 2025 Jan. Available from: https://www.ncbi.nlm.nih.gov/books/NBK541141/
16. Ball M, Falkson SR, Fakoya AO, et al. Anatomy, Angle of Louis. [Updated 2023 Dec 10]. In: StatPearls [Internet]. Treasure Island (FL): StatPearls Publishing; 2025 Jan. Available from: https://www.ncbi.nlm.nih.gov/books/NBK459336/
17. Carrier G, Fréchette E, Ugalde P, Deslauriers J. Correlative anatomy for the sternum and ribs, costovertebral angle, chest wall muscles and intercostal spaces, thoracic outlet. Thorac Surg Clin. 2007 Nov;17(4):521–8. doi: 10.1016/j.thorsurg.2007.04.003. PMID: 18271166.
18. Kollmeier BR, Keenaghan M. Aspiration Risk. [Updated 2023 Mar 16]. In: StatPearls [Internet]. Treasure Island (FL): StatPearls Publishing; 2025 Jan. Available from: https://www.ncbi.nlm.nih.gov/books/NBK470169/
19. Chen J, Lai X, Song Y, Su X. Neuroimmune recognition and regulation in the respiratory system. Eur Respir Rev. 2024 Jun;33(172):240008. doi: 10.1183/16000617.0008-2024. PMID: 38925790; PMCID: PMC11216688.
20. Ganesan S, Comstock AT, Sajjan US. Barrier function of airway tract epithelium. Tissue Barriers. 2013 Oct;1(4):e24997. doi: 10.4161/tisb.24997. Epub 2013 May 30. PMID: 24665407; PMCID: PMC3783221.
21. Brody AR. The brush cell. Am J Respir Crit Care Med. 2005 Nov;172(10):1349. doi: 10.1164/ajrccm.172.10.1349. PMID: 16275741.
22. Drozdov I, Modlin IM, Kidd M, Goloubinov VV. From Leningrad to London: the saga of Kulchitsky and the legacy of the enterochromaffin cell. Neuroendocrinology. 2009;89(1):1 12. doi: 10.1159/000140663. Epub 2008 Jun 19. PMID: 18562785.
23. Lung K, St Lucia K, Lui F. Anatomy, Thorax, Serratus Anterior Muscles. [Updated 2024 Sep 10]. In: StatPearls [Internet]. Treasure Island (FL): StatPearls Publishing; 2025 Jan. Available from: https://www.ncbi.nlm.nih.gov/books/NBK531457/
24. Martin RM, Fish DE. Scapular winging: anatomical review, diagnosis, and treatments. Curr Rev Musculoskelet Med. 2008 Mar;1(1):1–11. doi: 10.1007/s12178-007-9000-5. PMID: 19468892; PMCID: PMC2684151.
25. Farrell C, Kiel J. Anatomy, Back, Rhomboid Muscles. [Updated 2023 May 16]. In: StatPearls [Internet]. Treasure Island (FL): StatPearls Publishing; 2025 Jan. Available from: https://www.ncbi.nlm.nih.gov/books/NBK534856/
26. Bains KNS, Kashyap S, Lappin SL. Anatomy, Thorax: Diaphragm. [Updated 2023 Jul 24]. In: StatPearls [Internet]. Treasure Island (FL): StatPearls Publishing; 2025 Jan. Available from: https://www.ncbi.nlm.nih.gov/books/NBK519558/
27. Terson de Paleville DG, McKay WB, Folz RJ, Ovechkin AV. Respiratory motor control disrupted by spinal cord injury: mechanisms, evaluation, and restoration. Transl Stroke Res. 2011 Dec;2(4):463–73. doi: 10.1007/s12975-011-0114-0. PMID: 22408690; PMCID: PMC3297359.
28. Rosen RD, Winters R. Physiology, Lower Esophageal Sphincter. [Updated 2023 Mar 17]. In: StatPearls [Internet]. Treasure Island (FL): StatPearls Publishing; 2025 Jan. Available from: https://www.ncbi.nlm.nih.gov/books/NBK557452/
29. Arora Y, Sapra A. Anatomy, Thorax, Superior Thoracic Arteries. [Updated 2023 Jul 24]. In: StatPearls [Internet]. Treasure Island (FL): StatPearls Publishing; 2025 Jan. Available from: https://www.ncbi.nlm.nih.gov/books/NBK553140/
30. Rehman I, Rehman A. Anatomy, Thorax, Heart. [Updated 2023 Aug 28]. In: StatPearls [Internet]. Treasure Island (FL): StatPearls Publishing; 2025 Jan. Available from: https://www.ncbi.nlm.nih.gov/books/NBK470256/
31. Saxton A, Tariq MA, Bordoni B. Anatomy, Thorax, Cardiac Muscle. [Updated 2023 Aug 8]. In: StatPearls [Internet]. Treasure Island (FL): StatPearls Publishing; 2025 Jan. Available from: https://www.ncbi.nlm.nih.gov/books/NBK535355/
32. Boyette LC, Burns B. Physiology, Pulmonary Circulation. [Updated 2022 Sep 19]. In: StatPearls [Internet]. Treasure Island (FL): StatPearls Publishing; 2025 Jan. PMID: 30085539.
33. Lakomkin VL, Abramov AA, Prosvirnin AV, et al. The structure of left ventricular relaxation in case of ventriculography. Kardiologiia. 2024 Aug;64(8):32–38. Russian, English. doi: 10.18087/cardio.2024.8.n2640. PMID: 39262351.
34. Ten Tusscher KHWJ, Panfilov AV. Modelling of the ventricular conduction system. Prog Biophys Mol Biol. 2008 Jan–Apr;96(1–3):152–70. doi: 10.1016/j.pbiomolbio.2007.07.026.

35. Felner JM. The Second Heart Sound. In: Walker HK, Hall WD, Hurst JW, editors. Clinical Methods: The History, Physical, and Laboratory Examinations. 3rd edition. Boston: Butterworths; 1990. Available from: https://www.ncbi.nlm.nih.gov/books/NBK341/.
36. Wei X, Yohannan S, Richards JR. Physiology, Cardiac Repolarization Dispersion and Reserve. [Updated 2023 Apr 17]. In: StatPearls [Internet]. Treasure Island (FL): StatPearls Publishing; 2025 Jan. Available from: https://www.ncbi.nlm.nih.gov/books/NBK537194/
37. Godwin L, Tariq MA, Crane JS. Histology, Capillary. [Updated 2023 Apr 24]. In: StatPearls [Internet]. Treasure Island (FL): StatPearls Publishing; 2025 Jan. Available from: https://www.ncbi.nlm.nih.gov/books/NBK546578/
38. Yuan SY, Rigor RR. Regulation of Endothelial Barrier Function. San Rafael (CA): Morgan & Claypool Life Sciences; 2010. Available from: https://www.ncbi.nlm.nih.gov/books/NBK54117/ doi: 10.4199/C00025ED1V01Y201101ISP013
39. Cheung SS. Responses of the hands and feet to cold exposure. Temperature (Austin). 2015 Feb;2(1):105–20. doi: 10.1080/23328940.2015.1008890. PMID: 27227009; PMCID: PMC4843861.
40. Grubb S, Cai C, Hald BO, Khennouf L, Murmu RP, Jensen AGK, Fordsmann J, Zambach S, Lauritzen M. Precapillary sphincters maintain perfusion in the cerebral cortex. Nat Commun. 2020 Jan;11(1):395. doi: 10.1038/s41467-020-14330-z. PMID: 31959752; PMCID: PMC6971292.
41. Daneman R, Prat A. The blood-brain barrier. Cold Spring Harb Perspect Biol. 2015 Jan;7(1):a020412. doi: 10.1101/cshperspect.a020412. PMID: 25561720; PMCID: PMC4292164.
42. Korthuis RJ. Skeletal Muscle Circulation. San Rafael (CA): Morgan & Claypool Life Sciences; 2011. Available from: https://www.ncbi.nlm.nih.gov/books/NBK57141/
43. Pittman RN. Regulation of Tissue Oxygenation. San Rafael (CA): Morgan & Claypool Life Sciences; 2011. Chapter 2, The Circulatory System and Oxygen Transport. Available from: https://www.ncbi.nlm.nih.gov/books/NBK54112/
44. Villa AD, Sammut E, Nair A, et al. Coronary artery anomalies overview: the normal and the abnormal. World J Radiol. 2016 Jun;8(6):537–55. doi: 10.4329/wjr.v8.i6.537. PMID: 27358682; PMCID: PMC4919754.
45. Panagouli E, Tsoucalas G, Papaioannou T, Fiska A, Venieratos D, Skandalakis P. Right and left common carotid arteries arising from the branchiocephalic, a rare variation of the aortic arch. Anat Cell Biol. 2018 Sep;51(3):215–17. doi: 10.5115/acb.2018.51.3.215. Epub 2018 Sep 28. PMID: 30310716; PMCID: PMC6172589.
46. Psillas G, Kekes G, Constantinidis J, Triaridis S, Vital V. Subclavian steal syndrome: neurotological manifestations. Acta Otorhinolaryngol Ital. 2007 Feb;27(1):33–7. PMID: 17601209; PMCID: PMC2640015.
47. Loukas M, Diala el-Z, Tubbs RS, Zhan L, Rhizek P, Monsekis A, Akiyama M. A review of the distribution of the arterial and venous vasculature of the diaphragm and its clinical relevance. Folia Morphol (Warsz). 2008 Aug;67(3):159–65. PMID: 18828095.
48. Bird JD, Lance ML, Bachasson D, Dominelli PB, Foster GE. Diaphragm blood flow: new avenues for human translation. J Appl Physiol (1985). 2025 Apr;138(4):909–25. doi: 10.1152/japplphysiol.00669.2024. Epub 2025 Mar 6. PMID: 40048319.
49. Klein AL, Abbara S, Agler DA, et al. American Society of Echocardiography clinical recommendations for multimodality cardiovascular imaging of patients with pericardial disease: endorsed by the Society for Cardiovascular Magnetic Resonance and Society of Cardiovascular Computed Tomography. J Am Soc Echocardiogr. 2013;26(9):965–1012.e15. doi:10.1016/j.echo.2013.06.023.
50. Reyaldeen R, Chan N, Lo Presti S, et al. Pericardial anatomy, interventions and therapeutics: a contemporary review. Struct Heart. 2021 Nov–Dec;5(6):556–69. doi: 10.1080/24748706.2021.1989531
51. Sternbach G. Claude Beck: cardiac compression triads. J Emerg Med. 1988 Sep–Oct;6(5):417–9. doi: 10.1016/0736-4679(88)90017-0. PMID: 3066820.
52. Hoit BD. Anatomy and physiology of the pericardium. Cardiol Clin. 2017;35(4):481–90. doi: 10.1016/j.ccl.2017.07.002.
53. Spodick DH. Macrophysiology, microphysiology, and anatomy of the pericardium: a synopsis. Am Heart J. 1992;124(4):1046–51. doi: 10.1016/0002-8703(92)90990-D.
54. Hayase J, Mori S, Shivkumar K, Bradfield JS. Anatomy of the pericardial space. Card Electrophysiol Clin. 2020;12(3):265–70. doi: 10.1016/j.ccep.2020.04.003.
55. Rodriguez ER, Tan CD. Structure and anatomy of the human pericardium. Prog Cardiovasc Dis. 2017 Jan–Feb; 59(4):327–40. doi: 10.1016/j.pcad.2016.12.010. Epub 2017 Jan 4. PMID: 28062264.
56. Xu B, Kwon DH, Klein AL. Imaging of the pericardium: a multimodality cardiovascular imaging update. Cardiol Clin. 2017;35(4):491–503. doi: 10.1016/j.ccl.2017.07.003.
57. Bhargava M, Wazni OM, Saliba WI. Interventional pericardiology. Curr Cardiol Rep. 2016;18(3):31. doi: 10.1007/s11886-016-0698-9.
58. Luis SA, Kane GC, Luis CR, Oh JK, Sinak LJ Overview of optimal techniques for pericardiocentesis in contemporary practice. Curr Cardiol Rep. 2020;22(8):60. doi: 10.1007/s11886-020-01324-y.

59. Kesieme EB, Okokhere PO, Iruolagbe CO, et al. Surgical management of massive pericardial effusion and predictors for development of constrictive pericarditis in a resource limited setting. Adv Med. 2016;2016:8917954. doi: 10.1155/2016/8917954. Epub 2016 Jul 19. PMID: 27517082; PMCID: PMC4969508.
60. Imazio M, Adler Y. Management of pericardial effusion. Eur Heart J. 2013 Apr;34(16):1186–97. doi: 10.1093/eurheartj/ehs372. Epub 2012 Nov 2. PMID: 23125278.

CHAPTERS 3 AND 11 BACK

1. Yousef H, Alhajj M, Fakoya AO, et al. Anatomy, Skin (Integument), Epidermis. [Updated 2024 Jun 8]. In: StatPearls [Internet]. Treasure Island (FL): StatPearls Publishing; 2025 Jan. Available from: https://www.ncbi.nlm.nih.gov/books/NBK470464/
2. Ryan TJ. The blood vessels of the skin. J Invest Dermatol. 1976 Jul;67(1):110–8. doi: 10.1111/1523-1747.ep12512516. PMID: 778283.
3. Rzepka K, Schaarschmidt G, Nagler M, Wohlrab J. Epidermale Stammzellen [Epidermal stem cells]. J Dtsch Dermatol Ges. 2005 Dec;3(12):962–73. German. doi: 10.1111/j.1610-0387.2005.05071.x. PMID: 16405712.
4. Ravara B, Hofer C, Kern H, et al. Dermal papillae flattening of thigh skin in *conus cauda* Syndrome. Eur J Transl Myol. 2018 Dec;28(4):7914. doi: 10.4081/ejtm.2018.7914. PMID: 30662702; PMCID: PMC6317141.
5. Mahanty S, Setty SRG. Epidermal lamellar body biogenesis: insight into the roles of golgi and lysosomes. Front Cell Dev Biol. 2021 Aug;9:701950. doi: 10.3389/fcell.2021.701950. PMID: 34458262; PMCID: PMC8387949.
6. Oren A, Ganz T, Liu L, Meerloo T. In human epidermis, β-defensin 2 is packaged in lamellar bodies. Exp Mol Pathol. 2003;74(2):180–2. doi: 10.1016/S0014-4800(02)00023-0.
7. Ganz T, Selsted ME, Lehrer RI. Defensins. Eur J Haematol. 1990 Jan;44(1):1–8. doi: 10.1111/j.1600-0609.1990.tb00339.x. PMID: 2407547.
8. Murphrey MB, Miao JH, Zito PM. Histology, Stratum Corneum. [Updated 2022 Nov 14]. In: StatPearls [Internet]. Treasure Island (FL): StatPearls Publishing; 2025 Jan. Available from: https://www.ncbi.nlm.nih.gov/books/NBK513299/
9. Freeman SC, Sonthalia S. Histology, Keratohyalin Granules. [Updated 2023 May 1]. In: StatPearls [Internet]. Treasure Island (FL): StatPearls Publishing; 2025 Jan. Available from: https://www.ncbi.nlm.nih.gov/books/NBK537049/
10. Ashworth ET. Sweat evaporation in humans: a molecular and thermodynamic perspective. Exp Physiol. 2026 Mar;111:643–52. doi: 10.1113/EP093011. Epub ahead of print. PMID: 40719527.
11. Gagnon D, Crandall CG. Sweating as a heat loss thermoeffector. Handb Clin Neurol. 2018;156:211–32. doi: 10.1016/B978-0-444-63912-7.00013-8. PMID: 30454591.
12. Varkey M, Ding J, Tredget EE. Advances in skin substitutes—potential of tissue engineered skin for facilitating anti-fibrotic healing. J Funct Biomater. 2015;6(3):547–63. doi: 10.3390/jfb6030547.
13. Piccinin MA, Miao JH, Schwartz J. Histology, Meissner Corpuscle. [Updated 2023 Mar 6]. In: StatPearls [Internet]. Treasure Island (FL): StatPearls Publishing; 2025 Jan. Available from: https://www.ncbi.nlm.nih.gov/books/NBK518980/
14. Schmitt CM, Schoen S. Interoception: a multi-sensory foundation of participation in daily life. Front Neurosci. 2022 Jun;16:875200. doi: 10.3389/fnins.2022.875200. PMID: 35757546; PMCID: PMC9220286.
15. Vega JA, García-Suárez O, Montaño JA, Pardo B, Cobo JM. The Meissner and Pacinian sensory corpuscles revisited new data from the last decade. Microsc Res Tech. 2009 Apr;72(4):299–309. doi: 10.1002/jemt.20651. PMID: 19012318.
16. Germann C, Sutter R, Nanz D. Novel observations of Pacinian corpuscle distribution in the hands and feet based on high-resolution 7-T MRI in healthy volunteers. Skeletal Radiol. 2021 Jun;50(6):1249–55. doi: 10.1007/s00256-020-03667-7. Epub 2020 Nov 6. PMID: 33156397; PMCID: PMC8035111.
17. Riegler G, Brugger PC, Gruber GM, et al. High-resolution ultrasound visualization of Pacinian corpuscles. Ultrasound Med Biol. 2018 Dec;44(12):2596–601. doi: 10.1016/j.ultrasmedbio.2018.08.001. Epub 2018 Sep 14. PMID: 30220423.
18. Kholinne E, Lee HJ, Lee YM, et al. Mechanoreceptor profile of the lateral collateral ligament complex in the human elbow. Asia Pac J Sports Med Arthrosc Rehabil Technol. 2018 May;14:17–21. doi: 10.1016/j.asmart.2018.04.001. PMID: 30302315; PMCID: PMC6170793.
19. Juneja P, Munjal A, Hubbard JB. Anatomy, Joints. [Updated 2024 Apr 21]. In: StatPearls [Internet]. Treasure Island (FL): StatPearls Publishing; 2025 Jan. Available from: https://www.ncbi.nlm.nih.gov/books/NBK507893/
20. Waxenbaum JA, Reddy V, Futterman B. Anatomy, Back, Intervertebral Discs. [Updated 2023 Dec 9]. In: StatPearls [Internet]. Treasure Island (FL): StatPearls Publishing; 2025 Jan. Available from: https://www.ncbi.nlm.nih.gov/books/NBK470583/

 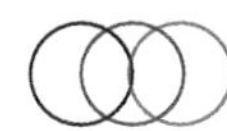

21. Velnar T, Gradisnik L. Endplate role in the degenerative disc disease: a brief review. World J Clin Cases. 2023 Jan;11(1):17–29. doi: 10.12998/wjcc.v11.i1.17. PMID: 36687189; PMCID: PMC9846967.
22. Simion G, Eckardt N, Ullrich BW, Senft C, Schwarz F. Bone density of the cervical, thoracic and lumbar spine measured using Hounsfield units of computed tomography: results of 4350 vertebras. BMC Musculoskelet Disord. 2024 Mar;25(1):200. doi: 10.1186/s12891-024-07324-1. PMID: 38443864; PMCID: PMC10916010.
23. Jackowe DJ, Biener MG. Atlas and talus. J Anat. 2022 Jun;240(6):1174–8. doi: 10.1111/joa.13613. Epub 2021 Dec 16. PMID: 34914100; PMCID: PMC9119609.
24. Kaiser JT, Reddy V, Launico MV, et al. Anatomy, Head and Neck: Cervical Vertebrae. [Updated 2023 Oct 24]. In: StatPearls [Internet]. Treasure Island (FL): StatPearls Publishing; 2025 Jan. Available from: https://www.ncbi.nlm.nih.gov/books/NBK539734/
25. Jung B, Black AC, Bhutta BS. Anatomy, Head and Neck, Neck Movements. [Updated 2023 Nov 9]. In: StatPearls [Internet]. Treasure Island (FL): StatPearls Publishing; 2025 Jan. Available from: https://www.ncbi.nlm.nih.gov/books/NBK557555/
26. Olivier T, Kasprzak K, Herteleer M, Demondion X, Jacques T, Cotten A. Anatomical study of the sterno-clavicular joint using high-frequency ultrasound. Insights Imaging. 2022 Apr;13(1):66. doi: 10.1186/s13244-022-01167-x. PMID: 35380281; PMCID: PMC8982694.
27. DeSai C, Reddy V, Agarwal A. Anatomy, Back, Vertebral Column. [Updated 2023 Aug 8]. In: StatPearls [Internet]. Treasure Island (FL): StatPearls Publishing; 2025 Jan. PMID: 30247844.
28. Green K, Reddy V, Hogg JP. Neuroanatomy, Spinal Cord Veins. [Updated 2023 Jul 24]. In: StatPearls [Internet]. Treasure Island (FL): StatPearls Publishing; 2025 Jan, Available from: https://www.ncbi.nlm.nih.gove/books/NBK542181/
29. Kaplan KM, Spivak JM, Bendo JA. Embryology of the spine and associated congenital abnormalities. Spine J. 2005 Sep–Oct;5(5):564–76. doi: 10.1016/j.spinee.2004.10.044. PMID: 16153587.
30. Kalamchi L, Valle C. Embryology, Vertebral Column Development. [Updated 2023 May 1]. In: StatPearls [Internet]. Treasure Island (FL): StatPearls Publishing; 2025 Jan. Available from: https://www.ncbi.nlm.nih.gov/books/NBK549917/
31. Karsonovich T, Alruwaili AA, Das JM. Myelomeningocele. [Updated 2024 Nov 21]. In: StatPearls [Internet]. Treasure Island (FL): StatPearls Publishing; 2025 Jan. PMID: 31536302.
32. Dop D, Pădureanu V, Pădureanu R, et al. Risk factors involved in postural disorders in children and adolescents. Life (Basel). 2024 Nov;14(11):1463. doi: 10.3390/life14111463. PMID: 39598261; PMCID: PMC11595710.
33. Doganay S, Yikilmaz A, Kahriman G, Tuna IS, Coskun A. Scheuermann's disease of the thoracolumbar spine in a boy. Eurasian J Med. 2010 Aug;42(2):104. doi: 10.5152/eajm.2010.30. PMID: 25610136; PMCID: PMC4261336.
34. Yoon YS, Lee JH, Lee M, et al. Mechanical changes of the lumbar intervertebral space and lordotic angle caused by posterior-to-anterior traction using a spinal thermal massage device in healthy people. Healthcare (Basel). 2021 Jul;9(7):900. doi: 10.3390/healthcare9070900. PMID: 34356278; PMCID: PMC8307674.
35. Yoseph ET, Taiwo R, Kiapour A, et al. Pregnancy-related spinal biomechanics: a review of low back pain and degenerative spine disease. Bioengineering (Basel). 2025 Aug;12(8):858. doi: 10.3390/bioengineering12080858. PMID: 40868371; PMCID: PMC12383562.
36. Lippa L, Lippa L, Cacciola F. Loss of cervical lordosis: what is the prognosis? J Craniovertebr Junction Spine. 2017 Jan–Mar;8(1):9–14. doi: 10.4103/0974-8237.199877. PMID: 28250631; PMCID: PMC5324370.
37. Zhu Z, Zhao Q, Wang B, et al. Scoliotic posture as the initial symptom in adolescents with lumbar disc herniation: its curve pattern and natural history after lumbar discectomy. BMC Musculoskelet Disord. 2011 Sep;12:216. doi: 10.1186/1471-2474-12-216. PMID: 21962233; PMCID: PMC3196737.
38. Dydyk AM, Khan MZ, Singh P. Radicular Back Pain. [Updated 2022 Oct 24]. In: StatPearls [Internet]. Treasure Island (FL): StatPearls Publishing; 2025 Jan. PMID: 31536200.
39. De Cicco FL, Camino Willhuber GO. Nucleus Pulposus Herniation. [Updated 2023 Aug 7]. In: StatPearls [Internet]. Treasure Island (FL): StatPearls Publishing; 2025 Jan. Available from: https://www.ncbi.nlm.nih.gov/books/NBK542307/
40. Tenny S, Gillis CC. Annular Disc Tear. [Updated 2023 Aug 7]. In: StatPearls [Internet]. Treasure Island (FL): StatPearls Publishing; 2025 Jan. Available from: https://www.ncbi.nlm.nih.gov/books/NBK459235/
41. Nedelea DG, Vulpe DE, Gherghiceanu F, et al. Surgical and non-surgical management of spondylolisthesis: a comprehensive review. J Med Life. 2025 Mar;18(3):196–207. doi: 10.25122/jml-2025-0039. PMID: 40291940; PMCID: PMC12022737.
42. Munakomi S, Foris LA, Varacallo MA. Spinal Stenosis and Neurogenic Claudication. [Updated 2023 Aug 13]. In: StatPearls [Internet]. Treasure Island (FL): StatPearls Publishing; 2025 Jan. Available from: https://www.ncbi.nlm.nih.gov/books/NBK430872/
43. Simkin PA. Simian stance: a sign of spinal stenosis. Lancet. 1982 Sep;2(8299):652–3. doi: 10.1016/s0140-6736(82)92751-9. PMID: 6125787.

44. Lee BH, Moon SH, Suk KS, et al. Lumbar spinal stenosis: pathophysiology and treatment principle: a narrative review. Asian Spine J. 2020 Oct;14(5):682–93. doi: 10.31616/asj.2020.0472. Epub 2020 Oct 14. PMID: 33108834; PMCID: PMC7595829.
45. Prakash D, Prabhu SM, Irodi A. Seronegative spondyloarthropathy-related sacroiliitis: CT, MRI features and differentials. Indian J Radiol Imaging. 2014 Jul;24(3):271–8. doi: 10.4103/0971-3026.137046. PMID: 25114391; PMCID: PMC4126143.
46. Sattar MH, Guthrie ST. Anatomy, Back, Sacral Vertebrae. [Updated 2023 Jul 30]. In: StatPearls [Internet]. Treasure Island (FL): StatPearls Publishing; 2025 Jan. Available from: https://www.ncbi.nlm.nih.gov/books/NBK551653/
47. Figueroa C, Jozsa F, Le PH. Anatomy, Bony Pelvis and Lower Limb: Pelvis Bones. [Updated 2023 Jul 30]. In: StatPearls [Internet]. Treasure Island (FL): StatPearls Publishing; 2025 Jan. Available from: https://www.ncbi.nlm.nih.gov/books/NBK545204/
48. Siccardi MA, Imonugo O, Arbor TC, et al. Anatomy, Abdomen and Pelvis, Pelvic Inlet. [Updated 2023 Mar 5]. In: StatPearls [Internet]. Treasure Island (FL): StatPearls Publishing; 2025 Jan. Available from: https://www.ncbi.nlm.nih.gov/books/NBK519068/
49. Poilliot AJ, Zwirner J, Doyle T, Hammer N. A Systematic review of the normal sacroiliac joint anatomy and adjacent tissues for pain physicians. Pain Physician. 2019 Jul;22(4):E247–74. PMID: 31337164.
50. Chaudhry SR, Imonugo O, Jozsa F, et al. Anatomy, Abdomen and Pelvis: Ligaments. [Updated 2023 Jan 13]. In: StatPearls [Internet]. Treasure Island (FL): StatPearls Publishing; 2025 Jan. Available from: https://www.ncbi.nlm.nih.gov/books/NBK493215/
51. Raj MA, Ampat G, Varacallo MA. Sacroiliac Joint Pain. [Updated 2023 Aug 14]. In: StatPearls [Internet]. Treasure Island (FL): StatPearls Publishing; 2025 Jan. Available from: https://www.ncbi.nlm.nih.gov/books/NBK470299/
52. Du Plessis AM, Greyling LM, Page BJ. Differentiation and classification of thoracolumbar transitional vertebrae. J Anat. 2018 May;232(5):850–6. doi: 10.1111/joa.12781. Epub 2018 Jan 23. PMID: 29363131; PMCID: PMC5879990.
53. Kim SR, Lee MJ, Lee SJ, Suh YS, Kim DH, Hong JH. Thoracolumbar junction syndrome causing pain around posterior iliac crest: a case report. Korean J Fam Med. 2013 Mar;34(2):152–5. doi: 10.4082/kjfm.2013.34.2.152. Epub 2013 Mar 20. PMID: 23560215; PMCID: PMC3611104.
54. Donnally III CJ, Margetis K, Varacallo MA. Vertebral Compression Fractures. [Updated 2025 May 4]. In: StatPearls [Internet]. Treasure Island (FL): StatPearls Publishing; 2025 Jan. Available from: https://www.ncbi.nlm.nih.gov/books/NBK448171/
55. Leonard MK, Blumberg HM. Musculoskeletal tuberculosis. Microbiol Spectr. 2017 Apr;5(2). doi: 10.1128/microbiolspec.TNMI7-0046-2017. PMID: 28409551; PMCID: PMC11687488.
56. Siddiqi A, Siddiqi A, Almohsen H, et al. Gibbus deformity: lessons from incompletely treated osteomyelitis. Radiol Case Rep. 2022 Feb;17(4):1054–6. doi: 10.1016/j.radcr.2022.01.028. PMID: 35154552; PMCID: PMC8822296.
57. Rider LS, Marra EM. Cauda Equina and Conus Medullaris Syndromes. [Updated 2023 Aug 7]. In: StatPearls [Internet]. Treasure Island (FL): StatPearls Publishing; 2025 Jan. Available from: https://www.ncbi.nlm.nih.gov/books/NBK537200/
58. Waxenbaum JA, Reddy V, Bordoni B. Anatomy, Head and Neck: Cervical Nerves. [Updated 2025 Apr 6]. In: StatPearls [Internet]. Treasure Island (FL): StatPearls Publishing; 2025 Jan. Available from: https://www.ncbi.nlm.nih.gov/books/NBK538136/
59. Loughenbury PR, Wadhwani S, Soames RW. The posterior longitudinal ligament and peridural (epidural) membrane. Clin Anat. 2006 Sep;19(6):487–92. doi: 10.1002/ca.20200. PMID: 16283649.
60. Shahidi B, Hubbard JC, Gibbons MC, et al. Lumbar multifidus muscle degenerates in individuals with chronic degenerative lumbar spine pathology. J Orthop Res. 2017 Dec;35(12):2700–06. doi: 10.1002/jor.23597. Epub 2017 May 23. PMID: 28480978; PMCID: PMC5677570.
61. Bordoni B, Sina RE, Varacallo MA. Anatomy, Abdomen and Pelvis, Quadratus Lumborum. [Updated 2024 Jul 17]. In: StatPearls [Internet]. Treasure Island (FL): StatPearls Publishing; 2025 Jan. Available from: https://www.ncbi.nlm.nih.gov/books/NBK535407/

CHAPTERS 4 AND 12 PELVIS AND PERINEUM

1. Rosner J, Samardzic T, Sarao MS. Physiology, Female Reproduction. [Updated 2024 Mar 20]. In: StatPearls [Internet]. Treasure Island (FL): StatPearls Publishing; 2025 Jan. Available from: https://www.ncbi.nlm.nih.gov/books/NBK537132/

2. Achinger L, Kluczynski DF, Gladwell A, et al. The known and unknown about female reproductive tract mucus rheological properties. Bioessays. 2025 Jun;47(6):e70002. doi: 10.1002/bies.70002. Epub 2025 Mar 22. PMID: 40119784; PMCID: PMC12101046.
3. Soulsbury CD, Humphries S. Biophysical determinants and constraints on sperm swimming velocity. Cells. 2022;11(21):3360. doi: 10.3390/cells11213360
4. Fisher HS, Roldan ERS, Avidor-Reiss T, Rowe M. On the origin and evolution of sperm cells. Cells. 2022 Dec;12(1):159. doi: 10.3390/cells12010159. PMID: 36611950; PMCID: PMC9818235.
5. Alves K, Katz JN, Sabatini CS. Gluteal fibrosis and its surgical treatment. J Bone Joint Surg Am. 2019 Feb;101(4):361–8. doi: 10.2106/JBJS.17.01670. PMID: 30801376; PMCID: PMC6738551.
6. Elzanie A, Borger J. Anatomy, Bony Pelvis and Lower Limb, Gluteus Maximus Muscle. [Updated 2023 Apr 1]. In: StatPearls [Internet]. Treasure Island (FL): StatPearls Publishing; 2025 Jan. Available from: https://www.ncbi.nlm.nih.gov/books/NBK538193/
7. Wobser AM, Adkins Z, Wobser RW. Anatomy, Abdomen and Pelvis: Bones (Ilium, Ischium, and Pubis). [Updated 2023 Jul 24]. In: StatPearls [Internet]. Treasure Island (FL): StatPearls Publishing; 2025 Jan. Available from: https://www.ncbi.nlm.nih.gov/books/NBK519524/
8. Haque M, Faruqi NA, Yunus SM. Morphometric study of subpubic angle in human fetuses. J Clin Diagn Res. 2016 Jan;10(1):AC01–4. doi: 10.7860/JCDR/2016/17699.7051. Epub 2016 Jan 1. PMID: 26894049; PMCID: PMC4740576.
9. Siccardi MA, Imonugo O, Arbor TC, et al. Anatomy, Abdomen and Pelvis, Pelvic Inlet. [Updated 2023 Mar 5]. In: StatPearls [Internet]. Treasure Island (FL): StatPearls Publishing; 2025 Jan. Available from: https://www.ncbi.nlm.nih.gov/books/NBK519068/
10. Selçuk İ, Yassa M, Tatar İ, Huri E. Anatomic structure of the internal iliac artery and its educative dissection for peripartum and pelvic hemorrhage. Turk J Obstet Gynecol. 2018 Jun;15(2):126–9. doi: 10.4274/tjod.23245. Epub 2018 Jun 21. PMID: 29971190; PMCID: PMC6022419.
11. Craig ME, Sudanagunta S, Billow M. Anatomy, Abdomen and Pelvis: Broad Ligaments. [Updated 2023 Jul 24]. In: StatPearls [Internet]. Treasure Island (FL): StatPearls Publishing; 2025 Jan. Available from: https://www.ncbi.nlm.nih.gov/books/NBK499943/
12. Lescay HA, Jiang J, Leslie SW, et al. Anatomy, Abdomen and Pelvis Ureter. [Updated 2024 May 5]. In: StatPearls [Internet]. Treasure Island (FL): StatPearls Publishing; 2025 Jan. Available from: https://www.ncbi.nlm.nih.gov/books/NBK532980/
13. Kenig J, Richter P. Definition of the rectum and level of the peritoneal reflection: still a matter of debate? Wideochir Inne Tech Maloinwazyjne. 2013 Sep;8(3):183–6. doi: 10.5114/wiitm.2011.34205. Epub 2013 Mar 26. PMID: 24130630; PMCID: PMC3796725.
14. Jiang J, Koay J. Anatomy, Abdomen and Pelvis: Conjoint Tendon (Inguinal Aponeurotic Falx). [Updated 2023 Jul 24]. In: StatPearls [Internet]. Treasure Island (FL): StatPearls Publishing; 2025 Jan. [Figure, Arcuate Line of Ilium, Linea.... Available from: https://www.ncbi.nlm.nih.gov/books/NBK549772/figure/article-19884.image.f2/
15. Reitter A, Daviss BA, Bisits A, Schollenberger A, Vogl T, Herrmann E, Louwen F, Zangos S. Does pregnancy and/or shifting positions create more room in a woman's pelvis? Am J Obstet Gynecol. 2014 Dec;211(6):662.e1-9. doi: 10.1016/j.ajog.2014.06.029. Epub 2014 Jun 17. PMID: 24949546.
16. Chaudhry SR, Nahian A, Chaudhry K. Anatomy, Abdomen and Pelvis, Pelvis. [Updated 2023 Jul 25]. In: StatPearls [Internet]. Treasure Island (FL): StatPearls Publishing; 2025 Jan. PMID: 29489173.
17. Tuma F, Lopez RA, Varacallo MA. Anatomy, Abdomen and Pelvis: Inguinal Region (Inguinal Canal). [Updated 2023 Jul 24]. In: StatPearls [Internet]. Treasure Island (FL): StatPearls Publishing; 2025 Jan. Available from: https://www.ncbi.nlm.nih.gov/books/NBK470204/
18. Humes DJ, Simpson J. Acute appendicitis. BMJ. 2006 Sep;333(7567):530–4. doi: 10.1136/bmj.38940.664363.AE. PMID: 16960208; PMCID: PMC1562475.
19. Aihara T, Takahashi K, Yamagata M, Moriya H, Tamaki T. Biomechanical functions of the iliolumbar ligament in L5 spondylolysis. J Orthop Sci. 2000;5(3):238–42. doi: 10.1007/s007760050158. PMID: 10982664.
20. Albatati AS, Khalifa AFM, El-Sherbiny M, et al. Deferent anatomical presentations of iliolumbar ligament: a cadaveric study. Biomed Res Int. 2022 Nov;2022:5992510. doi: 10.1155/2022/5992510. PMID: 36452060; PMCID: PMC9705086.
21. Sattar MH, Guthrie ST. Anatomy, Back, Sacral Vertebrae. [Updated 2023 Jul 30]. In: StatPearls [Internet]. Treasure Island (FL): StatPearls Publishing; 2025 Jan. Available from: https://www.ncbi.nlm.nih.gov/books/NBK551653/
22. Aldabe D, Ribeiro DC, Milosavljevic S, Dawn Bussey M. Pregnancy-related pelvic girdle pain and its relationship with relaxin levels during pregnancy: a systematic review. Eur Spine J. 2012 Sep;21(9):1769–76. doi: 10.1007/s00586-012-2162-x. Epub 2012 Feb 4. PMID: 22310881; PMCID: PMC3459115.
23. Kesikburun S, Güzelküçük Ü, Fidan U, Demir Y, Ergün A, Tan AK. Musculoskeletal pain and symptoms in pregnancy: a descriptive study. Ther Adv Musculoskelet Dis. 2018 Nov;10(12):229–34. doi: 10.1177/1759720X18812449. PMID: 30515249; PMCID: PMC6262502.

24. Petersen LK, Vogel I, Agger AO, Westergård J, Nils M, Uldbjerg N. Variations in serum relaxin (hRLX-2) concentrations during human pregnancy. Acta Obstet Gynecol Scand. 1995 Apr;74(4):251–6. doi: 10.3109/00016349509024444. PMID: 7732796.
25. Owens K, Pearson A, Mason G. Symphysis pubis dysfunction: a cause of significant obstetric morbidity. Eur J Obstet Gynecol Reprod Biol. 2002 Nov;105(2):143–6. doi: 10.1016/s0301-2115(02)00192-6. PMID: 12381476.
26. Becker I, Woodley SJ, Stringer MD. The adult human pubic symphysis: a systematic review. J Anat. 2010 Nov;217(5):475–87. doi: 10.1111/j.1469-80.2010.01300.x. Epub 2010 Sep 14. PMID: 20840351; PMCID: PMC3035856.
27. Daniel M, Iglic A, Kralj-Iglic V. The shape of acetabular cartilage optimizes hip contact stress distribution. J Anat. 2005 Jul;207(1):85–91. doi: 10.1111/j.1469-7580.2005.00425.x. PMID: 16011547; PMCID: PMC1571495.
28. Shimodaira H, Tensho K, Akaoka Y, et al. The acetabular fossa may not be located at the true center of the acetabulum: a detailed analysis using preoperative CT images. J Bone Joint Surg Am. 2018 Mar;100(5):e27. doi: 10.2106/JBJS.17.00362. PMID: 29509621.
29. Lee SH, Yang M, Won HS, Kim YD. Coccydynia: anatomic origin and considerations regarding the effectiveness of injections for pain management. Korean J Pain. 2023 Jul;36(3):272–80. doi: 10.3344/kjp.23175. PMID: 37394271; PMCID: PMC10322656.
30. Pomian A, Lisik W, Kosieradzki M, Barcz E. Obesity and pelvic floor disorders: a review of the literature. Med Sci Monit. 2016 Jun;22:1880–6. doi: 10.12659/msm.896331. PMID: 27255341; PMCID: PMC4907402.
31. National Guideline Alliance (UK). Risk factors for pelvic floor dysfunction: Pelvic floor dysfunction: prevention and non-surgical management: Evidence review B. London: National Institute for Health and Care Excellence (NICE); 2021 Dec. (NICE Guideline, No. 210.) Available from: https://www.ncbi.nlm.nih.gov/books/NBK579611/
32. Bump RC, Mattiasson A, Bø K, et al. The standardization of terminology of female pelvic organ prolapse and pelvic floor dysfunction. Am J Obstet Gynecol. 1996 Jul;175(1):10–7. doi: 10.1016/s0002-9378(96)70243-0. PMID: 8694033.
33. Jelovsek JE, Maher C, Barber MD. Pelvic organ prolapse. Lancet. 2007 Mar;369(9566):1027–38. doi: 10.1016/S0140-6736(07)60462-0. PMID: 17382829.
34. Nygaard I, Barber MD, Burgio KL, et al. Pelvic Floor Disorders Network. Prevalence of symptomatic pelvic floor disorders in US women. JAMA. 2008 Sep;300(11):1311–6. doi: 10.1001/jama.300.11.1311. PMID: 18799443; PMCID: PMC2918416.
35. Kuo CH, Martingano DJ, Mikes BA. Pelvic Organ Prolapse. [Updated 2025 Sep 21]. In: StatPearls [Internet]. Treasure Island (FL): StatPearls Publishing; 2025 Jan. Available from: https://www.ncbi.nlm.nih.gov/books/NBK563229/
36. Mikes BA, Adamski JJ. Chandelier Sign. [Updated 2025 Feb 6]. In: StatPearls [Internet]. Treasure Island (FL): StatPearls Publishing; 2025 Jan. Available from: https://www.ncbi.nlm.nih.gov/books/NBK545286/
37. Karena ZV, Mehta AD. Sonography Female Pelvic Pathology Assessment, Protocols, and Interpretation. [Updated 2023 Aug 14]. In: StatPearls [Internet]. Treasure Island (FL): StatPearls Publishing; 2025 Jan. Available from: https://www.ncbi.nlm.nih.gov/books/NBK585034/
38. Dobaria DG, Tafti D, Cohen HL. Pelvic Ultrasound. [Updated 2025 Jan 22]. In: StatPearls [Internet]. Treasure Island (FL): StatPearls Publishing; 2025 Jan. Available from: https://www.ncbi.nlm.nih.gov/books/NBK470360/
39. Kieserman-Shmokler C, Swenson CW, Chen L, et al. From molecular to macro: the key role of the apical ligaments in uterovaginal support. Am J Obstet Gynecol. 2020 May;222(5):427–36. doi: 10.1016/j.ajog.2019.10.006. Epub 2019 Oct 19. PMID: 31639371; PMCID: PMC7166152.
40. Gasner A, Aatsha PA. Physiology, Uterus. [Updated 2023 Jul 30]. In: StatPearls [Internet]. Treasure Island (FL): StatPearls Publishing; 2025 Jan. Available from: https://www.ncbi.nlm.nih.gov/books/NBK557575/
41. Ameer MA, Peterson DC. Anatomy, Abdomen and Pelvis: Uterus. [Updated 2025 Jun 3]. In: StatPearls [Internet]. Treasure Island (FL): StatPearls Publishing; 2025 Jan. PMID: 29262069.
42. Toumi D, Medemagh M, Ghaddab I, et al. Torsion of distal right hydrosalpinx in a primiparous woman at term: a case report. Int J Surg Case Rep. 2024 Oct;123:110255. doi: 10.1016/j.ijscr.2024.110255. Epub 2024 Sep 7. PMID: 39255729; PMCID: PMC11413677.
43. Kjer JJ, Mogensen AM. The arterial blood supply of the parametrium. Eur J Obstet Gynecol Reprod Biol. 1989 Mar;30(3):275–8. doi: 10.1016/0028-2243(89)90012-9. PMID: 2714508.
44. Gibson E, Mahdy H. Anatomy, Abdomen and Pelvis, Ovary. [Updated 2023 Jul 24]. In: StatPearls [Internet]. Treasure Island (FL): StatPearls Publishing; 2025 Jan. Available from: https://www.ncbi.nlm.nih.gov/books/NBK545187/
45. Williams CJ, Erickson GF. Morphology and Physiology of the Ovary. [Updated 2012 Jan 30]. In: Feingold KR, Ahmed SF, Anawalt B, et al., editors. Endotext [Internet]. South Dartmouth (MA): MDText.com, Inc.; 2000. Available from: https://www.ncbi.nlm.nih.gov/books/NBK278951/

46. Han J, Sadiq NM. Anatomy, Abdomen and Pelvis: Fallopian Tube. [Updated 2023 Jul 24]. In: StatPearls [Internet]. Treasure Island (FL): StatPearls Publishing; 2025 Jan. Available from: https://www.ncbi.nlm.nih.gov/books/NBK547660/
47. Thurmond AS, Machan LS, Maubon AJ, et al. A review of selective salpingography and fallopian tube catheterization. Radiographics. 2000 Nov–Dec;20(6):1759–68. doi: 10.1148/radiographics.20.6.g00nv211759. PMID: 11112827.
48. Holstein AF, Schulze W, Davidoff M. Understanding spermatogenesis is a prerequisite for treatment. Reprod Biol Endocrinol. 2003 Nov;1:107. doi: 10.1186/1477-7827-1-107. PMID: 14617369; PMCID: PMC293421.
49. Suede SH, Malik A, Sapra A. Histology, Spermatogenesis. [Updated 2023 Mar 6]. In: StatPearls [Internet]. Treasure Island (FL): StatPearls Publishing; 2025 Jan. Available from: https://www.ncbi.nlm.nih.gov/books/NBK553142/
50. Gilbert SF. Developmental Biology. 6th edition. Sunderland (MA): Sinauer Associates; 2000. Spermatogenesis. Available from: https://www.ncbi.nlm.nih.gov/books/NBK10095/.
51. Zirkin BR, Papadopoulos V. Leydig cells: formation, function, and regulation. Biol Reprod. 2018 Jul;99(1):101–11. doi: 10.1093/biolre/ioy059. PMID: 29566165; PMCID: PMC6044347.
52. O'Donnell L, Stanton P, de Kretser DM. Endocrinology of the Male Reproductive System and Spermatogenesis. [Updated 2017 Jan 11]. In: Feingold KR, Adler RA, Ahmed SF, et al., editors. Endotext [Internet]. South Dartmouth (MA): MDText.com, 2000. Available from: https://www.ncbi.nlm.nih.gov/books/NBK279031/
53. McKay AC, Odeluga N, Jiang J, et al. Anatomy, Abdomen and Pelvis, Seminal Vesicle. [Updated 2023 Jul 24]. In: StatPearls [Internet]. Treasure Island (FL): StatPearls Publishing; 2025 Jan. Available from: https://www.ncbi.nlm.nih.gov/books/NBK499854/
54. Sam P, Nassereddin A, LaGrange CA. Anatomy, Abdomen and Pelvis: Bladder Detrusor Muscle. [Updated 2023 Aug 8]. In: StatPearls [Internet]. Treasure Island (FL): StatPearls Publishing; 2025 Jan. Available from: https://www.ncbi.nlm.nih.gov/books/NBK482181/
55. Flores JL, Cortes GA, Leslie SW. Physiology, Urination. [Updated 2023 Sep 13]. In: StatPearls [Internet]. Treasure Island (FL): StatPearls Publishing; 2025 Jan. Available from: https://www.ncbi.nlm.nih.gov/books/NBK562181/
56. Singh O, Bolla SR. Anatomy, Abdomen and Pelvis, Prostate. [Updated 2023 Jul 17]. In: StatPearls [Internet]. Treasure Island (FL): StatPearls Publishing; 2025 Jan. Available from: https://www.ncbi.nlm.nih.gov/books/NBK540987/
57. Ng M, Leslie SW, Baradhi KM. Benign Prostatic Hyperplasia. [Updated 2024 Oct 20]. In: StatPearls [Internet]. Treasure Island (FL): StatPearls Publishing; 2025 Jan. Available from: https://www.ncbi.nlm.nih.gov/books/NBK558920/
58. Raychaudhuri B, Cahill D. Pelvic fasciae in urology. Ann R Coll Surg Engl. 2008 Nov;90(8):633–7. doi: 10.1308/003588408X321611. Epub 2008 Sep 22. PMID: 18828961; PMCID: PMC2727803.
59. Wang YHW, Wiseman J. Anatomy, Abdomen and Pelvis, Rectum. [Updated 2023 Jul 25]. In: StatPearls [Internet]. Treasure Island (FL): StatPearls Publishing; 2025 Jan. Available from: https://www.ncbi.nlm.nih.gov/books/NBK537245/
60. Azzouz LL, Sharma S. Physiology, Large Intestine. [Updated 2023 Jul 31]. In: StatPearls [Internet]. Treasure Island (FL): StatPearls Publishing; 2025 Jan. Available from: https://www.ncbi.nlm.nih.gov/books/NBK507857/
61. Czepiel J, Dróżdż M, Pituch H, et al. *Clostridium difficile* infection: review. Eur J Clin Microbiol Infect Dis. 2019 Jul;38(7):1211–21. doi: 10.1007/s10096-019-03539-6. Epub 2019 Apr 3. PMID: 30945014; PMCID: PMC6570665.
62. McFarlane MJ. The Rectal Examination. In: Walker HK, Hall WD, Hurst JW, editors. Clinical Methods: The History, Physical, and Laboratory Examinations. 3rd edition. Boston: Butterworths; 1990. Chapter 97. Available from: https://www.ncbi.nlm.nih.gov/books/NBK424/.
63. Bowdino CS, Owens J, Shaw PM. Anatomy, Abdomen and Pelvis, Renal Veins. [Updated 2023 Jan 2]. In: StatPearls [Internet]. Treasure Island (FL): StatPearls Publishing; 2025 Jan. Available from: https://www.ncbi.nlm.nih.gov/books/NBK538298/
64. Joseph A, Scharbach S, Samant H. Anatomy, Anterolateral Abdominal Wall Veins. [Updated 2023 Aug 28]. In: StatPearls [Internet]. Treasure Island (FL): StatPearls Publishing; 2025 Jan. Available from: https://www.ncbi.nlm.nih.gov/sites/books/NBK507909/
65. Dao DPD, Le PH. Anatomy, Abdomen and Pelvis: Veins. [Updated 2023 Mar 5]. In: StatPearls [Internet]. Treasure Island (FL): StatPearls Publishing; 2025 Jan. Available from: https://www.ncbi.nlm.nih.gov/sites/books/NBK554574/
66. Mühlberger D, Morandini L, Brenner E. Venous valves and major superficial tributary veins near the saphenofemoral junction. J Vasc Surg. 2009 Jun;49(6):1562–9.

67. Oelrich TM. The striated urogenital sphincter muscle in the female. Anat Rec. 1983 Feb;205(2):223–32. doi: 10.1002/ar.1092050213. PMID: 6846873.
68. Sam P, Jiang J, Leslie SW, et al. Anatomy, Abdomen and Pelvis, Sphincter Urethrae. [Updated 2023 Jun 4]. In: StatPearls [Internet]. Treasure Island (FL): StatPearls Publishing; 2025 Jan. Available from: https://www.ncbi.nlm.nih.gov/books/NBK482438/
69. Gowda SN, Bordoni B. Anatomy, Abdomen and Pelvis: Levator Ani Muscle. [Updated 2022 Oct 26]. In: StatPearls [Internet]. Treasure Island (FL): StatPearls Publishing; 2025 Jan. Available from: https://www.ncbi.nlm.nih.gov/books/NBK556078/
70. Bordoni B, Launico MV. Anatomy, Abdomen and Pelvis, Perineal Body. [Updated 2024 Dec 11]. In: StatPearls [Internet]. Treasure Island (FL): StatPearls Publishing; 2025 Jan. Available from: https://www.ncbi.nlm.nih.gov/books/NBK537345/
71. Stein TA, DeLancey JO. Structure of the perineal membrane in females: gross and microscopic anatomy. Obstet Gynecol. 2008 Mar;111(3):686–93. doi: 10.1097/AOG.0b013e318163a9a5. PMID: 18310372; PMCID: PMC2775042.
72. Haider MZ, Annamaraju P. Bladder Catheterization. [Updated 2023 Aug 8]. In: StatPearls [Internet]. Treasure Island (FL): StatPearls Publishing; 2025 Jan. Available from: https://www.ncbi.nlm.nih.gov/books/NBK560748/
73. Stoddard N, Leslie SW. Histology, Male Urethra. [Updated 2023 May 1]. In: StatPearls [Internet]. Treasure Island (FL): StatPearls Publishing; 2025 Jan. Available from: https://www.ncbi.nlm.nih.gov/books/NBK542238/
74. Chughtai B, Sawas A, O'Malley RL, et al. A neglected gland: a review of Cowper's gland. Int J Androl. 2005 Apr;28(2):74–7. doi: 10.1111/j.1365-2605.2005.00499.x. PMID: 15811067.
75. Weech D, Ameer MA, Ashurst JV. Anatomy, Abdomen and Pelvis, Penis Dorsal Nerve. [Updated 2023 Aug 8]. In: StatPearls [Internet]. Treasure Island (FL): StatPearls Publishing; 2025 Jan. Available from: https://www.ncbi.nlm.nih.gov/books/NBK525966/
76. Boyce L, Omole AE, Varacallo MA. Anatomy, Abdomen and Pelvis: Deep Perineal Space. [Updated 2025 Dec 1]. In: StatPearls [Internet]. Treasure Island (FL): StatPearls Publishing; 2025 Jan. Available from: https://www.ncbi.nlm.nih.gov/books/NBK538272/
77. Filipoiu FM, Ion RT, Filipoiu ZF, et al. Septum of the penis: dissection, anatomical description and functional relevance. Basic Clin Androl. 2024 Nov;34(1):19. doi: 10.1186/s12610-024-00235-0. PMID: 39528924; PMCID: PMC11555820.
78. Dwyer ME, Salgado CJ, Lightner DJ. Normal penile, scrotal, and perineal anatomy with reconstructive considerations. Semin Plast Surg. 2011 Aug;25(3):179–88. doi: 10.1055/s-0031-1281487. PMID: 22851909; PMCID: PMC3312188.

CHAPTERS 5 AND 13 UPPER LIMB

1. Yousef H, Alhajj M, Fakoya AO, et al. Anatomy, Skin (Integument), Epidermis. [Updated 2024 Jun 8]. In: StatPearls [Internet]. Treasure Island (FL): StatPearls Publishing; 2025 Jan. Available from: https://www.ncbi.nlm.nih.gov/books/NBK470464/
2. Mort RL, Jackson IJ, Patton EE. The melanocyte lineage in development and disease. Development. 2015 Feb;142(4):620–32. doi: 10.1242/dev.106567. Erratum in: Development. 2015 Apr 1;142(7):1387. doi: 10.1242/dev.123729. PMID: 25670789; PMCID: PMC4325379.
3. Fakoya AO, Hohman MH, Westbrook KE, et al. Anatomy, Head and Neck: Facial Muscles. [Updated 2024 Apr 20]. In: StatPearls [Internet]. Treasure Island (FL): StatPearls Publishing; 2025 Jan. Available from: https://www.ncbi.nlm.nih.gov/books/NBK493209/
4. Garcia RA, Sajjad H. Anatomy, Abdomen and Pelvis, Scrotum. [Updated 2023 Jul 24]. In: StatPearls [Internet]. Treasure Island (FL): StatPearls Publishing; 2025 Jan. Available from: https://www.ncbi.nlm.nih.gov/books/NBK549893/
5. InformedHealth.org [Internet]. Cologne, Germany: Institute for Quality and Efficiency in Health Care (IQWiG); 2006. In brief: Structure of the Nails. [Updated 2024 Jul 29]. Available from: https://www.ncbi.nlm.nih.gov/books/NBK513133/
6. Martel JL, Miao JH, Badri T, et al. Anatomy, Hair Follicle. [Updated 2024 Jun 22]. In: StatPearls [Internet]. Treasure Island (FL): StatPearls Publishing; 2025 Jan. Available from: https://www.ncbi.nlm.nih.gov/books/NBK470321/
7. Hoover E, Alhajj M, Flores JL. Physiology, Hair. [Updated 2023 Jul 30]. In: StatPearls [Internet]. Treasure Island (FL): StatPearls Publishing; 2025 Jan. Available from: https://www.ncbi.nlm.nih.gov/books/NBK499948/

8. Verhave BL, Nassereddin A, Lappin SL. Embryology, Lanugo. [Updated 2022 Oct 10]. In: StatPearls [Internet]. Treasure Island (FL): StatPearls Publishing; 2025 Jan. PMID: 30252348.
9. Nguyen JD, Fakoya AO, Duong H. Anatomy, Abdomen and Pelvis: Female External Genitalia. [Updated 2025 Feb 15]. In: StatPearls [Internet]. Treasure Island (FL): StatPearls Publishing; 2025 Jan. Available from: https://www.ncbi.nlm.nih.gov/books/NBK547703/
10. Relhan V, Garg VK, Ghunawat S, Mahajan K (Eds.). Comprehensive Textbook on Vitiligo, 1st edition. London: CRC Press; 2020. doi: 10.1201/9781315112183.
11. Malkud S. Telogen effluvium: a review. J Clin Diagn Res. 2015 Sep;9(9): WE01–3. doi: 10.7860/JCDR/2015/15219.6492. Epub 2015 Sep 1. PMID: 26500992; PMCID: PMC4606321.
12. Jackson EA. Hair disorders. Prim Care. 2000 Jun;27(2):319–32. doi: 10.1016/s0095-4543(05)70198-6. PMID: 10815046.
13. Wolff H, Fischer TW, Blume-Peytavi U. The diagnosis and treatment of hair and scalp diseases. Dtsch Arztebl Int. 2016 May 27;113(21):377–86. doi: 10.3238/arztebl.2016.0377. PMID: 27504707; PMCID: PMC4908932.
14. Gilmore A, Roller J, Dyer JA. Leprosy (Hansen's disease): an update and review. Mo Med. 2023 Jan–Feb;120(1):39–44. PMID: 36860602; PMCID: PMC9970335.
15. Russo CR. The effects of exercise on bone. Basic concepts and implications for the prevention of fractures. Clin Cases Miner Bone Metab. 2009 Sep;6(3):223–8. PMID: 22461250; PMCID: PMC2811354.
16. Juneja P, Munjal A, Hubbard JB. Anatomy, Joints. [Updated 2024 Apr 21]. In: StatPearls [Internet]. Treasure Island (FL): StatPearls Publishing; 2025 Jan. Available from: https://www.ncbi.nlm.nih.gov/books/NBK507893/
17. Sharma AR, Jagga S, Lee SS, Nam JS. Interplay between cartilage and subchondral bone contributing to pathogenesis of osteoarthritis. Int J Mol Sci. 2013 Sep;14(10):19805–30. doi: 10.3390/ijms141019805. PMID: 24084727; PMCID: PMC3821588.
18. Ralphs JR, Benjamin M. The joint capsule: structure, composition, ageing and disease. J Anat. 1994 Jun;184 (Pt 3) (Pt 3):503–9. PMID: 7928639; PMCID: PMC1259958.
19. McCausland C, Sawyer E, Eovaldi BJ, et al. Anatomy, Shoulder and Upper Limb, Shoulder Muscles. [Updated 2023 Aug 8]. In: StatPearls [Internet]. Treasure Island (FL): StatPearls Publishing; 2025 Jan. Available from: https://www.ncbi.nlm.nih.gov/books/NBK534836/
20. Hik F, Ackland DC. The moment arms of the muscles spanning the glenohumeral joint: a systematic review. J Anat. 2019 Jan;234(1):1–15. doi: 10.1111/joa.12903. Epub 2018 Nov 8. PMID: 30411350; PMCID: PMC6284439.
21. Card RK, Lowe JB. Anatomy, Shoulder and Upper Limb, Elbow Joint. [Updated 2023 Jul 24]. In: StatPearls [Internet]. Treasure Island (FL): StatPearls Publishing; 2025 Jan. Available from: https://www.ncbi.nlm.nih.gov/books/NBK532948/
22. Morris MS, Ozer K. Elbow dislocations in contact sports. Hand Clin. 2017 Feb;33(1):63–72. doi: 10.1016/j.hcl.2016.08.003. PMID: 27886840.
23. Chang LR, Anand P, Varacallo MA. Anatomy, Shoulder and Upper Limb, Glenohumeral Joint. [Updated 2025 Mar 3]. In: StatPearls [Internet]. Treasure Island (FL): StatPearls Publishing; 2025 Jan. Available from: https://www.ncbi.nlm.nih.gov/books/NBK537018/
24. Wong M, Kiel J. Anatomy, Shoulder and Upper Limb, Acromioclavicular Joint. [Updated 2023 Jul 24]. In: StatPearls [Internet]. Treasure Island (FL): StatPearls Publishing; 2025 Jan. Available from: https://www.ncbi.nlm.nih.gov/books/NBK499858/
25. Streilein JW. Skin-associated lymphoid tissues (SALT): origins and functions. J Invest Dermatol. 1983 Jun;80(Suppl):12s–16s. doi: 10.1111/1523-1747.ep12536743. PMID: 6602189.
26. Araki T, Nishino M, Gao W, et al. Normal thymus in adults: appearance on CT and associations with age, sex, BMI and smoking. Eur Radiol. 2016 Jan;26(1):15–24. doi: 10.1007/s00330-015-3796-y. Epub 2015 Apr 30. PMID: 25925358; PMCID: PMC4847950.
27. Park S. Robot-assisted thoracic surgery thymectomy. J Chest Surg. 2021 Aug;54(4):319–24. doi: 10.5090/jcs.21.059. PMID: 34353974; PMCID: PMC8350461.
28. Yan F, Mo X, Liu J, et al. Thymic function in the regulation of T cells, and molecular mechanisms underlying the modulation of cytokines and stress signaling (Review). Mol Med Rep. 2017 Nov;16(5):7175–84. doi: 10.3892/mmr.2017.7525. Epub 2017 Sep 19. PMID: 28944829; PMCID: PMC5865843.
29. Savvidis S, Ragazzini R, de Rafael VC, et al. Advanced three-dimensional X-ray imaging unravels structural development of the human thymus compartments. Commun Med (Lond). 2024 Oct;4(1):204. doi: 10.1038/s43856-024-00623-7. PMID: 39438572; PMCID: PMC11496816.
30. Remien K, Jozsa F, Jan A. Anatomy, Head and Neck, Thymus. [Updated 2025 Jun 23]. In: StatPearls [Internet]. Treasure Island (FL): StatPearls Publishing; 2025 Jan. Available from: https://www.ncbi.nlm.nih.gov/books/NBK539748/
31. Safieddine N, Keshavjee S. Anatomy of the thymus gland. Thorac Surg Clin. 2011 May;21(2):191–5, viii. doi: 10.1016/j.thorsurg.2010.12.011. PMID: 21477769.

32. Bujoreanu I, Gupta V. Anatomy, Lymph Nodes. [Updated 2023 Jul 25]. In: StatPearls [Internet]. Treasure Island (FL): StatPearls Publishing; 2025 Jan. Available from: https://www.ncbi.nlm.nih.gov/books/NBK557717/
33. Suami H, Taylor GI, Pan WR. The lymphatic territories of the upper limb: anatomical study and clinical implications. Plast Reconstr Surg. 2007 May;119(6):1813–22. doi: 10.1097/01.prs.0000246516.64780.61. PMID: 17440362.
34. Kyriacou H, Khan YS. Anatomy, Shoulder and Upper Limb, Axillary Lymph Nodes. [Updated 2023 Jul 24]. In: StatPearls [Internet]. Treasure Island (FL): StatPearls Publishing; 2025 Jan. Available from: https://www.ncbi.nlm.nih.gov/books/NBK559188/
35. Khan YS, Fakoya AO, Sajjad H. Anatomy, Thorax: Mammary Gland. [Updated Feb 18]. In: StatPearls [Internet]. Treasure Island (FL): StatPearls Publishing; 2025 Jan. PMID: 31613446.
36. Capobianco SM, Fahmy MW, Sicari V. Anatomy, Thorax, Subclavian Veins. [Updated 2023 Jul 24]. In: StatPearls [Internet]. Treasure Island (FL): StatPearls Publishing; 2025 Jan. PMID: 30422480.
37. Gordon A, Alsayouri K. Anatomy, Shoulder and Upper Limb, Axilla. [Updated 2023 Jul 24]. In: StatPearls [Internet]. Treasure Island (FL): StatPearls Publishing; 2025 Jan. Available from: https://www.ncbi.nlm.nih.gov/books/NBK547723/
38. Thiel R, Munjal A, Daly DT. Anatomy, Shoulder and Upper Limb, Axillary Artery. [Updated 2025 Jan 20]. In: StatPearls [Internet]. Treasure Island (FL): StatPearls Publishing; 2025 Jan. PMID: 29489298.
39. Herekar R, Bordoni B, Daly DT. Anatomy, Shoulder and Upper Limb, Intercostobrachial Nerves. [Updated 2023 Jul 17]. In: StatPearls [Internet]. Treasure Island (FL): StatPearls Publishing; 2025 Jan. Available from: https://www.ncbi.nlm.nih.gov/books/NBK557619/
40. Polcaro L, Charlick M, Daly DT. Anatomy, Head and Neck: Brachial Plexus. [Updated 2023 Aug 14]. In: StatPearls [Internet]. Treasure Island (FL): StatPearls Publishing; 2025 Jan. Available from: https://www.ncbi.nlm.nih.gov/books/NBK531473/
41. Kaiser JT, Lugo-Pico JG. Neuroanatomy, Spinal Nerves. [Updated 2023 Aug 14]. In: StatPearls [Internet]. Treasure Island (FL): StatPearls Publishing; 2025 Jan. Available from: https://www.ncbi.nlm.nih.gov/books/NBK542218/
42. Abdullah S, Bowden RE. The blood supply of the brachial plexus. Proc R Soc Med. 1960 Mar;53(3):203–5. doi: 10.1177/003591576005300311. PMID: 13791417; PMCID: PMC1870934.
43. Patel M, Varacallo MA. Anatomy, Shoulder and Upper Limb, Arm Nerves. [Updated 2024 Mar 13]. In: StatPearls [Internet]. Treasure Island (FL): StatPearls Publishing; 2025 Jan. Available from: https://www.ncbi.nlm.nih.gov/books/NBK547735/
44. Johnson EO, Vekris M, Demesticha T, Soucacos PN. Neuroanatomy of the brachial plexus: normal and variant anatomy of its formation. Surg Radiol Anat. 2010 Mar;32(3):291–7. doi: 10.1007/s00276-010-0646-0. Epub 2010 Mar 17. PMID: 20237781.
45. Kuhn JE, Lebus V GF, Bible JE. Thoracic outlet syndrome. J Am Acad Orthop Surg. 2015 Apr;23(4):222–32. doi: 10.5435/JAAOS-D-13-00215. PMID: 25808686.
46. Ruchelsman DE, Pettrone S, Price AE, Grossman JA. Brachial plexus birth palsy: an overview of early treatment considerations. Bulletin of the NYU Hospital for Joint Diseases. 2009;67(1):83–89. PMID: 19302062.
47. Lovaglio AC, Socolovsky M, Di Masi G, Bonilla G. Treatment of neuropathic pain after peripheral nerve and brachial plexus traumatic injury. Neurol India. 2019 Jan–Feb;67(Supplement):S32–37. doi: 10.4103/0028-3886.250699. PMID: 30688230.
48. Mostafa E, Imonugo O, Varacallo MA. Anatomy, Shoulder and Upper Limb, Humerus. [Updated 2023 Aug 7]. In: StatPearls [Internet]. Treasure Island (FL): StatPearls Publishing; 2025 Jan. Available from: https://www.ncbi.nlm.nih.gov/books/NBK534821/
49. Jeno SH, Varacallo MA. Anatomy, Back, Latissimus Dorsi. [Updated 2023 Mar 5]. In: StatPearls [Internet]. Treasure Island (FL): StatPearls Publishing; 2025 Jan. Available from: https://www.ncbi.nlm.nih.gov/books/NBK448120/
50. Plantz MA, Bordoni B. Anatomy, Shoulder and Upper Limb, Brachialis Muscle. [Updated 2023 Feb 21]. In: StatPearls [Internet]. Treasure Island (FL): StatPearls Publishing; 2025 Jan. Available from: https://www.ncbi.nlm.nih.gov/books/NBK551630/
51. Melaku T, Wondmagegn H, Gebremickael A, Tadesse A. Patterns of superficial veins in the cubital fossa and its clinical implications among southern Ethiopian population. Anat Cell Biol. 2022 Jun;55(2):148–54. doi: 10.5115/acb.21.217. Epub 2022 Apr 6. PMID: 35383135; PMCID: PMC9256478.
52. Darabi MR, Shams A, Bayat P, et al. A case report: variation of the cephalic and external jugular veins. ASJ 2015; 12 (4):203–5. URL: http://anatomyjournal.ir/article-1-90-en.html.
53. Sheen JR, Khan YS. Anatomy, Shoulder and Upper Limb, Cubital Fossa. [Updated 2023 Jul 24]. In: StatPearls [Internet]. Treasure Island (FL): StatPearls Publishing; 2025 Jan. Available from: https://www.ncbi.nlm.nih.gov/books/NBK551674/

54. Bordoni B, Omole AE. Anatomy, Thorax, Brachiocephalic (Innominate) Veins. [Updated 2025 Dec 9]. In: StatPearls [Internet]. Treasure Island (FL): StatPearls Publishing; 2025 Jan. Available from: https://www.ncbi.nlm.nih.gov/books/NBK544339/
55. Nguyen JD, Duong H. Anatomy, Shoulder and Upper Limb, Veins. [Updated 2023 Aug 14]. In: StatPearls [Internet]. Treasure Island (FL): StatPearls Publishing; 2025 Jan. Available from: https://www.ncbi.nlm.nih.gov/books/NBK546676/
56. Javed O, Maldonado KA, Ashmyan R. Anatomy, Shoulder and Upper Limb, Muscles. [Updated 2023 Jul 24]. In: StatPearls [Internet]. Treasure Island (FL): StatPearls Publishing; 2025 Jan. Available from: https://www.ncbi.nlm.nih.gov/books/NBK482410/
57. Ambike S, Paclet F, Zatsiorsky VM, Latash ML. Factors affecting grip force: anatomy, mechanics, and referent configurations. Exp Brain Res. 2014 Apr;232(4):1219–31. doi: 10.1007/s00221-014-3838-8. Epub 2014 Jan 31. PMID: 24477762; PMCID: PMC4013148.
58. Okwumabua E, Sinkler MA, Bordoni B. Anatomy, Shoulder and Upper Limb, Hand Muscles. [Updated 2023 Jul 24]. In: StatPearls [Internet]. Treasure Island (FL): StatPearls Publishing; 2025 Jan. Available from: https://www.ncbi.nlm.nih.gov/books/NBK537229/
59. Lung BE, Burns B. Anatomy, Shoulder and Upper Limb, Hand Flexor Digitorum Profundus Muscle. [Updated 2023 Nov 13]. In: StatPearls [Internet]. Treasure Island (FL): StatPearls Publishing; 2025 Jan. Available from: https://www.ncbi.nlm.nih.gov/books/NBK526046/
60. Cooney WP 3rd, Chao EY. Biomechanical analysis of static forces in the thumb during hand function. J Bone Joint Surg Am. 1977 Jan;59(1):27–36. PMID: 833171.
61. Figueroa-Jacinto R, Armstrong T, Zhou W. An investigation on normal force distribution and posture of a hand pressing on a flat surface. J Biomech. 2018 Oct;79:164–72. doi:10.1016/j.jbiomech.2018.08.002.

CHAPTERS 6 AND 14 LOWER LIMB

1. Lopez-Ojeda W, Pandey A, Alhajj M, et al. Anatomy, Skin (Integument). [Updated 2022 Oct 17]. In: StatPearls [Internet]. Treasure Island (FL): StatPearls Publishing; 2025 Jan. Available from: https://www.ncbi.nlm.nih.gov/books/NBK441980/
2. Dodia P, Arida MA. Dermatopathology Epidermis Histology. [Updated 2023 May 6]. In: StatPearls [Internet]. Treasure Island (FL): StatPearls Publishing; 2025 Jan. Available from: https://www.ncbi.nlm.nih.gov/books/NBK592423/
3. Institute of Medicine (US) Committee to Review Dietary Reference Intakes for Vitamin D and Calcium; Ross AC, Taylor CL, Yaktine AL, et al., editors. Dietary Reference Intakes for Calcium and Vitamin D. Washington (DC): National Academies Press (US); 2011. Available from: https://www.ncbi.nlm.nih.gov/books/NBK56061/
4. Losquadro WD. Anatomy of the skin and the pathogenesis of nonmelanoma skin cancer. Facial Plast Surg Clin North Am. 2017 Aug;25(3):283–9. doi: 10.1016/j.fsc.2017.03.001. Epub 2017 May 30. PMID: 28676156.
5. Wilson TE, Crandall CG. Effect of thermal stress on cardiac function. Exerc Sport Sci Rev. 2011 Jan;39(1): 12–7. doi: 10.1097/JES.0b013e318201eed6. PMID: 21088607; PMCID: PMC3076691.
6. Casa DJ, Cheuvront SN, Galloway SD, Shirreffs SM. Fluid needs for training, competition, and recovery in track-and-field athletes. Int J Sport Nutr Exerc Metab. 2019 Mar;29(2):175–80. doi: 10.1123/ijsnem.2018-0374. Epub 2019 Apr 4. PMID: 30943836.
7. Cramer MN, Gagnon D, Laitano O, Crandall CG. Human temperature regulation under heat stress in health, disease, and injury. Physiol Rev. 2022 Oct;102(4):1907–89. doi: 10.1152/physrev.00047.2021. Epub 2022 Jun 9. PMID: 35679471; PMCID: PMC9394784.
8. Hoover E, Aslam S, Krishnamurthy K. Physiology, Sebaceous Glands. [Updated 2022 Oct 10]. In: StatPearls [Internet]. Treasure Island (FL): StatPearls Publishing; 2025 Jan. Available from: https://www.ncbi.nlm.nih.gov/books/NBK499819/
9. Patel BC, Treister AD, McCausland C, Lio PA, Jozsa F. Anatomy, Skin, Sudoriferous Gland. [Updated 2023 Apr 24]. In: StatPearls [Internet]. Treasure Island (FL): StatPearls Publishing; 2025 Jan. PMID: 30020616.
10. Baker LB. Physiology of sweat gland function: the roles of sweating and sweat composition in human health. Temperature (Austin). 2019 Jul;6(3):211–59. doi: 10.1080/23328940.2019.1632145. PMID: 31608304; PMCID: PMC6773238.
11. Sato K, Leidal R, Sato F. Morphology and development of an apoeccrine sweat gland in human axillae. Am J Physiol. 1987 Jan;252(1 Pt 2):R166–80. doi: 10.1152/ajpregu.1987.252.1.R166. PMID: 3812728.
12. Lee MM, Anand S, Loyd JW. Saphenous Vein Cutdown. [Updated 2023 Sep 4]. In: StatPearls [Internet]. Treasure Island (FL): StatPearls Publishing; 2025 Jan. Available from: https://www.ncbi.nlm.nih.gov/books/NBK532880/

13. Khan A, Arain A. Anatomy, Bony Pelvis and Lower Limb: Anterior Thigh Muscles. [Updated 2023 Mar 17]. In: StatPearls [Internet]. Treasure Island (FL): StatPearls Publishing; 2025 Jan. Available from: https://www.ncbi.nlm.nih.gov/books/NBK538425/
14. Gladden JD, Gulati R, Sandoval Y. Contemporary techniques for femoral and radial arterial access in the cardiac catheterization laboratory. Rev Cardiovasc Med. 2022 Sep;23(9):316. doi: 10.31083/j.rcm2309316. PMID: 39077689; PMCID: PMC11262397.
15. Haleem SM, Collier SA, Agasthi P. Femoral Vascular Closure Devices After Catheterization Procedure. [Updated 2025 Aug 2]. In: StatPearls [Internet]. Treasure Island (FL): StatPearls Publishing; 2025 Jan. Available from: https://www.ncbi.nlm.nih.gov/books/NBK557472/
16. Azam M, Wehrle CJ, Shaw PM. Anatomy, Bony Pelvis and Lower Limb: Tibial Artery. [Updated 2023 Aug 8]. In: StatPearls [Internet]. Treasure Island (FL): StatPearls Publishing; 2025 Jan. Available from: https://www.ncbi.nlm.nih.gov/books/NBK532871/
17. Bowers Z, Nassereddin A, Sinkler MA, et al. Anatomy, Bony Pelvis and Lower Limb: Popliteal Artery. [Updated 2023 Jul 24]. In: StatPearls [Internet]. Treasure Island (FL): StatPearls Publishing; 2025 Jan. Available from: https://www.ncbi.nlm.nih.gov/books/NBK537125/
18. Tajran J, Gosman AA. Anatomy, Head and Neck, Scalp. [Updated 2023 Jul 24]. In: StatPearls [Internet]. Treasure Island (FL): StatPearls Publishing; 2025 Jan. Available from: https://www.ncbi.nlm.nih.gov/books/NBK551565/
19. Callese TE, Cusumano L, Redwood KD, et al. Classification of genicular artery anatomic variants using intraoperative cone-beam computed tomography. Cardiovasc Intervent Radiol. 2023 May;46(5):628–34. doi: 10.1007/s00270-023-03411-3. Epub 2023 Mar 22. PMID: 36949185; PMCID: PMC10156764.
20. Torkian P, Golzarian J, Chalian M, et al. Osteoarthritis-related knee pain treated with genicular artery embolization: a systematic review and meta-analysis. Orthop J Sports Med. 2021 Jul;9(7):23259671211021356. doi: 10.1177/23259671211021356. PMID: 34350303; PMCID: PMC8287378.
21. Casadaban LC, Mandell JC, Epelboym Y. Genicular artery embolization for osteoarthritis related knee pain: a systematic review and qualitative analysis of clinical outcomes. Cardiovasc Intervent Radiol. 2021 Jan;44(1):1–9. doi: 10.1007/s00270-020-02687-z. Epub 2020 Nov 1. PMID: 33135117; PMCID: PMC8025891.
22. Goodfellow J, Hungerford DS, Zindel M. Patello-femoral joint mechanics and pathology. 1. Functional anatomy of the patello-femoral joint. J Bone Joint Surg Br. 1976 Aug;58(3):287–90. doi: 10.1302/0301-620X.58B3.956243. PMID: 956243.
23. Wendt PP, Johnson RP. A study of quadriceps excursion, torque, and the effect of patellectomy on cadaver knees. J Bone Joint Surg Am. 1985 Jun;67(5):726–32. PMID: 3997925.
24. Loudon JK. Biomechanics and pathomechanics of the patellofemoral joint. Int J Sports Phys Ther. 2016 Dec;11(6):820–30. PMID: 27904787; PMCID: PMC5095937.
25. Falkson SR, Hinson JW. Westphal Sign. [Updated 2023 Feb 6]. In: StatPearls [Internet]. Treasure Island (FL): StatPearls Publishing; 2025 Jan. Available from: https://www.ncbi.nlm.nih.gov/books/NBK553214/
26. Brinkman JC, Reeson E, Chhabra A. Acute Patellar Tendon Ruptures: An Update on Management. J Am Acad Orthop Surg Glob Res Rev. 2024 Apr;8(4):e24.00060. doi: 10.5435/JAAOSGlobal-D-24-00060. PMID: 38569093; PMCID: PMC10994452.
27. Mendiguchia J, Alentorn-Geli E, Idoate F, Myer GD. Rectus femoris muscle injuries in football: a clinically relevant review of mechanisms of injury, risk factors and preventive strategies. Br J Sports Med. 2013 Apr;47(6):359–66. doi: 10.1136/bjsports-2012-091250. Epub 2012 Aug 3. PMID: 22864009.
28. Ma C, Wang X, Li J. Assessment in location of sciatic nerve between the ischial tuberosity and the greater trochanter of the femur: a cadaveric study. Heliyon. 2023 Dec;10(1):e23751. doi: 10.1016/j.heliyon.2023.e23751. PMID: 38192877; PMCID: PMC10772174.
29. Murdock CJ, Mudreac A, Agyeman K. Anatomy, Abdomen and Pelvis, Rectus Femoris Muscle. [Updated 2023 Nov 13]. In: StatPearls [Internet]. Treasure Island (FL): StatPearls Publishing; 2025 Jan. Available from: https://www.ncbi.nlm.nih.gov/books/NBK539897/
30. Yu JS, Oh JS. Greater trochanter location measurement using a three-dimensional motion capture system during prone hip extension. J Phys Ther Sci. 2017 Feb;29(2):250 –54. doi: 10.1589/jpts.29.250. Epub 2017 Feb 24. PMID: 28265151; PMCID: PMC5332982.
31. Grant C, Pajaczkowski J. Conservative management of femoral anterior glide syndrome: a case series. J Can Chiropr Assoc. 2018 Dec;62(3):182–92. PMID: 30662073; PMCID: PMC6319433.
32. Craxford S, Vris A, Ahluwalia R, et al. Fracture related infection in open tibial fractures. J Orthop. 2024 Jan;51:98–02. doi: 10.1016/j.jor.2024.01.010. PMID: 38357441; PMCID: PMC10862397.
33. Barr L, Hatch N, Roque J, Wu TS. Basic ultrasound-guided procedures. Critical Care Clinics. 2014 Apr;30(2):275–04. doi: 10.1016/j.ccc.2013.10.004.
34. Pomposelli FB Jr, Marcaccio EJ, Gibbons GW, et al. Dorsalis pedis arterial bypass: durable limb salvage for foot ischemia in patients with diabetes mellitus. J Vasc Surg. 1995 Mar;21(3):375–84. doi: 10.1016/s0741-5214(95)70279-2. PMID: 7877219.

 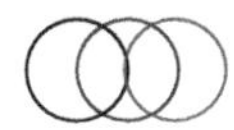

35. Ntuli S, Nalla S, Kiter A. Anatomical variation of the dorsalis pedis artery in a South African population: a cadaveric study. Foot (Edinb). 2018 Jun;35:16–27. doi: 10.1016/j.foot.2018.01.002. Epub 2018 May 10. PMID: 29753997.
36. Mavili E, Dönmez H, Kahriman G, et al. Popliteal artery branching patterns detected by digital subtraction angiography. Diagn Interv Radiol. 2011 Mar;17(1):80–3. doi: 10.4261/1305-3825.DIR.3141-09.1. Epub 2010 Aug 13. PMID: 20706978.
37. Chitra R. The relationship between the deep fibular nerve and the dorsalis pedis artery and its surgical importance. Indian J Plast Surg. 2009 Jan–Jun;42(1):18–21. doi: 10.4103/0970-0358.53007. PMID: 19881015; PMCID: PMC2772271.
38. McDermott MM, Criqui MH. Ankle-brachial index screening and improving peripheral artery disease detection and outcomes. JAMA. 2018 Jul;320(2):143–5. doi: 10.1001/jama.2018.8953. PMID: 29998324.
39. Noussios G, Theologou K, Chouridis P, et al. A rare morphological study concerning the longest bone of the human anatomy in the population of the northern greece. J Clin Med Res. 2019 Nov;11(11):740–4. doi: 10.14740/jocmr3986. Epub 2019 Oct 29. PMID: 31803316; PMCID: PMC6879022.
40. Tsutsumi M, Nimura A, Utsunomiya H, Kudo S, Akita K. Capsular attachment on the anterosuperior femoral head-neck junction: a hypothesis about femoroacetabular impingement. J Anat. 2024 Aug;245(2):231–9. doi: 10.1111/joa.14046. Epub 2024 Apr 8. PMID: 38590168; PMCID: PMC11259747.
41. Landin D, Thompson M, Reid M. Knee and ankle joint angles influence the plantarflexion torque of the gastrocnemius. J Clin Med Res. 2015 Aug;7(8):602–6. doi: 10.14740/jocmr2107w. Epub 2015 Jun 9. PMID: 26124905; PMCID: PMC4471746.
42. Bordoni B, Varacallo MA. Anatomy, Bony Pelvis and Lower Limb, Gastrocnemius Muscle. [Updated 2023 Apr 17]. In: StatPearls [Internet]. Treasure Island (FL): StatPearls Publishing; 2025 Jan. Available from: https://www.ncbi.nlm.nih.gov/books/NBK532946/
43. Lung K, Lui F. Anatomy, Abdomen and Pelvis: Superior Gluteal Nerve. [Updated 2023 Aug 14]. In: StatPearls [Internet]. Treasure Island (FL): StatPearls Publishing; 2025 Jan. Available from: https://www.ncbi.nlm.nih.gov/books/NBK535408/
44. DeJong AF, Mangum LC, Resch JE, Saliba SA. Detection of gluteal changes using ultrasound imaging during phases of gait in individuals with medial knee displacement. J Sport Rehabil. 2019 Jul;28(5):494–04. doi: 10.1123/jsr.2017-0336. Epub 2018 Dec 17. PMID: 29543116.
45. Willard FH, Vleeming A, Schuenke MD, Danneels L, Schleip R. The thoracolumbar fascia: anatomy, function and clinical considerations. J Anat. 2012 Dec;221(6):507–36. doi: 10.1111/j.1469-7580.2012.01511.x. Epub 2012 May 27. PMID: 22630613; PMCID: PMC3512278.
46. Barker PJ, Hapuarachchi KS, Ross JA, et al. Anatomy and biomechanics of gluteus maximus and the thoracolumbar fascia at the sacroiliac joint. Clin Anat. 2014 Mar;27(2):234–40. doi: 10.1002/ca.22233. Epub 2013 Aug 20. PMID: 23959791.
47. Rocos B, Ward A. Gluteal compartment syndrome with sciatic nerve palsy caused by traumatic rupture of the inferior gluteal artery: a successful surgical treatment. BMJ Case Rep. 2017 Jan;2017:bcr2016216709. doi: 10.1136/bcr-2016-216709. PMID: 28122800; PMCID: PMC5278333.
48. Elzanie A, Borger J. Anatomy, Bony Pelvis and Lower Limb, Gluteus Maximus Muscle. [Updated 2023 Apr 1]. In: StatPearls [Internet]. Treasure Island (FL): StatPearls Publishing; 2025 Jan. Available from: https://www.ncbi.nlm.nih.gov/books/NBK538193/
49. Gallego-Izquierdo T, Vidal-Aragón G, Calderón-Corrales P, et al. Effects of a gluteal muscles specific exercise program on the vertical jump. Int J Environ Res Public Health. 2020 Jul;17(15):5383. doi: 10.3390/ijerph17155383. PMID: 32726899; PMCID: PMC7432749.
50. Lieberman DE, Raichlen DA, Pontzer H, Bramble DM, Cutright-Smith E. The human gluteus maximus and its role in running. J Exp Biol. 2006 Jun;209(Pt 11):2143–55. doi: 10.1242/jeb.02255. PMID: 16709916.
51. Ipaktchi R, Boyce MK, Mett TR, Vogt PM. Defektdeckung mit Musculus-tensor-fasciae-latae-Lappen [Reconstruction using the tensor fasciae latae muscle flap]. Oper Orthop Traumatol. 2018 Aug;30(4):228–35. German. doi: 10.1007/s00064-018-0556-6. Epub 2018 Jun 27. PMID: 29951749.
52. Walters BB, Varacallo MA. Anatomy, Bony Pelvis and Lower Limb: Thigh Sartorius Muscle. [Updated 2023 Aug 28]. In: StatPearls [Internet]. Treasure Island (FL): StatPearls Publishing; 2025 Jan. Available from: https://www.ncbi.nlm.nih.gov/books/NBK532889/
53. Polguj M, Bliźniewska K, Jędrzejewski K, Majos A, Topol M. Morphological study of linea aspera variations: proposal of classification and sexual dimorphism. Folia Morphol (Warsz). 2013 Feb;72(1):72–7. doi: 10.5603/fm.2013.0012. PMID: 23749715.
54. Hyland S, Sinkler MA, Varacallo MA. Anatomy, Bony Pelvis and Lower Limb: Popliteal Region. [Updated 2023 Jul 25]. In: StatPearls [Internet]. Treasure Island (FL): StatPearls Publishing; 2025 Jan. PMID: 30422486.
55. Yeung AY, Arbor TC, Garg R. Anatomy, Sesamoid Bones. [Updated 2023 Apr 4]. In: StatPearls [Internet]. Treasure Island (FL): StatPearls Publishing; 2025 Jan. Available from: https://www.ncbi.nlm.nih.gov/books/NBK578171/

56. Melvin JS, Mehta S. Patellar fractures in adults. J Am Acad Orthop Surg. 2011 Apr;19(4):198–07. doi: 10.5435/00124635-201104000-00004. PMID: 21464213.
57. Hallinan JTPD, Wang W, Pathria MN, Smitaman E, Huang BK. The peroneus longus muscle and tendon: a review of its anatomy and pathology. Skeletal Radiol. 2019 Sep;48(9):1329–44. doi: 10.1007/s00256-019-3168-9. Epub 2019 Feb 15. PMID: 30770941.
58. Benjamin M, Ralphs JR. Fibrocartilage in tendons and ligaments: an adaptation to compressive load. J Anat. 1998 Nov;193 (Pt 4):481–94. doi: 10.1046/j.1469-7580.1998.19340481.x. PMID: 10029181; PMCID: PMC1467873.
59. Wood VE. The sesamoid bones of the hand and their pathology. J Hand Surg Br. 1984 Oct;9(3):261–4. doi: 10.1016/0266-7681(84)90038-x. PMID: 6512360.
60. Chatra PS. Bursae around the knee joints. Indian J Radiol Imaging. 2012 Jan;22(1):27–30. doi: 10.4103/0971-3026.95400. PMID: 22623812; PMCID: PMC3354353.
61. Koh WL, Kwek JW, Quek ST, Peh WC. Clinics in diagnostic imaging (77). Pes anserine bursitis. Singapore Med J. 2002 Sep;43(9):485–91. PMID: 12568429.
62. McCarthy CL, McNally EG. The MRI appearance of cystic lesions around the knee. Skeletal Radiol. 2004 Apr;33(4):187–209. doi: 10.1007/s00256-003-0741-y. Epub 2004 Feb 27. PMID: 14991250.
63. Basinger H, Hogg JP. Anatomy, Abdomen and Pelvis: Femoral Triangle. [Updated 2023 Mar 11]. In: StatPearls [Internet]. Treasure Island (FL): StatPearls Publishing; 2025 Jan. Available from: https://www.ncbi.nlm.nih.gov/books/NBK541140/
64. Migirov A, Arbor TC, Vilella RC. Anatomy, Abdomen and Pelvis: Adductor Canal (Subsartorial Canal, Hunter Canal). [Updated 2024 Jan 9]. In: StatPearls [Internet]. Treasure Island (FL): StatPearls Publishing; 2025 Jan. Available from: https://www.ncbi.nlm.nih.gov/books/NBK556046/
65. Jeno SH, Launico MV, Schindler GS. Anatomy, Bony Pelvis and Lower Limb: Thigh Adductor Magnus Muscle. [Updated 2023 Oct 24]. In: StatPearls [Internet]. Treasure Island (FL): StatPearls Publishing; 2025 Jan. Available from: https://www.ncbi.nlm.nih.gov/books/NBK534842/
66. Hyland S, Sinkler MA, Varacallo MA. Anatomy, Bony Pelvis and Lower Limb: Popliteal Region. [Updated 2023 Jul 25]. In: StatPearls [Internet]. Treasure Island (FL): StatPearls Publishing; 2025 Jan. Available from: https://www.ncbi.nlm.nih.gov/books/NBK532891/
67. Gupton M, Imonugo O, Black AC, et al. Anatomy, Bony Pelvis and Lower Limb, Knee. [Updated 2023 Nov 5]. In: StatPearls [Internet]. Treasure Island (FL): StatPearls Publishing; 2025 Jan. Available from: https://www.ncbi.nlm.nih.gov/books/NBK500017/
68. Golanó P, Vega J, de Leeuw PA, et al. Anatomy of the ankle ligaments: a pictorial essay. Knee Surg Sports Traumatol Arthrosc. 2010 May;18(5):557–69. doi: 10.1007/s00167-010-1100-x. Epub 2010 Mar 23. PMID: 20309522; PMCID: PMC2855022.
69. Volpon JB, de Carvalho Filho G. Calcaneal apophysitis: a quantitative radiographic evaluation of the secondary ossification center. Arch Orthop Trauma Surg. 2002 Jul;122(6):338–41. doi: 10.1007/s00402-002-0410-y. Epub 2002 Apr 30. PMID: 12136298.
70. Smith JM, Varacallo MA. Osgood-Schlatter Disease. [Updated 2023 Aug 4]. In: StatPearls [Internet]. Treasure Island (FL): StatPearls Publishing; 2025 Jan. Available from: https://www.ncbi.nlm.nih.gov/books/NBK441995/
71. Medina McKeon JM, Hoch MC. The ankle-joint complex: a kinesiologic approach to lateral ankle sprains. J Athl Train. 2019 Jun;54(6):589–602. doi: 10.4085/1062-6050-472-17. Epub 2019 Jun 11. PMID: 31184957; PMCID: PMC6602390.
72. Bowley MP, Doughty CT. Entrapment neuropathies of the lower extremity. Med Clin North Am. 2019 Mar;103(2):371–82. doi: 10.1016/j.mcna.2018.10.013. Epub 2018 Dec 3. PMID: 30704688.
73. Takebe K, Nakagawa A, Minami H, Kanazawa H, Hirohata K. Role of the fibula in weight-bearing. Clin Orthop Relat Res. 1984;184:289–92. PMID: 6705357. doi: 10.1097/00003086-198404000-00047.
74. Zhao W, Wang Q, Cui Z, et al. A retrospective assessment of the clinical efficacy of different internal fixation methods in the treatment of distal fibula fractures in the elderly. Medicine (Baltimore). 2022 Oct;101(43):e30973. doi: 10.1097/MD.0000000000030973. PMID: 36316934; PMCID: PMC9622573.
75. Le Minor JM, Mousson JF, de Mathelin P, Bierry G. Non-metric variation of the middle phalanges of the human toes (II-V): long/short types and their evolutionary significance. J Anat. 2016 Jun;228(6):965–74. doi: 10.1111/joa.12462. Epub 2016 Mar 31. PMID: 27031825; PMCID: PMC5341584.
76. Keener BJ, Sizensky JA. The anatomy of the calcaneus and surrounding structures. Foot Ankle Clin. 2005 Sep;10(3):413–24. doi: 10.1016/j.fcl.2005.04.003. PMID: 16081012.
77. MacGregor R, Byerly DW. Anatomy, Bony Pelvis and Lower Limb: Foot Bones. [Updated 2023 May 23]. In: StatPearls [Internet]. Treasure Island (FL): StatPearls Publishing; 2025 Jan. Available from: https://www.ncbi.nlm.nih.gov/books/NBK557447/
78. Ficke J, Byerly DW. Anatomy, Bony Pelvis and Lower Limb: Foot. [Updated 2023 Aug 7]. In: StatPearls [Internet]. Treasure Island (FL): StatPearls Publishing; 2025 Jan. Available from: https://www.ncbi.nlm.nih.gov/books/NBK546698/

 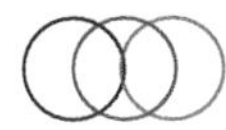

79. Melenevsky Y, Mackey RA, Abrahams RB, Thomson NB 3rd. Talar fractures and dislocations: a radiologist's guide to timely diagnosis and classification. Radiographics. 2015 May–Jun;35(3):765–79. doi: 10.1148/rg.2015140156. PMID: 25969933.
80. Manganaro D, Alsayouri K. Anatomy, Bony Pelvis and Lower Limb: Ankle Joint. [Updated 2023 May 23]. In: StatPearls [Internet]. Treasure Island (FL): StatPearls Publishing; 2025 Jan. PMID: 31424742.
81. Brockett CL, Chapman GJ. Biomechanics of the ankle. Orthop Trauma. 2016 Jun;30(3):232–8. doi: 10.1016/j.mporth.2016.04.015. PMID: 27594929; PMCID: PMC4994968.
82. Resnick D. Talar ridges, osteophytes, and beaks: a radiologic commentary. Radiology. 1984 May;151(2):329–32. doi: 10.1148/radiology.151.2.6709899. PMID: 6709899.
83. Gefen A. Biomechanical analysis of fatigue-related foot injury mechanisms in athletes and recruits during intensive marching. Med Biol Eng Comput. 2002 May;40(3):302–10. doi: 10.1007/BF02344212. PMID: 12195977.
84. Agrawal U, Tiwari V. Metatarsal Fractures. [Updated 2023 Aug 3]. In: StatPearls [Internet]. Treasure Island (FL): StatPearls Publishing; 2025 Jan. Available from: https://www.ncbi.nlm.nih.gov/books/NBK574512/
85. Prapto D, Dreyer MA. Anatomy, Bony Pelvis and Lower Limb: Navicular Bone. [Updated 2023 Aug 21]. In: StatPearls [Internet]. Treasure Island (FL): StatPearls Publishing; 2025 Jan. Available from: https://www.ncbi.nlm.nih.gov/books/NBK547675/
86. Chauhan HM, Taqi M. Anatomy, Bony Pelvis and Lower Limb: Arches of the Foot. [Updated 2025 Aug 27]. In: StatPearls [Internet]. Treasure Island (FL): StatPearls Publishing; 2025 Jan. [Figure, Lateral Longitudinal Arch of the.... Available from: https://www.ncbi.nlm.nih.gov/books/NBK587361/figure/article-149120.image.f4/
87. Gutiérrez-Vilahú L, Guerra-Balic M. Footprint measurement methods for the assessment and classification of foot types in subjects with Down syndrome: a systematic review. J Orthop Surg Res. 2021 Aug;16(1):537. doi: 10.1186/s13018-021-02667-0. PMID: 34452620; PMCID: PMC8393714.
88. Gutiérrez-Vilahú L, Massó-Ortigosa N, Rey-Abella F, Costa-Tutusaus L, Guerra-Balic M. Reliability and validity of the footprint assessment method using Photoshop CS5 software in young people with Down syndrome. J Am Podiatr Med Assoc. 2016 May;106(3):207–13. doi: 10.7547/15-012. PMID: 27269976.
89. Allam AE, Chang KV. Plantar Heel Pain. [Updated 2024 Jan 4]. In: StatPearls [Internet]. Treasure Island (FL): StatPearls Publishing; 2025 Jan. Available from: https://www.ncbi.nlm.nih.gov/books/NBK499868/

CHAPTERS 7 AND 15 HEAD AND NECK

1. Boes KM, Durham AC. Bone Marrow, Blood Cells, and the Lymphoid/Lymphatic System. In: Pathologic Basis of Veterinary Disease. 2017, 724–804.e2. doi: 10.1016/B978-0-323-35775-3.00013-8. Epub 2017 Feb 17. PMCID: PMC7158316.
2. Rindy LJ, Chambers AR. Bone Marrow Aspiration and Biopsy. [Updated 2023 May 29]. In: StatPearls [Internet]. Treasure Island (FL): StatPearls Publishing; 2025 Jan. Available from: https://www.ncbi.nlm.nih.gov/books/NBK559232/
3. Wang H, Leng Y, Gong Y. Bone marrow fat and hematopoiesis. Front Endocrinol (Lausanne). 2018 Nov;9:694. doi: 10.3389/fendo.2018.00694. PMID: 30546345; PMCID: PMC6280186.
4. Juneja P, Munjal A, Hubbard JB. Anatomy, Joints. [Updated 2024 Apr 21]. In: StatPearls [Internet]. Treasure Island (FL): StatPearls Publishing; 2025 Jan. Available from: https://www.ncbi.nlm.nih.gov/books/NBK507893/
5. Chijimatsu R, Saito T. Mechanisms of synovial joint and articular cartilage development. Cell Mol Life Sci. 2019 Oct;76(20):3939–52. doi: 10.1007/s00018-019-03191-5. Epub 2019 Jun 14. PMID: 31201464; PMCID: PMC11105481.
6. Breeland G, Sinkler MA, Menezes RG. Embryology, Bone Ossification. [Updated 2023 May 1]. In: StatPearls [Internet]. Treasure Island (FL): StatPearls Publishing; 2025 Jan. Available from: https://www.ncbi.nlm.nih.gov/books/NBK539718/
7. Cope PJ, Ourradi K, Li Y, Sharif M. Models of osteoarthritis: the good, the bad and the promising. Osteoarthritis Cartilage. 2019 Feb;27(2):230–9. doi: 10.1016/j.joca.2018.09.016. Epub 2018 Oct 25. PMID: 30391394; PMCID: PMC6350005.
8. Tu C, He J, Wu B, Wang W, Li Z. An extensive review regarding the adipokines in the pathogenesis and progression of osteoarthritis. Cytokine. 2019 Jan;113:1–12. doi: 10.1016/j.cyto.2018.06.019. Epub 2018 Jun 28. PMID: 30539776.
9. Kim TH, Lee SH, Kim DH, et al. The suprasternal notch as a landmark of chest compression depth in CPR. Am J Emerg Med. 2016 Mar;34(3):433–6. doi: 10.1016/j.ajem.2015.11.026. Epub 2015 Dec 1. PMID: 26682672.

10. Murphy MC, O'Donnell CPF. The suprasternal notch: a surface landmark for endotracheal tube tip position in newborns? Arch Dis Child Fetal Neonatal Ed. 2017 Jul;102(4):F371–2. doi: 10.1136/archdischild-2016-312555. Epub 2017 May 3. PMID: 28468897.
11. Claus I, Van Bael K, Speybrouck S, Van Der Tempel G. Subclavian artery stenosis caused by a prominent first rib. SAGE Open Med Case Rep. 2015 Apr;3. doi: 10.1177/2050313X15578319. PMID: 27489685; PMCID: PMC4857319.
12. Demondion X, Herbinet P, Van Sint Jan S, et al. Imaging assessment of thoracic outlet syndrome. Radiographics. 2006 Nov–Dec;26(6):1735–50. doi: 10.1148/rg.266055079. PMID: 17102047.
13. Plewa MC, Hall WA. Cavernous Sinus Thrombosis. [Updated 2025 Jun 16]. In: StatPearls [Internet]. Treasure Island (FL): StatPearls Publishing; 2025 Jan. Available from: https://www.ncbi.nlm.nih.gov/books/NBK448177/
14. Bechmann S, Rahman S, Kashyap V. Anatomy, Head and Neck, External Jugular Veins. [Updated 2023 Aug 8]. In: StatPearls [Internet]. Treasure Island (FL): StatPearls Publishing; 2025 Jan. Available from: https://www.ncbi.nlm.nih.gov/books/NBK538222/
15. Zeledón RA. Hemoflagellates. In: Baron S, editor. Medical Microbiology. 4th edition. Galveston (TX): University of Texas Medical Branch at Galveston; 1996. Chapter 82. Available from: https://www.ncbi.nlm.nih.gov/books/NBK8434/.
16. Allen E, Fingeret A. Anatomy, Head and Neck, Thyroid. [Updated 2025 Jun 23]. In: StatPearls [Internet]. Treasure Island (FL): StatPearls Publishing; 2025 Jan. Available from: https://www.ncbi.nlm.nih.gov/books/NBK470452/
17. Bunea MC, Rusali LM, Tudorache SI, Bratu IC, Bordei P. Considerations on the morphology of the thyroid ima artery. Surg Radiol Anat. 2024 Jan;46(1):91–9. doi: 10.1007/s00276-023-03268-8. Epub 2023 Nov 22. PMID: 37991506.
18. Saylam CY, Ozgiray E, Orhan M, Cagli S, Zileli M. Neuroanatomy of cervical sympathetic trunk: a cadaveric study. Clin Anat. 2009 Apr;22(3):324–30. doi: 10.1002/ca.20764. PMID: 19173257.
19. Casale J, Geiger Z. Anatomy, Head and Neck, Posterior Neck Triangle. [Updated 2023 Apr 28]. In: StatPearls [Internet]. Treasure Island (FL): StatPearls Publishing; 2025 Jan. Available from: https://www.ncbi.nlm.nih.gov/books/NBK537289/
20. Toth J, Lappin SL. Anatomy, Head and Neck, Mylohyoid Muscle. [Updated 2023 Jun 5]. In: StatPearls [Internet]. Treasure Island (FL): StatPearls Publishing; 2025 Jan. Available from: https://www.ncbi.nlm.nih.gov/books/NBK545293/
21. Bhaskar P, John J, Lone RA, Sallehuddin A. Selective use of superficial temporal artery cannulation in infants undergoing cardiac surgery. Ann Card Anaesth. 2015 Oct–Dec;18(4):606–8. doi: 10.4103/0971-9784.166486. PMID: 26440256; PMCID: PMC4881661.
22. Gardner S, Garber L, Grossi J. Bell's palsy: description, diagnosis, and current management. Cureus. 2025 Jan;17(1):e77656. doi: 10.7759/cureus.77656. PMID: 39974265; PMCID: PMC11835628.
23. Newadkar UR, Chaudhari L, Khalekar YK. Facial palsy, a disorder belonging to influential neurological dynasty: review of literature. N Am J Med Sci. 2016 Jul;8(7):263–7. doi: 10.4103/1947-2714.187130. PMID: 27583233; PMCID: PMC4982354.
24. Chason HM, Downs BW. Anatomy, Head and Neck, Parotid Gland. [Updated 2024 Sep 10]. In: StatPearls [Internet]. Treasure Island (FL): StatPearls Publishing; 2025 Jan. PMID: 30480958.
25. Ghannam MG, Singh P. Anatomy, Head and Neck, Salivary Glands. [Updated 2023 May 29]. In: StatPearls [Internet]. Treasure Island (FL): StatPearls Publishing; 2025 Jan. Available from: https://www.ncbi.nlm.nih.gov/books/NBK538325/
26. Tong J, Lopez MJ, Fakoya AO, Patel BC. Anatomy, Head and Neck: Orbicularis Oculi Muscle. [Updated May 25]. In: StatPearls [Internet]. Treasure Island (FL): StatPearls Publishing; 2025 Jan. PMID: 28722936.
27. Kitagawa N, Iwanaga J, Tubbs RS, Kim H, Moon YS, Hur MS. Variant muscle fibers connecting the orbicularis oculi to the orbicularis oris: case report. Anat Cell Biol. 2022 Dec;55(4):497–500. doi: 10.5115/acb.22.108. Epub 2022 Sep 1. PMID: 36044997; PMCID: PMC9747335.
28. Henry JP, Munakomi S. Anatomy, Head and Neck, Levator Scapulae Muscles. [Updated 2023 Aug 28]. In: StatPearls [Internet]. Treasure Island (FL): StatPearls Publishing; 2025 Jan. Available from: https://www.ncbi.nlm.nih.gov/books/NBK553120/
29. Bordoni B, Jozsa F, Varacallo MA. Anatomy, Head and Neck, Sternocleidomastoid Muscle. [Updated 2023 Apr 4]. In: StatPearls [Internet]. Treasure Island (FL): StatPearls Publishing; 2025 Jan. Available from: https://www.ncbi.nlm.nih.gov/books/NBK532881/
30. Downey RP, Samra NS. Anatomy, Thorax, Tracheobronchial Tree. [Updated 2023 Jul 24]. In: StatPearls [Internet]. Treasure Island (FL): StatPearls Publishing; 2025 Jan. Available from: https://www.ncbi.nlm.nih.gov/books/NBK556044/
31. Amador C, Weber C, Varacallo MA. Anatomy, Thorax, Bronchial. [Updated 2023 Aug 8]. In: StatPearls [Internet]. Treasure Island (FL): StatPearls Publishing; 2025 Jan. Available from: https://www.ncbi.nlm.nih.gov/books/NBK537353/

32. Miniato MA, Anand P, Varacallo MA. Anatomy, Shoulder and Upper Limb, Shoulder. [Updated 2023 Jul 24]. In: StatPearls [Internet]. Treasure Island (FL): StatPearls Publishing; 2025 Jan. Available from: https://www.ncbi.nlm.nih.gov/books/NBK536933/
33. Lofgren DH, McGuire D, Gotlib A. Frontal Sinus Fractures. [Updated 2023 Jun 30]. In: StatPearls [Internet]. Treasure Island (FL): StatPearls Publishing; 2025 Jan. Available from: https://www.ncbi.nlm.nih.gov/books/NBK557519/
34. Shaikh FH, Shumway KR, Soni A. Physiology, Taste. [Updated 2023 Jul 30]. In: StatPearls [Internet]. Treasure Island (FL): StatPearls Publishing; 2025 Jan. Available from: https://www.ncbi.nlm.nih.gov/books/NBK557768/
35. Breeland G, Aktar A, Patel BC. Anatomy, Head and Neck, Mandible. [Updated 2023 Apr 1]. In: StatPearls [Internet]. Treasure Island (FL): StatPearls Publishing; 2025 Jan. PMID: 30335325.
36. Rehman I, Mahabadi N, Motlagh M, et al. Anatomy, Head and Neck, Eye Fovea. [Updated 2023 Aug 28]. In: StatPearls [Internet]. Treasure Island (FL): StatPearls Publishing; 2025 Jan. Available from: https://www.ncbi.nlm.nih.gov/books/NBK482301/
37. Falkson SR, Sutton AE, Tadi P. Otoscopy. [Updated 2025 Jan 20]. In: StatPearls [Internet]. Treasure Island (FL): StatPearls Publishing; 2025 Jan. Available from: https://www.ncbi.nlm.nih.gov/books/NBK556090/
38. Chen CH, Huang CY, Cheng HL, et al. Smartphone-enabled versus conventional otoscopy in detecting middle ear disease: a meta-analysis. Diagnostics (Basel). 2022 Apr;12(4):972. doi: 10.3390/diagnostics12040972. PMID: 35454020; PMCID: PMC9029949.
39. Baratela MC, Mayer WP, Baptista JDS. Development and cross-sectional morphology of the recurrent laryngeal nerves in human fetuses. Anat Cell Biol. 2024 Sep;57(3):392–9. doi: 10.5115/acb.24.052. Epub 2024 Jul 17. PMID: 39013797; PMCID: PMC11424565.
40. Suárez-Quintanilla J, Fernández Cabrera A, Sharma S. Anatomy, Head and Neck: Larynx. [Updated 2023 Sep 4]. In: StatPearls [Internet]. Treasure Island (FL): StatPearls Publishing; 2025 Jan. Available from: https://www.ncbi.nlm.nih.gov/books/NBK538202/
41. Bui T, Fakoya AO, Das JM. Anatomy, Head and Neck: Pharyngeal Muscles. [Updated 2024 May 25]. In: StatPearls [Internet]. Treasure Island (FL): StatPearls Publishing; 2025 Jan. Available from: https://www.ncbi.nlm.nih.gov/books/NBK551654/
42. Collins JT, Nguyen A, Omole AE, et al. Anatomy, Abdomen and Pelvis, Small Intestine. [Updated 2025 Feb 18]. In: StatPearls [Internet]. Treasure Island (FL): StatPearls Publishing; 2025 Jan. Available from: https://www.ncbi.nlm.nih.gov/books/NBK459366/
43. Ogobuiro I, Gonzales J, Shumway KR, et al. Physiology, Gastrointestinal. [Updated 2023 Apr 8]. In: StatPearls [Internet]. Treasure Island (FL): StatPearls Publishing; 2025 Jan. Available from: https://www.ncbi.nlm.nih.gov/books/NBK537103/
44. Sumida K, Yamashita K, Kitamura S. Gross anatomical study of the human palatopharyngeus muscle throughout its entire course from origin to insertion. Clin Anat. 2012 Apr;25(3):314–23. doi: 10.1002/ca.21233. Epub 2011 Jul 28. PMID: 21800375.
45. Perta K, Kalmar E, Bae Y. A Cadaveric and magnetic resonance imaging investigation of the salpingopharyngeus. J Speech Lang Hear Res. 2021 May;64(5):1436–46. doi: 10.1044/2021_JSLHR-20-00483. Epub 2021 Apr 8. PMID: 33831310.
46. Jain P, Rathee M. Anatomy, Head and Neck, Stylopharyngeus Muscles. [Updated 2023 Jun 5]. In: StatPearls [Internet]. Treasure Island (FL): StatPearls Publishing; 2025 Jan. Available from: https://www.ncbi.nlm.nih.gov/books/NBK547719/
47. Jung B, Black AC, Bhutta BS. Anatomy, Head and Neck, Neck Movements. [Updated 2023 Nov 9]. In: StatPearls [Internet]. Treasure Island (FL): StatPearls Publishing; 2025 Jan. Available from: https://www.ncbi.nlm.nih.gov/books/NBK557555/
48. Choi IS. Functional vascular anatomy of the head and neck. Interv Neuroradiol. 2003 Oct;9(Suppl 2):29–30. doi: 10.1177/15910199030090S202. Epub 2004 Oct 22. PMID: 20591274; PMCID: PMC3556659.
49. Andani R, Khan YS. Anatomy, Head and Neck: Carotid Sinus. [Updated 2023 Jul 24]. In: StatPearls [Internet]. Treasure Island (FL): StatPearls Publishing; 2025 Jan. Available from: https://www.ncbi.nlm.nih.gov/books/NBK554378/
50. Bordoni B, Jozsa F, Varacallo MA. Anatomy, Head and Neck, Scalenus Muscle. [Updated 2025 Mar 25]. In: StatPearls [Internet]. Treasure Island (FL): StatPearls Publishing; 2025 Jan. Available from: https://www.ncbi.nlm.nih.gov/books/NBK519058/
51. Feigl G, Hammer GP, Litz R, Kachlik D. The intercarotid or alar fascia, other cervical fascias, and their adjacent spaces: a plea for clarification of cervical fascia and spaces terminology. J Anat. 2020 Jul;237(1):197–207. doi: 10.1111/joa.13175. Epub 2020 Feb 20. PMID: 32080853; PMCID: PMC7309289.
52. Harry WG, Bennett JD, Guha SC. Scalene muscles and the brachial plexus: anatomical variations and their clinical significance. Clin Anat. 1997;10(4):250–2. doi: 10.1002/(SICI)1098-2353(1997)10:4<250::AID-CA6>3.0.CO;2-W. PMID: 9213042.

53. Roesch ZK, Tadi P. Anatomy, Head and Neck, Neck. [Updated 2023 Jul 24]. In: StatPearls [Internet]. Treasure Island (FL): StatPearls Publishing; 2025 Jan. Available from: https://www.ncbi.nlm.nih.gov/books/NBK542313/

CHAPTERS 8 AND 16 NEUROANATOMY

1. Franklin RJ, French-Constant C. Remyelination in the CNS: from biology to therapy. Nat Rev Neurosci. 2008 Nov;9(11):839–55. doi: 10.1038/nrn2480. PMID: 18931697.
2. Baumann N, Pham-Dinh D. Biology of oligodendrocyte and myelin in the mammalian central nervous system. Physiol Rev. 2001 Apr;81(2):871–927. doi: 10.1152/physrev.2001.81.2.871. PMID: 11274346.
3. al-Ali SY, al-Hussain SM. An ultrastructural study of the phagocytic activity of astrocytes in adult rat brain. J Anat. 1996 Apr;188 (Pt 2):257–62. PMID: 8621323; PMCID: PMC1167560.
4. Harrow-Mortelliti M, Reddy V, Jimsheleishvili G. Physiology, Spinal Cord. [Updated 2023 Mar 17]. In: StatPearls [Internet]. Treasure Island (FL): StatPearls Publishing; 2025 Jan. Available from: https://www.ncbi.nlm.nih.gov/books/NBK544267/
5. Ludwig PE, Reddy V, Varacallo MA. Neuroanatomy, Neurons. [Updated 2023 Jul 24]. In: StatPearls [Internet]. Treasure Island (FL): StatPearls Publishing; 2025 Jan. Available from: https://www.ncbi.nlm.nih.gov/books/NBK441977/
6. Ahimsadasan N, Reddy V, Khan Suheb MZ, et al. Neuroanatomy, Dorsal Root Ganglion. [Updated 2022 Sep 21]. In: StatPearls [Internet]. Treasure Island (FL): StatPearls Publishing; 2025 Jan. Available from: https://www.ncbi.nlm.nih.gov/books/NBK532291/
7. Cooper GM. The Cell: A Molecular Approach. In: The Nucleolus. 2nd edition. Sunderland (MA): Sinauer Associates; 2000. Available from: https://www.ncbi.nlm.nih.gov/books/NBK9939/.
8. Muzio MR, Fakoya AO, Cascella M. Histology, Axon. [Updated 2022 Nov 14]. In: StatPearls [Internet]. Treasure Island (FL): StatPearls Publishing; 2025 Jan. Available from: https://www.ncbi.nlm.nih.gov/books/NBK554388/
9. Spillane M, Ketschek A, Jones SL, et al. The actin nucleating Arp2/3 complex contributes to the formation of axonal filopodia and branches through the regulation of actin patch precursors to filopodia. Dev Neurobiol. 2011 Sep;71(9):747–58. doi: 10.1002/dneu.20907. PMID: 21557512; PMCID: PMC3154400.
10. Boonpirak N, Apinhasmit W. Length and caudal level of termination of the spinal cord in Thai adults. Acta Anat (Basel). 1994;149(1):74–8. doi: 10.1159/000147558. PMID: 8184662.
11. Ko HY, Park JH, Shin YB, Baek SY. Gross quantitative measurements of spinal cord segments in human. Spinal Cord. 2004 Jan;42(1):35–40. doi: 10.1038/sj.sc.3101538. PMID: 14713942.
12. Liu A, Yang K, Wang D, et al. Level of conus medullaris termination in adult population analyzed by kinetic magnetic resonance imaging. Surg Radiol Anat. 2017 Jul;39(7):759–65. doi: 10.1007/s00276-017-1813-3. Epub 2017 Jan 16. PMID: 28091734.
13. Nene Y, Jilani TN. Neuroanatomy, Conus Medullaris. [Updated 2023 Aug 7]. In: StatPearls [Internet]. Treasure Island (FL): StatPearls Publishing; 2025 Jan. Available from: https://www.ncbi.nlm.nih.gov/books/NBK545227/
14. Kang JH, Im S. Functional anatomy of the spinal tracts based on evolutionary perspectives. Korean J Neurotrauma. 2023 Sep;19(3):275–87. doi: 10.13004/kjnt.2023.19.e43. PMID: 37840623; PMCID: PMC10567534.
15. Bui T, Das JM. Neuroanatomy, Cerebral Hemisphere. [Updated 2023 Jul 24]. In: StatPearls [Internet]. Treasure Island (FL): StatPearls Publishing; 2025 Jan. Available from: https://www.ncbi.nlm.nih.gov/books/NBK549789/
16. Stinnett TJ, Reddy V, Zabel MK. Neuroanatomy, Broca Area. [Updated 2023 Aug 8]. In: StatPearls [Internet]. Treasure Island (FL): StatPearls Publishing; 2025 Jan. Available from: https://www.ncbi.nlm.nih.gov/books/NBK526096/
17. Flinker A, Korzeniewska A, Shestyuk AY, et al. Redefining the role of Broca's area in speech. Proc Natl Acad Sci USA. 2015 Mar;112(9):2871–5. doi: 10.1073/pnas.1414491112. Epub 2015 Feb 17. PMID: 25730850; PMCID: PMC4352780.
18. Margetis K, Weisbrod LJ, Launico MV. Neuroanatomy, Cerebrospinal Fluid. [Updated 2025 Jul 7]. In: StatPearls [Internet]. Treasure Island (FL): StatPearls Publishing; 2025 Jan. Available from: https://www.ncbi.nlm.nih.gov/books/NBK470578/
19. Lechan RM, Toni R. Functional Anatomy of the Hypothalamus and Pituitary. [Updated 2016 Nov 28]. In: Feingold KR, Ahmed SF, Anawalt B, et al., editors. Endotext [Internet]. South Dartmouth (MA): MDText.com, Inc.; 2000. Available from: https://www.ncbi.nlm.nih.gov/books/NBK279126/

20. Torrico TJ, Abdijadid S. Neuroanatomy, Limbic System. [Updated 2023 Jul 17]. In: StatPearls [Internet]. Treasure Island (FL): StatPearls Publishing; 2025 Jan. Available from: https://www.ncbi.nlm.nih.gov/sites/books/NBK538491/
21. Damasio A, Damasio H, Tranel D. Persistence of feelings and sentience after bilateral damage of the insula. Cereb Cortex. 2013 Apr;23(4):833–46. doi: 10.1093/cercor/bhs077. Epub 2012 Apr 3. PMID: 22473895; PMCID: PMC3657385.
22. Ludwig PE, Das JM. Histology, Glial Cells. [Updated 2023 May 1]. In: StatPearls [Internet]. Treasure Island (FL): StatPearls Publishing; 2025 Jan. Available from: https://www.ncbi.nlm.nih.gov/books/NBK441945/
23. Reemst K, Noctor SC, Lucassen PJ, Hol EM. The indispensable roles of microglia and astrocytes during brain development. Front Hum Neurosci. 2016 Nov;10:566. doi: 10.3389/fnhum.2016.00566. PMID: 27877121; PMCID: PMC5099170.
24. Salzer JL. Schwann cell myelination. Cold Spring Harb Perspect Biol. 2015 Jun;7(8):a020529. doi: 10.1101/cshperspect.a020529. PMID: 26054742; PMCID: PMC4526746.
25. Nelles DG, Hazrati LN. Ependymal cells and neurodegenerative disease: outcomes of compromised ependymal barrier function. Brain Commun. 2022 Nov;4(6):fcac288. doi: 10.1093/braincomms/fcac288. PMID: 36415662; PMCID: PMC9677497.
26. Del Bigio MR. The ependyma: a protective barrier between brain and cerebrospinal fluid. Glia. 1995 May;14(1):1–13. doi: 10.1002/glia.440140102. PMID: 7615341.
27. Nualart-Marti A, Solsona C, Fields RD. Gap junction communication in myelinating glia. Biochim Biophys Acta. 2013 Jan;1828(1):69–78. doi: 10.1016/j.bbamem.2012.01.024. Epub 2012 Feb 3. PMID: 22326946; PMCID: PMC4474145.
28. Abrams CK. Mechanisms of diseases associated with mutation in GJC2/connexin 47. Biomolecules. 2023 Apr;13(4):712. doi: 10.3390/biom13040712. PMID: 37189458; PMCID: PMC10135871.
29. Gibbins I. Functional organization of autonomic neural pathways. Organogenesis. 2013 Jul–Sep;9(3):169–75. doi: 10.4161/org.25126. Epub 2013 Jun 6. PMID: 23872517; PMCID: PMC3896588.
30. LeBouef T, Yaker Z, Whited L. Physiology, Autonomic Nervous System. [Updated 2023 May 1]. In: StatPearls [Internet]. Treasure Island (FL): StatPearls Publishing; 2025 Jan. Available from: https://www.ncbi.nlm.nih.gov/sites/books/NBK538516/
31. Alshak MN, Das JM. Neuroanatomy, Sympathetic Nervous System. [Updated 2023 May 8]. In: StatPearls [Internet]. Treasure Island (FL): StatPearls Publishing; 2025 Jan. Available from: https://www.ncbi.nlm.nih.gov/books/NBK542195/
32. Shibasaki M, Crandall CG. Mechanisms and controllers of eccrine sweating in humans. Front Biosci (Schol Ed). 2010 Jan;2(2):685–96. doi: 10.2741/s94. PMID: 20036977; PMCID: PMC2866164.
33. Strosberg AD. Structure, function, and regulation of the three beta-adrenergic receptors. Obes Res. 1995 Nov;3(Suppl 4):501S–5S. doi: 10.1002/j.1550-8528.1995.tb00219.x. PMID: 8697050.
34. Biaggioni I. The pharmacology of autonomic failure: from hypotension to hypertension. Pharmacol Rev. 2017 Jan;69(1):53–62. doi: 10.1124/pr.115.012161. PMID: 28011746; PMCID: PMC6047298.
35. Shahid Z, Asuka E, Singh G. Physiology, Hypothalamus. [Updated 2023 May 1]. In: StatPearls [Internet]. Treasure Island (FL): StatPearls Publishing; 2025 Jan. Available from: https://www.ncbi.nlm.nih.gov/books/NBK535380/
36. Waxenbaum JA, Reddy V, Varacallo MA. Anatomy, Autonomic Nervous System. [Updated 2023 Jul 24]. In: StatPearls [Internet]. Treasure Island (FL): StatPearls Publishing; 2025 Jan. Available from: https://www.ncbi.nlm.nih.gov/books/NBK539845/
37. Tindle J, Tadi P. Neuroanatomy, Parasympathetic Nervous System. [Updated 2022 Oct 31]. In: StatPearls [Internet]. Treasure Island (FL): StatPearls Publishing; 2025 Jan. Available from: https://www.ncbi.nlm.nih.gov/books/NBK553141/
38. Sharkey KA, Mawe GM. The enteric nervous system. Physiol Rev. 2023 Apr;103(2):1487–564. doi: 10.1152/physrev.00018.2022. Epub 2022 Dec 15. PMID: 36521049; PMCID: PMC9970663.
39. Esposito G. Introducing enteric glial cells. Methods Mol Biol. 2026;2971:1–5. doi: 10.1007/978-1-0716-4795-0_1. PMID: 41028619.
40. Nwako JG, McCauley HA. Enteroendocrine cells regulate intestinal homeostasis and epithelial function. Mol Cell Endocrinol. 2024 Nov;593:112339. doi: 10.1016/j.mce.2024.112339. Epub 2024 Aug 5. PMID: 39111616; PMCID: PMC11401774.
41. Kim SY, Motlagh M, Naqvi IA. Neuroanatomy, Cranial Nerve 4 (Trochlear) [Updated 2023 Jul 15]. In: StatPearls [Internet]. Treasure Island (FL): StatPearls Publishing; 2025 Jan. Available from: https://www.ncbi.nlm.nih.gov/books/NBK537244/
42. Peterson DC, Hamel RN. Corneal Reflex. [Updated 2023 Jul 25]. In: StatPearls [Internet]. Treasure Island (FL): StatPearls Publishing; 2025 Jan. Available from: https://www.ncbi.nlm.nih.gov/books/NBK534247/

43. Ghatak RN, Helwany M, Ginglen JG. Anatomy, Head and Neck, Mandibular Nerve. [Updated 2023 May 1]. In: StatPearls [Internet]. Treasure Island (FL): StatPearls Publishing; 2025 Jan-. Available from: https://www.ncbi.nlm.nih.gov/books/NBK507820/
44. Payne T, Kronenbuerger M, Wong G. Gustatory Testing. [Updated 2023 Jan 16]. In: StatPearls [Internet]. Treasure Island (FL): StatPearls Publishing; 2025 Jan. Available from: https://www.ncbi.nlm.nih.gov/books/NBK567734/
45. Kopala W, Kukwa A. Evaluation of the acoustic (stapedius) reflex test in children and adolescents with peripheral facial nerve palsy. Int J Pediatr Otorhinolaryngol. 2016 Oct;89:102–6. doi: 10.1016/j.ijporl.2016.08.001. Epub 2016 Aug 4. PMID: 27619038.
46. Subramanian NS, Mahalakshmi B, Chiragkumar DD, et al. Effectiveness of balloon blowing on respiratory parameters among children with lower respiratory tract infection: a quasi-experimental study. J Pharm Bioallied Sci. 2025 Jun;17(Suppl 2):S1239–41. doi: 10.4103/jpbs.jpbs_1978_24. Epub 2025 Jun 18. PMID: 40655645; PMCID: PMC12244867.
47. Brandt JP, Winters R. Bone Conduction Evaluation. [Updated 2023 Jan 30]. In: StatPearls [Internet]. Treasure Island (FL): StatPearls Publishing; 2025 Jan. Available from: https://www.ncbi.nlm.nih.gov/books/NBK578177/
48. Helwany M, Rathee M. Anatomy, Head and Neck, Palate. [Updated 2023 Jun 5]. In: StatPearls [Internet]. Treasure Island (FL): StatPearls Publishing; 2025 Jan. Available from: https://www.ncbi.nlm.nih.gov/books/NBK557817/
49. Reese V, Das JM, Al Khalili Y. Cranial Nerve Testing. [Updated 2023 May 6]. In: StatPearls [Internet]. Treasure Island (FL): StatPearls Publishing; 2025 Jan. Available from: https://www.ncbi.nlm.nih.gov/books/NBK585066/
50. National Research Council (US) Committee on Recognition and Alleviation of Pain in Laboratory Animals. Recognition and Alleviation of Pain in Laboratory Animals. Washington (DC): National Academies Press (US); 2009. 2, Mechanisms of Pain. Available from: https://www.ncbi.nlm.nih.gov/books/NBK32659/.
51. Ong WY, Stohler CS, Herr DR. Role of the prefrontal cortex in pain processing. Mol Neurobiol. 2019 Feb;56(2):1137–66. doi: 10.1007/s12035-018-1130-9. Epub 2018 Jun 6. PMID: 29876878; PMCID: PMC6400876.
52. Gaillard D, Kinnamon SC. New evidence for fat as a primary taste quality. Acta Physiol (Oxf). 2019 May;226(1):e13246. doi: 10.1111/apha.13246. Epub 2019 Jan 16. PMID: 30588748; PMCID: PMC6800056.
53. Spence C. The tongue map and the spatial modulation of taste perception. Curr Res Food Sci. 2022 Mar;5: 598–10. doi: 10.1016/j.crfs.2022.02.004. PMID: 35345819; PMCID: PMC8956797.
54. Wooding SP, Ramirez VA, Behrens M. Bitter taste receptors: genes, evolution and health. Evol Med Public Health. 2021 Oct;9(1):431–47. doi: 10.1093/emph/eoab031. PMID: 35154779; PMCID: PMC8830313.
55. Dutt M, Ng Y-K, Molendijk J, et al. Western diet induced remodelling of the tongue proteome. Proteomes. 2021;9:22. doi: 10.3390/proteomes9020022.
56. Branigan B, Tadi P. Physiology, Olfactory. [Updated 2023 May 1]. In: StatPearls [Internet]. Treasure Island (FL): StatPearls Publishing; 2025 Jan. Available from: https://www.ncbi.nlm.nih.gov/books/NBK542239/
57. Melis M, Tomassini Barbarossa I, Sollai G. The implications of taste and olfaction in nutrition and health. Nutrients. 2023 Jul;15(15):3412. doi: 10.3390/nu15153412. PMID: 37571348; PMCID: PMC10421496.
58. Câmara R, Griessenauer GJ. Anatomy of the Vagus Nerve. In: Shane Tubbs ERR, Shoja MM, Loukas M, Barbaro N, Spinner RJ, editors. Nerves and Nerve Injuries. London: Academic Press; 2015, 385–97.
59. Browning KN, Verheijden S, Boeckxstaens GE. The Vagus nerve in appetite regulation, mood, and intestinal inflammation. Gastroenterology. 2017;152:730–44. doi: 10.1053/j.gastro.2016.10.046
60. Chayer C, Freedman M. Frontal lobe functions. Curr Neurol Neurosci Rep. 2001 Nov;1(6):547–52. doi: 10.1007/s11910-001-0060-4. PMID: 11898568.
61. Smith EE, Jonides J. Storage and executive processes in the frontal lobes. Science. 1999 Mar;283(5408): 1657–61. doi: 10.1126/science.283.5408.1657. PMID: 10073923.
62. Maldonado KA, Alsayouri K. Physiology, Brain. [Updated 2023 Mar 17]. In: StatPearls [Internet]. Treasure Island (FL): StatPearls Publishing; 2025 Jan. Available from: https://www.ncbi.nlm.nih.gov/books/NBK551718/
63. Brem AK, Ran K, Pascual-Leone A. Learning and memory. Handb Clin Neurol. 2013;116:693–37. doi: 10.1016/B978-0-444-53497-2.00055-3. PMID: 24112934; PMCID: PMC4248571.
64. Cohen NJ, Squire LR. Preserved learning and retention of pattern-analyzing skill in amnesia: dissociation of knowing how and knowing that. Science. 1980;210:207–10. doi: 10.1126/science.7414331.
65. Young CB, Reddy V, Sonne J. Neuroanatomy, Basal Ganglia. [Updated 2023 Jul 24]. In: StatPearls [Internet]. Treasure Island (FL): StatPearls Publishing; 2025 Jan. Available from: https://www.ncbi.nlm.nih.gov/books/NBK537141/
66. DiGuiseppi J, Tadi P. Neuroanatomy, Postcentral Gyrus. [Updated 2023 Jul 24]. In: StatPearls [Internet]. Treasure Island (FL): StatPearls Publishing; 2025 Jan. PMID: 31751015.

 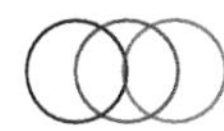

67. Raju H, Tadi P. Neuroanatomy, Somatosensory Cortex. [Updated 2022 Nov 7]. In: StatPearls [Internet]. Treasure Island (FL): StatPearls Publishing; 2025 Jan. Available from: https://www.ncbi.nlm.nih.gov/books/NBK555915/
68. Hsiao S, Gomez-Ramirez M. Touch. In: Gottfried JA, editor. Neurobiology of Sensation and Reward. Boca Raton (FL): CRC Press/Taylor & Francis; 2011. Chapter 7. Available from: https://www.ncbi.nlm.nih.gov/books/NBK92803/.
69. Cano LA, Albarracín AL, Farfán FD, Fernández E. Brain-hemispheric differences in the premotor area for motor planning: an approach based on corticomuscular connectivity during motor decision-making. Neuroimage. 2025 May;312:121230. doi: 10.1016/j.neuroimage.2025.121230. Epub 2025 Apr 17. PMID: 40252879; PMCID: PMC12055607.
70. Abusrair AH, Elsekaily W, Bohlega S. Tremor in Parkinson's disease: from pathophysiology to advanced therapies. Tremor Other Hyperkinet Mov (NY). 2022 Sep;12:29. doi: 10.5334/tohm.712. PMID: 36211804; PMCID: PMC9504742.
71. Kovács A, Kiss M, Pintér N, Szirmai I, Kamondi A. Characteristics of tremor induced by lesions of the cerebellum. Cerebellum. 2019 Aug;18(4):705–20. doi: 10.1007/s12311-019-01027-3. PMID: 30963396.
72. Shenoy SS, Lui F. Neuroanatomy, Ventricular System. [Updated 2023 Jul 24]. In: StatPearls [Internet]. Treasure Island (FL): StatPearls Publishing; 2025 Jan. Available from: https://www.ncbi.nlm.nih.gov/books/NBK532932/
73. Margetis K, Baker S. Physiology, Cerebral Spinal Fluid. [Updated 2025 Aug 9]. In: StatPearls [Internet]. Treasure Island (FL): StatPearls Publishing; 2025 Jan. Available from: https://www.ncbi.nlm.nih.gov/books/NBK519007/
74. Wessels T, Möller-Hartmann W, Noth J, Klötzsch C. CT findings and clinical features as markers for patient outcome in primary pontine hemorrhage. AJNR Am J Neuroradiol. 2004 Feb;25(2):257–60. PMID: 14970027; PMCID: PMC7974614.
75. Jeong JH, Yoon SJ, Kang SJ, Choi KG, Na DL. Hypertensive pontine microhemorrhage. Stroke. 2002 Apr;33(4):925–9. doi: 10.1161/01.str.0000013563.73522.cb. PMID: 11935038.
76. Jimsheleishvili S, Dididze M. Neuroanatomy, Cerebellum. [Updated 2023 Jul 24]. In: StatPearls [Internet]. Treasure Island (FL): StatPearls Publishing; 2025 Jan. Available from: https://www.ncbi.nlm.nih.gov/books/NBK538167/
77. Ganapathy MK, Tadi P. Anatomy, Head and Neck, Pituitary Gland. [Updated 2023 Jul 24]. In: StatPearls [Internet]. Treasure Island (FL): StatPearls Publishing; 2025 Jan. Available from: https://www.ncbi.nlm.nih.gov/books/NBK551529/
78. Williams LS, Schmalfuss IM, Sistrom CL, et al. MR imaging of the trigeminal ganglion, nerve, and the perineural vascular plexus: normal appearance and variants with correlation to cadaver specimens. AJNR Am J Neuroradiol. 2003 Aug;24(7):1317–23. PMID: 12917119; PMCID: PMC7973681.
79. O'Driscoll J, Minarro JC, Sanchez-Sotelo J. Paralysis of the trapezius muscle: evaluation and surgical management. JSES Rev Rep Tech. 2024 Apr;4(3):329–40. doi: 10.1016/j.xrrt.2024.03.014. PMID: 39157246; PMCID: PMC11329012.
80. Purves D, Augustine GJ, Fitzpatrick D, et al., editors. Neuroscience. The Subdivisions of the Central Nervous System. 2nd edition. Sunderland (MA): Sinauer Associates; 2001. Available from: https://www.ncbi.nlm.nih.gov/books/NBK10926/.
81. Sonne J, Omole AE, Lopez-Ojeda W. Neuroanatomy, Cranial Nerve. [Updated 2025 Jan 24]. In: StatPearls [Internet]. Treasure Island (FL): StatPearls Publishing; 2025 Jan. Available from: https://www.ncbi.nlm.nih.gov/books/NBK470353/

INDEX

A

B

C

D

E

F

G

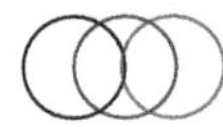

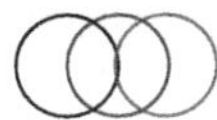

N

O

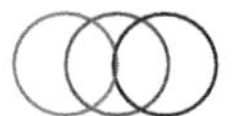

P

Q

R

S

T

 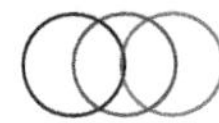

U

V

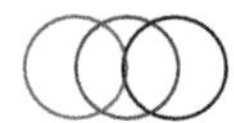

W

X

Z

For Product Safety Concerns and Information please contact our EU representative GPSR@taylorandfrancis.com Taylor & Francis Verlag GmbH, Kaufingerstraße 24, 80331 München, Germany